Profiles in Gerontology

PROFILES IN GERONTOLOGY

A Biographical Dictionary

W. ANDREW ACHENBAUM AND
DANIEL M. ALBERT

Foreword by Carol Ann Schutz

Greenwood Press
Westport, Connecticut • London

ACV 7633

Library of Congress Cataloging-in-Publication Data

Achenbaum, W. Andrew.
    Profiles in gerontology : a biographical dictionary / W. Andrew
Achenbaum and Daniel M. Albert; foreword by Carol Ann Schutz.
      p.   cm.
    Includes indexes.
    ISBN 0–313–29274–4
    1. Gerontologists—United States—Biography—Dictionaries.
    2. Gerontologists—Biography—Dictionaries. I. Albert, Daniel M.
II. Title.
HQ1064.U5A624   1995
305.26'092'2—dc20   95–8002

British Library Cataloguing in Publication Data is available.

Library of Congress Catalog Card Number: 95–8002

First published in 1995
Greenwood Press, 88 Post Road West, Westport, CT 06881
An imprint of Greenwood Publishing Group, Inc.

Printed in The United States of America

The paper used in this book complies with the
Permanent Paper Standard issued by the National
Information Standards Organization (Z39.48–1984).

10 9 8 7 6 5 4 3 2 1

CONTENTS

FOREWORD ⎯⎯⎯⎯⎯⎯⎯⎯⎯

Profiles in Gerontology: A Biographical Dictionary is an important and needed book. It complements Dr. Achenbaum's previous book, *Crossing Frontiers: Gerontology Emerges as a Science*, on the history of gerontology by identifying the individuals who made that history and charting the field's future. In doing so, the authors have provided historians and future researchers a valuable knowledge base for understanding the development of a complex scientific field and for advancing a body of knowledge crucial to the well-being of future generations.

In the introductory article of the first issue of the *Journal of Gerontology*, Lawrence K. Frank, a founder and early president of The Gerontological Society of America, wrote, "Gerontology . . . is not just one more highly specialized discipline, . . . but reflects the recognition of a new kind of problem . . . that transcends the knowledge and methods of any one discipline or profession, and demands the focussing of the findings of many separate investigators into a synthesized, coherent whole."

The challenge of building that coherent whole is as important and difficult today as it was fifty years ago when the Society was established.

The field has grown rapidly in the past half century. There are now gerontological research and education programs in many colleges and universities, with some institutions offering degrees in the field. There is a National Institute on Aging and numerous other aging research centers. Even so, most researchers and professionals come from and maintain their identities in basic disciplines, which is both a strength and difficulty.

As a science, gerontology is only as strong as its research base is sound.

Disciplinary rigor is crucial. Yet, the multidisciplinary nature of the field means the body of researchers is disperse; the body of knowledge broad and difficult to synthesize. Syntheses comes through cross-dicipline discourses, jointly authored articles, eclectic collections of essays, and publications bringing together the works of scholars from different disciplines, as well as through a limited amount of multi- and interdisciplinary research.

The development of gerontology then can only be understood and advanced by identifying and drawing on the work of the disperse body of researchers and professionals who have contributed critical bits and pieces to the search for a coherent whole. Hence, the great importance of this book is that it identifies and describes many of the key contributors to that search. Students of gerontology, researchers seeking to advance new theories, and future historians will be indebted to the work of Dr. Achenbaum and Mr. Albert.

The timing of the book is fortuitous, for it coincides with the fiftieth anniversary of the founding of The Gerontological Society of America. Since the development of the Society closely parallels the development of the field, and since many of the people described in the book were or are members of the Society, the observance of the anniversary and publication of the book reinforce the recognition owed those persons who have brought a relatively new field to a place of deserved prominence and who have had impacts far beyond their numbers.

And finally, and on a personal note, the book is particularly welcomed, for I have had the good fortune to know many of the people listed. It has been exciting working with them and a privilege to know them. They deserve to be so recognized.

Carol Ann Schutz
Executive Director
The Gerontological Society of America

ACKNOWLEDGMENTS ⸻

Jeanne Bader deserves her colleagues' heartfelt gratitude for initially conceiving of this biographical dictionary. She designed the original questionnaire and has remained keenly interested in seeing this project completed.

Although she chose not to accept credit or blame by assuming editorial responsibilities, Patricia Blackman made sure that all of the pieces of papers and electronic disks finally coalesced into a publishable volume. Pat, Dan, and I discovered that the task of managing a venture of this sort, which depends on the good will and good humor of many people, is far more complex than completing a monograph or even editing a collection of papers. We owe Pat much more than we can say.

During the summer of 1994, while feverishly putting together the last set of entries, Dan and I were lucky to have the assistance of Hajj Womach from Morehouse College. Hajj claims that playing detective was good preparation for graduate work in history. That he actually found "facts" that eluded us speaks well for his potential success.

Thanks, too, to the staff of the libraries of the University of Michigan and those senior officials who invested so much in the electronic retrieval of information. Despite cutbacks and hard times, the library has remained a wonderfully accessible place. Without it, this dictionary would not be as rich in detail as it is.

Finally, we wish to salute members, past and present, of The Gerontological Society of America on the fiftieth anniversary of that organization's founding. Not all researchers on aging are gerontologists, much less active in the Society. But through its meetings and publications this Society has been indispensable in promoting work in this area. Friendships and ideas generated by its activities animate these pages.

INTRODUCTION _____

In May 1945, five U.S. physicians, scientists, and academics interested in promoting research into the problems of aging filed the necessary legal papers in New York City to incorporate a Gerontological Society for professionals. According to their statement of purpose, the men were interested in creating an organization that would promote studies of senescence that were grounded in the biological, medical, psychological, and social sciences. The Gerontological Society, they hoped, would provide an institutional structure that facilitated the exchange of ideas, data, methods, and applications among researchers, scientists, and scholars who came together from different disciplines.

> The purposes for which the corporation is to be formed are to promote the scientific study of aging, in order to advance public health and mental hygiene, the science and art of medicine, and the cure of disease; to foster the growth and diffusion knowledge relating to problems of aging and of the sciences contributing to an understanding thereof; to afford a common meeting ground for representation of the various scientific fields interested in such problems and those responsible for care and treatment of the aged.[1]

No single theoretical orientation sufficiently captured all of the dynamic interactions. No research paradigm could explain all the cumulative changes among genetic, environmental, and developmental factors affecting living organisms as they grew older and died. Different problems, practical and intellectual, required different perspectives and methods. "Gerontology is an enterprise calling for many and diversified studies, for pooled and concerted investigations, indeed, for the orchestration of all relevant disciplines and professional practices," declared Lawrence K. Frank, one of the five incorporators.[2]

The choice of the term "gerontological" for the society's name was equally deliberate. Despite its classical Greek roots, the word was coined in the twentieth century: Elie Metchnikoff of the Pasteur Institute in Paris first used the word "gerontology" to describe the *science* of biological senescence.[3] Ever since, people who consider themselves gerontologists have wrestled with definitional issues. The Gerontological Society in 1959 formulated a working definition— "Gerontology is that branch of science which is concerned with situations and changes inherent in increments of time, with particular reference to post-maturational stages"—but issuing that statement hardly settled the matter.[4] To this day, gerontologists disagree about when "aging" begins. (For instance, some contend it starts at conception, not in post-maturational stages.) And increasing numbers of researchers on aging question whether the field has yet become—or ever will emerge—as a science. The very fuzziness of gerontology's boundaries, however, gives some credence to its practitioner's claims that they are experts doing specialized research.

During the Society's formative years, most of its members came from the bio-medical sciences. Of the eighty members on the rolls in 1946, forty-three joined the Clinical Medicine section, nine came from anatomy and physiology, seven from physiology, four from biochemistry, and one from botany. There were six psychologists, five sociologists, and two from social work; three people were listed in the "general" category. Six years later, clinicians and medical researchers made up nearly half of the membership, and biological scientists another quarter.[5] By 1991, social scientists and health care professionals, not bench scientists, dominated the organization. Roughly 46 percent of the 7,000 total membership belonged to the Behavioral and Social Sciences section; only 7 percent were affiliated with the Biological Sciences section. Nearly a third of the Society's members were nurses or physicians; another 13 percent were social workers.[6] No subset of the membership could claim to represent the overall interests and priorities of the Society. For our purposes, in preparing *Profiles in Gerontology: A Biographical Dictionary,* it makes sense to adhere to the National Institute on Aging's definition of gerontologists as those who "examine not only the clinical and biological aspects of aging but also psychosocial, economic, and historical conditions."[7]

Over the years, The Gerontological Society of America (GSA) has made it possible for professionals trained in a variety of disciplines to pursue knowledge consistent with their training, to facilitate interactions with kindred spirits, and to attempt to apply empirical insights into older people's behavior in efforts to ameliorate the aged's conditions. Those who join GSA are invited to belong to one of four relatively autonomous sections, now called Biological Sciences; Clinical Medicine; Behavioral and Social Sciences; and Social Research, Policy, and Practice. At the same time, GSA's leadership has taken great pains to produce high-quality journals and to conduct annual meetings so as to foster the founders' original vision of people sharing ideas across intellectual and professional boundaries. Hence the original *Journal of Gerontology* included not only bio-medical articles but also contributions from the humanities. Over the decades, editors-in-chief delegated more and more responsibility for evaluating quality to specialists and peer reviewers. Since 1986, the journal has been the four-part *Journals of Gerontology*, volumes for the biological sciences, clinical medicine, behavioral sciences, and the social sciences. To appeal to a broader audience, the Society authorized a second periodical, *The Gerontologist*, in 1960, which was to provide "a multidisciplinary perspective on human aging through publication of articles, on research and analysis in gerontology, including social policy, program development, and service delivery.[8]

The Gerontological Society has provided the impetus for many initiatives that have advanced research, education, and practical innovations in the area of aging. Starting in 1965, the Society honored with the Robert Kleemeier Award those who have done "outstanding research in the field of gerontology." The Donald P. Kent Award was established eight years later to recognize those "exemplifying the highest standards of professional leadership in gerontology through teaching, service, and the interpretation of gerontology to the larger society." Sections created their own prizes. Special opportunities were created under GSA's aegis to recruit minorities to the field. Graduate students and post-doctoral graduates with a practical bent were invited to compete for internships in applied gerontology. In addition to its scholarly journals and annual meetings, GSA members have given advice about the federal government's role in research on aging. In an attempt to anticipate "emerging issues," the Society issued special reports, such as *Ties That Bind* (1986), which focused on the policy choices before aging societies.

As The Gerontological Society approached the fiftieth anniversary of its founding, it seemed appropriate to produce some historical records that would celebrate the occasion. Creating such documents also might enable future researchers on aging to take stock of where gerontologists have been and where they are heading. Jeanne Bader deserves credit for conceiving of this biographical dictionary and for designing the original questionnaire used to construct the sketches in this volume.

Selection criteria were straightforward. Bader and W. Andrew Achenbaum drew up a core list of all GSA presidents, editors, and Kleemeier and Kent Award winners. We then added to this the names of people in various GSA membership directories who we felt should be included in the volume because of their longstanding contributions as gerontologists to the field of aging. Hence, to pick one example, we did not add William Graebner to our list, although his monograph, *A History of Retirement* (New Haven: Yale University, 1980) is arguably the best available treatment of the evolution of retirement as an institution in the United States. Graebner has never done any more research on aging; he considers himself a historian, not a gerontologist.

In the fall of 1991, Bader and Achenbaum mailed a four-page questionnaire to roughly 650 men and women; we intended to add several dozen figures whose importance to the field had not been diminished by death. We received back about 200 surveys, which were filled out to varying degrees of completeness. Some forms never did reach their intended recipients. Several prominent gerontologists told us that they did not wish to participate. (One senior official at the National Institute on Aging dismissed the entire venture as narcissistic.) But as Bader and Achenbaum reviewed the forms they received back, it became increasingly evident why it is so difficult to define the scope of gerontology. Pathologists, nurses, government officials, English teachers, clinical psychologists, and service providers operate in different professional cultures. Respondents seemed to have little in common, except that they served on committees together and built networks.

Job relocations and family responsibilities forced Bader to withdraw from the enterprise, and the project stalled. Achenbaum was in the midst of completing a history of developments in the United States, which Cambridge University Press issued as *Crossing Frontiers: Gerontology Emerges as a Science* in 1995. As he began writing chapters of his monograph, Achenbaum realized that *Crossing Frontiers* would focus on institutional developments and not very much on the countless individuals who had contributed to the network building and intellectual growth of the field. Accordingly, he decided that it was important to revive Bader's efforts; clearly, the history of the Gerontological Society is as much a history of its individual members as it is of cross-multi-interdisciplinary collaborations. He recruited the assistance of a graduate student in the history of science to complete *Profiles in Gerontology*. Together, Daniel M. Albert and Achenbaum collected more information about various entrants' views on aging, which would supplement the biographical facts gathered by Bader. They read selected publications by those who had submitted the original questionnaire to give a fuller sense of the contributors' ideas and accomplishments than is usually afforded in works of this sort. We asked figures who had declined our earlier invitation to participate to reconsider their decision; in a few instances, we went ahead and composed sketches on our own. To this list was added three dozen historical figures, most of whom were once associated with the Gerontological Society.

Most of the 300 people profiled live in the United States; a few come from Canada. Only Europeans who have interacted extensively with the U.S. gerontologists in this volume have been included. The editors bear the responsibility for any inconsistencies in style that have resulted in some instances, due to an early decision to invite as many of those who would be included in the volume to have a chance to review the sketch that we had prepared of them. (We sent out profiles during the fall of 1994; most people responded in a timely, constructive manner.) A surprising number of gerontologists, young and old, preferred not to have their birthdates listed. Some academics wished us to emphasize aspects of their careers that we did not expect them to accentuate; for the most part, we honored their request without abandoning our editorial responsibilities. Remaining errors, as well as sins of commission and omission, thus remain with Achenbaum and Albert.

Originally, we had hoped to try to "interpret" the data. This proved too daunting a task. But we cannot resist noting several patterns that emerge in these pages:

- Few of the nation's leading gerontologists over the age of fifty originally trained to become researchers on aging. Many of the field's "senior" figures fell into the field because of unexpected opportunities. While this is less true of younger gerontologists, many people's decisions to do research in aging seem serendipitous.

- Certain figures, such as James E. Birren, Wilma Donahue, George Maddox, Bernice L. Neugarten, and Nathan W. Shock, have trained many students who have gone on to achieve prominence. These figures were associated with gerontological centers of excellence—at the National Institute on Aging, Duke University, and the universities of Chicago, Michigan, and Southern California—that form the basis for those intellectual networks and professional ties so vital for sustaining fields.

- The growth of federal sponsorship of research and training in gerontology since the 1960s has made it possible for many men and women to pursue careers in the field. It also has lured middle-aged and more senior scholars from other fields to do research on aging.

- The commitment of so many distinguished gerontologists to remain actively engaged colleagues in one place (or no more than several sites simultaneously) and to work with the elderly has had a positive impact on research. This underscores the importance of "local" cultures.

- The gap between the biological and the social scientific approach to senescence remains wide, but the synergism between the two has been productive. In fact, this tension, not to mention a demographic juggernaut, promises a bright future for the field.

Others doubtless will discern various trends and idiosyncrasies in these biographical sketches. To prompt such inquires, we have noted cross-references to other entrants with an asterisk (*) and have compiled fairly comprehensive subject and name indexes that will facilitate further research.

W. Andrew Achenbaum and Daniel M. Albert

NOTES

1. "Certificate of Incorporation of the Gerontological Society, Inc.," *Journal of Gerontology,* 1 (January 1946): 134–35.

2. Lawrence K. Frank, "Gerontology," *Journal of Gerontology,* 1 (January 1946): 7. As a foundation officer at the Laura Spelman Rockefeller Memorial and the Josiah Macy

Foundation, Frank had been instrumental in organizing research into the study of child development as well as cross-disciplinary studies of maturity.

3. For more, see the entry for "gerontology and geriatrics" in *Gerontological Keywords*, eds. W. Andrew Achenbaum, Carole Haber, and Steven Weiland (New York: Springer Publishing Company, 1995).

4. "Report on Gerontology by the Subcommittee on Biology and Medicine, Research and Fellowships Committee of the Gerontological Society, Inc.," *Journal of Gerontology*, 14, section C (July 1959): 366.

5. Figures come from 1950 and 1952 reports of the Membership Committee, filed in the Gerontological Society's archives.

6. "Elections are Coming: What are the Voters?," *Gerontology News*, April 1992, p. 4. To put these figures into perspective, it is worth noting that the American Psychological Association, which had 4,000 members in 1946, exceeded 60,000 four decades later.

7. National Institute on Aging, *Age Words: A Glossary on Health and Aging* (Bethesda, Md.: NIH Publication 86–1849, January 1986), 7.

8. "General Information and Instruction to Authors," *The Gerontologist*, rev. February 1993.

A _____

RONALD P. ABELES. Ronald P. Abeles, born in 1944, earned his B.A. and Phi Beta Kappa key in psychology from UCLA in 1966. He was trained as a social psychologist in an interdisciplinary graduate program (Harvard University Ph.D., 1971). He completed a postdoctoral fellowship in political science and psychology at Yale. After working at Boston University and the Social Science Research Council, Abeles made important contributions to the research direction of gerontology at the national level through his work as deputy associate director (1980–1991), acting associate director (1991–1994), and associate director (1994–present) for Behavioral and Social Research at the National Institute on Aging, National Institutes of Health. Previously, he worked at the Social Science Research Council (1974–1977), on the Committee on Work and Personality in the Middle Years and the Committee on Life-Course Development in Middle and Old Age (1977–1978). It was through this work—with Orville G. Brim, Jr., Paul B. Baltes,* and especially Matilda White Riley*—that Abeles developed an interest in the field. Riley has been his mentor and primary collaborator. Together they developed a broad and influential research agenda for the social and behavioral sciences at the National Institute on Aging.

Abeles has helped add a perspective on aging to health and behavior research and to social psychology. See R. P. Abeles and M. W. Riley, "A Life-Course Perspective on the Later Years of Life: Some Implications for Research," *Social Science Research Council Annual Report, 1976–77; Aging, Health and Behavior,* eds. M. G. Ory,* R. P. Abeles, and P. D. Lipman (Newbury Park, Calif.: Sage Publications, 1992); *Aging and Quality of Life,* eds. R. P. Abeles, H. Gift, and M. G. Ory (New York: Springer Publishing, 1994); *Life-Span Perspectives* *and Social Psychology,* ed. R. P. Abeles (Hillsdale, N.J.: Lawrence Erlbaum Associates, 1987); F. Blanchard-Fields and R. P. Abeles, "Social Influences on Behavior and Aging," *The Handbook of the Psychology of Aging,* 4th edn., eds., J. E. Birren* and K. W. Schaie* (New York: Van Nostrand Reinhold, in press).

Abeles's conceptual contributions to the field are mostly associated with the concept of "sense of control," particularly in terms of age-related changes and consequences of "sense of control." " 'Sense of control' addresses people's beliefs and expectancies about their ability to perform behaviors leading to desired outcomes and about the responsiveness of social and physical environments to their behaviors," Abeles explains. It is an important factor in a wide variety of behaviors ranging from stress management to intellectual achievement, as well as physical and mental health. Abeles has delineated a model of "sense of control" within a life-course framework and thereby charted a research agenda. See R. P. Abeles, "Sense of Control as a Factor in the Quality of Life of the Frail Elderly," *The Concept and Measurement of Quality of Life in the Later Year,* eds., J. E. Birren, D. E. Deutchman, J. Lubben, and J. Rowe* (New York: Academic Press, 1991); R. P. Abeles, "Social Schemes, Sense of Control, and Aging," *Self-Directedness and Efficacy: Causes and Effects Throughout the Life Course,* eds. J. Rodin, C. Schooler, and K. W. Schaie (Hillsdale, N.J.: Lawrence Erlbaum and Associates, 1990), 85–94.

He has also published on the influence of social structure on psychological attributes, abilities, motivations, and behaviors as people age. He points out that "macrosocial structures" (that is, the economy, polity, social class) affect psychological processes by allocating people to different kinds of "microsocial structures" (that is, the immediate social environments in which people interact, such as the workplace or home) in which particular social roles become open or closed as people grow older. The components and characteristics of the immediate social environment shape psychological processes. See R. P. Abeles and M. W. Riley, "Longevity, Social Structure, and Cognitive Aging," *Cognitive Functioning and Social Structure over the Life-Course,* eds. C. Schooler and K. W. Schaie (Norwood, N.J.: Ablex, 1987), 161–75; R. P. Abeles, "Social Structure as a Determinant of Environmental Experience," *Social Structure and Aging: Psychological Processes,* eds. K. W. Schaie and C. Schooler (Hillsdale, N.J.: Lawrence Erlbaum and Associates, 1989), 149–53; R. P. Abeles, "Social Stratification and Aging: Contemporaneous and Cumulative Effects," *Social Stratification of Age and Health,* eds. K. W. Schaie, J. S. House, and D. Blazer* (Hillsdale, N.J.: Lawrence Erlbaum and Associates, 1991), 33–37.

ITAMAR B. ABRASS. Itamar B. Abrass received his medical degree from the University of California, San Francisco in 1966. He completed his internal medicine residency at Columbia-Presbyterian Hospital in New York, and spent two years at the National Institutes of Health (NIH), where he studied with Bert O'Malley. Most of his research has been directed to defining mechanisms of decreased beta-adrenergic responsiveness in aging. To this end, Abrass's laboratory was the first to demonstrate the receptor characteristics and adenylate cyclase activity that characterize age differences in rats, as a model system, and humans. His primary collaborators have been Philip Scarpace, James Allen, and Robert Schwartz. Among his early research papers are I. B. Abrass and P. Scarpace, "Human Lymphocyte Beta-Adrenergic Receptors Are Unaltered with Age," *Journal of Gerontology,* 36 (1981): 298–301; I. B. Abrass and P. Scarpace, "Catalytic Unit of Adenylate Cyclase: Reduced Action in Aged Human Lymphocytes," *Journal of Clinical, Endocrinological Metabolism,* 55 (1982): 1026–28; and P. Scarpace and I. B. Abrass, "Beta-Adrenergic Agonist-Mediated Desensitization in Senescent Rats," *Mechanical Ageing Development,* 35 (1986): 255–64. A new direction of Abrass' research, in collaboration with May Reed, is the definition of the basic mechanisms of wound healing in aging and the development of interventions to reverse the deficits associated with aging.

Abrass considers the development of junior faculty and fellows who make important contributions to gerontology and geriatric medicine to be his greatest professional service. In this regard it is not surprising that he considers John Beck and David Solomon to have been his role models; Laurence Z. Rubenstein* considers Abrass his mentor. Like Abrass, each has forged strong ties between a Department of Veterans Affairs medical center and a nearby university-based medical school. Abrass served as president of the Gerontological Society of America in 1993. He is now professor of medicine and head of the Division of Gerontology and Geriatric Medicine at the University of Washington School of Medicine.

REBECCA G. ADAMS. Rebecca G. Adams was born in 1952. Like many gerontologists, she was drawn to the field by Bernice Neugarten,* Stephan Golant and Gunhild Hagestad, with whom she studied at the University of Chicago. In particular, Golant's course on the spatial aspects of aging provided an outlet for Adams's fascination with the effects of residential mobility on friendship patterns. See R. Adams, "Emotional Closeness and Physical Distance Between Friends: Implications for Elderly Women Living in Age-Segregated and Age-Integrated Settings," *International Journal of Aging and Human Development* 22:1 (1985–1986), 55–76, an article that was based on her sociology dissertation in 1983.

When Adams began her work on friendship among older people, there were few empirical studies of the subject. Following the ground charted by the theoretical efforts of Beth Hess,* Adams explored the effects of geographical distance, social norms, and the role changes that accompany aging on the friendships of elderly women. Her findings departed from previous literature by treating changes in friendship networks as multidimensional, and by considering the effects of differing status groups on network evolution. "Old age is typically a period during which people have an opportunity to alter their earlier friendship patterns rather than a period during which choice is restricted," Adams argued.

While not ignoring the way age-related declines operate as constraints on the friendships of some people, Adams found other important, at times liberating, changes as well. See R. Adams, "Patterns of Network Change: A Longitudinal Study of Friendships of Elderly Women," *The Gerontologist*, 27:2 (1987): 222–27.

A growing body of empirical work on the subject has been collected and conceptually integrated by Adams and Rosemary Blieszner in *Older Adult Friendship: Structure and Process* (Newbury Park, Calif.: Sage Publications, 1989). A subsequent work, R. Adams, *Adult Friendship* (Newbury Park, Calif.: Sage Publications, 1992) develops an integrative model of friendship structure (for example, hierarchy, solidarity, homogeneity, density), processes (thoughts, feelings, and behaviors), and phases (formation, maintenance, dissolution). In "An Integrative Conceptual Framework for Friendship Research," *Journal of Social and Personal Relationships,* 11:2 (1994): 163–84, Adams and Blieszner subsequently developed the dynamic aspects of this model further. Adams is currently focusing on developing a contextual approach to the study of friendship, emphasizing the sociological factors that affect personal relationships. See R. Adams, "Activity as Structure and Process: Friendships of Older Adults," in *Activity and Aging,* ed. J. R. Kelly (Newbury Park, Calif.: Sage Publications, 1993), pp. 73–85.

Through this work Adams hopes to remind scholars that friendship plays an important role in the aging process, to encourage research on friendship as a distinct category of social relationships, and to remind friendship researchers that relationships are shaped by forces external to the individuals involved in them.

Adams currently teaches at the University of North Carolina at Greensboro.

RICHARD C. ADELMAN. Richard C. Adelman was born in Newark, New Jersey, in 1940. He went to Kenyon College with the intention of attending medical school but was lured by the excitement of bench science. His predoctoral adviser was Sidney Weinhouse, a professor of biochemistry at Temple Medical School and director of the Fels Research Institute in Philadelphia. Weinhouse was a member of the National Academy of Science, one of the "grand old men" in the areas of intermediary metabolism, diabetes, and cancer research. Weinhouse's administrative style, especially his willingness to give his colleagues free rein in identifying problems worthy of investigation, greatly influenced his student's subsequent approach to leadership. Adelman did postdoctoral work at Albert Einstein Medical School, working as an American Cancer Society Postdoctoral Fellow in the lab of Bernard Horecker, also a member of the National Academy of Sciences, who was at the time chairman of the department of molecular biology. Neither Horecker nor Weinhouse was a gerontologist, yet each, according to Adelman, had an "insatiable desire to instill in every one of his trainees the essence of the joy and honor of science."

Adelman was not attracted to gerontology by a particular body of work or "rising star." Rather, he was struck in the late 1960s by the absence of credible biochemical publications. Opportunities for advancement, he felt, lay in addressing regulatory aspects of oncogenesis, differentiation, and development, and aging. Building on his pre- and postdoctoral work on enzyme regulation, Adelman set out to document the adaptive sluggishness that generally characterizes aging organisms in the gross physiological sense. He felt that there were impaired abilities expressed at the molecular level, similar to the ways that older pedestrians approach and try to avoid oncoming cars.

More specifically, Adelman explored how the ability of certain cell populations (such as the liver) to respond *in vivo* to changes in nutrition by synthesizing specific gene products (such as enzyme molecules that catalyze metabolism of the challenging nutrient) is progressively delayed as host rats became older. Subsequent investigations also determined that the origin of such impaired responsiveness resides in the ability to secrete certain hormones, such as insulin, for which hepatic interaction is essential to expression of the enzyme response. The primary importance of this research is that it provides a means to identify specific molecular events, the modification of which, as an organism ages, is responsible directly for physiological expressions of aging. Such a line of reasoning was consistent with the bio-gerontological precept, best articulated by Nathan Shock at the Gerontology Research Center in Baltimore, that aging is a process rather than a pathological disorder. Adelman's most frequently cited research articles in this area include "An Age-Dependent Modification of Enzyme Regulation," *Journal of Biological Chemistry,* 245 (1970): 1032–35; "Loss of Adaptive Mechanisms During Aging," *Federal Proceedings,* 38 (1979): 1968–71; and "Secretion of Insulin During Aging," *Journal of American Geriatrics Society,* 37 (1989): 983–90.

Adelman was one of the first bench scientists to appreciate the importance of translating new biological knowledge into non-technical language so that non-biologists could understand it. He organized workshops on "biology for non-specialists" at annual meetings of the Gerontological Society. Adelman prepared a lengthy article on the biology of aging ("As the Body Ages") for the *Year-book of Science and the Future* for the *Encyclopaedia Britannica* (1982): 88–103, and stressed the importance of cross-disciplinary exchanges in *Higher Education in an Aging Society* (Washington, D.C.: Gerontological Society of America, 1990), 57–84. The Gerontological Society of America gave him the Donald P. Kent award in 1990 for his willingness to cross disciplinary boundaries in communicating research. In this effort, Adelman's approach has been parallel to that of George Maddox,* who has stressed the diversity and complementariness of research in geriatrics and gerontology, and Carroll E. Estes,* who explores the relationship between research and practice in policymaking.

After four years of directing the Institute of Aging at Temple, Adelman became director of the Institute of Gerontology at the University of Michigan in Ann Arbor in 1982. There, he has built a cadre of researchers with appointments in most of the university's professional schools, and helped Jeffrey B. Halter,

M.D.,* launch a geriatrics program now recognized by the Medical School as a "center of excellence." In addition to these administrative duties, Adelman has served as a president of the Gerontological Society of America. During his tenure as chair of the U.S. Department of Veterans Affairs Advisory Committee on Geriatrics and Gerontology, Adelman tenaciously and successfully demanded that greater priority be accorded the needs of elderly veterans.

Unlike most well-known bio-gerontologists, Adelman claims that he has had few research collaborators. That said, friendships forged with Vincent J. Cristofalo,* Edward J. Masoro,* George T. Baker,* and Jay Roberts during Adelman's Temple University years (1969–82) have proved remarkably enduring. These men gave one another mutual support and critical feedback at a time when research on the biology of aging had little credibility among biological researchers. Now geographically scattered, the group continues to exercise the leadership of the Gerontological Society with its demands that bio-gerontology be accorded a respect far exceeding the numerical strength of the section's size. Adelman also turns to this group as he thinks through ways to nurture and develop cooperative, productive research programs.

ARTHUR JOSEPH ALTMEYER. The nation's first Social Security commissioner was born in 1891 in De Pere, Wisconsin, the son of John G. Altmeyer and Carrie Smith. Altmeyer first became interested in social welfare and labor legislation when working as an office boy in his uncle's law firm. While sorting mail, he came across a pamphlet describing Wisconsin's landmark Workmen's Compensation Act, the first of its kind legislated in this country. Upon entering the University of Wisconsin, he took courses from John R. Commons, the dean of American labor economists, who believed that members of the academy should play an active role in policymaking. Altmeyer received his B.A. and Phi Beta Kappa key in 1914. He spent the next two years teaching high school and then, after marrying Ethel M. Thomas, served two years as a high school principal.

Altmeyer returned to the University of Wisconsin in 1918. While serving as Commons's research assistant, he co-authored a report, "The Health Insurance Movement in the United States," which greatly influenced the deliberations of the Illinois Health Insurance Commission and the Ohio Health and Old Age Insurance Commission. In 1920, Altmeyer became chief statistician of the Wisconsin Industrial Commission. In this capacity he launched a monthly publication, *Wisconsin Labor Market,* which became a prototype for employment indexes in the nation. In 1922, he became Secretary of the Wisconsin Industrial Commission, a post he held for eleven years. (In this period, he managed to earn his M.A. and Ph.D. (in 1931); he also took a six-month leave in 1927 to serve as deputy commissioner for the United States Employees' Compensation Commission for the Great Lakes region to put into effect the Longshoremen's and Harbor Workers' Compensation Act.) The highlight of his tenure was the enactment, in January 1932, of the Wisconsin Unemployment Reserves and Compensation Act, the first such Act passed in the United States.

Arthur Altmeyer's academic and administrative background caught the attention of New Deal architects, who hoped to model progressive federal social welfare and labor legislation on the so-called "Wisconsin Idea." On the recommendation of Sen. Robert LaFollette, Frances Perkins, the Secretary of Labor, invited Altmeyer in 1933 to come to Washington to assist in the development of working relationships with state labor departments. During the next year, while on leave from the Wisconsin Industrial Commission, he served as director of the Labor Compliance Division of the National Industrial Recovery Administration and assisted officials in organizing the Federal Emergency Relief Administration and the Civil Works Administration. In May 1934, Altmeyer became second Assistant Secretary of Labor, charged with reorganizing the department. A month later he was asked to chair the technical board advising the President's Cabinet Committee on Economic Security.

Altmeyer drew on his University of Wisconsin connections. He recruited Edwin Witte to be his staff director; Witte, in turn, brought along one of his recent graduates, Wilbur J. Cohen.* He worked closely with Thomas Eliot (who drafted the enabling legislation) and other federal officials in creating a omnibus bill that provided relief for the elderly poor, the blind, and families with dependent children; that collected money from employers and employees to underwrite old-age insurance; that coordinated a federal-state unemployment system; and that played a role in developing public health services, especially in rural areas. After signing the Social Security Act into law on August 14, 1935, President Roosevelt named Altmeyer to the three-member Social Security Board, assigned "the duty of studying and making recommendations as to the most effective methods of providing economic security through social insurance, and as to legislation and matters of administrative policy concerning old-age pensions, unemployment compensation, accident compensation, and related subjects."

Altmeyer became chairman of the board in 1937. In this capacity, he was instrumental in securing the enactment of the 1939 Social Security amendments, which expanded coverage for old-age insurance. "Social legislation," Altmeyer wrote at the time, "requires the development of new [governmental] techniques, calling for resourcefulness and imagination of a high order. Its success lies entirely in its administration."

During World War II, Altmeyer refused to scale down Social Security operations. He ridiculed the idea of finding "steel for the turrets of the Ship of State by prying a few plates off the bottom." Nonetheless, he took on other important tasks. Altmeyer was executive director of the War Manpower Commission from 1942 to 1945. Beginning in 1942, he chaired the American delegation to the first five biennial Inter-American conferences on Social Security. After the United Nations was chartered, he served for seven years as a consultant on social welfare legislation.

In 1946, Altmeyer became the first commissioner of Social Security, when his growing bureaucracy was transferred to the Federal Security Agency. For the next seven years he staved off attacks by conservatives, who hoped to rely on private initiatives and state-level schemes to provide a safety net for senior citizens and other beneficiaries. The passage of the 1950 amendments was Altmeyer's greatest legislative victory: Harry S Truman approved a 77 percent increase in old-age insurance benefits. But his greatest achievement was probably the recruitment of a cadre of men and women who would dedicate their careers to advancing social security in America by expanding coverage and liberalizing programs and benefits in an incremental manner.

Upon retiring from government in 1953, Altmeyer was lauded for his "remarkable gifts of patience and wisdom and understanding of human problems." Remaining active, he served as president of the National Conference on Social Work (1954–1955). He advised the governments of Iran and Turkey on social welfare matters, and advised private agencies in Colombia, Peru, and Pakistan. At the time of his death, Altmeyer was serving on the boards of the National Industrial Group Pension Plan and was chief appeals officer of the ILGWU National Retirement Fund. To honor his memory, the new Social Security Administration offices in Baltimore were named in his honor.

The best biographical sources are the accounts in *Who Was Who in America,* Vol. 5 (New York, 1973), p. 12; *Current Biography* (New York, 1946), p. 14; and Altmeyer's obituaries in the *New York Times,* October 18, 1972, p. 50, and the *Washington Post,* October 18, 1972, section C, p. 4. Altmeyer traces his early career in his preface to *The Formative Years of Social Security: A Chronicle of Social Security Legislation and Administration, 1934–1954* (Madison: University of Wisconsin Press, 1968). Valuable insights can be gleaned from Martha Derthick, *Policymaking for Social Security* (Washington, D.C.: Brookings, 1979); Carolyn Weaver, *The Real Crisis in Social Security* (Durham, N.C.: Duke Press, 1982), and W. Andrew Achenbaum, *Social Security: Visions and Revisions* (New York: Cambridge University Press, 1986).

JOHN E. ANDERSON. John Edward Anderson was born in Wyoming in 1893. He earned his A.B. at the University of Wyoming in 1914, and then went to Harvard, where he received his M.A. in 1915 and his Ph.D. in psychology (1917). From 1919 to 1925 he taught at Yale. Except for visiting appointments at the University of Chicago and at UCLA, Anderson was at the University of Minnesota for the rest of his career, where he was a professor of psychology and director of its world-renowned Institute of Child Welfare.

Anderson is primarily known for his experimental research in animal and child psychology and for designing tests and measurements that were used in developmental psychology. Among his best-known works were *Happy Childhood; The Development and Guidance of Children and Youth* (New York, London: D. Appleton-Century Co., 1933); and *A Handbook of Child Psychology,* ed. Carl Murchison (Worchester, Mass.: Clark University Press, 1931). Anderson chaired the committee on the infant and preschool child for the 1929 White

House Conference on Child Health and Protection; he also was a leader at the White House Conference on Children in a Democracy a decade later. Anderson was president of the American Psychological Association (1942–1943) and of the Society for Research in Child Development (1942–1944).

In the latter part of his career, Anderson turned his attention to the other end of the life-span. For the American Psychological Association, he edited *Psychological Aspects of Aging* (Washington, D.C.: American Psychological Association, 1956). In this endeavor he worked closely with James E. Birren,* Robert J. Havighurst,* and Harold E. Jones. Among the areas covered were personal and social adjustment; assessments of aging; perceptive and intellectual abilities; learning, motivation, and education; and functional efficiency, skills, and employment. Anderson summarized promising avenues for future work in a concluding chapter, "Research Problems in Aging." There, he made clear that a "double-barrelled approach" was necessary "first, through fundamental and basic research of a more abstract character and second, through functional and actional research growing out of practical situations" (p. 289).

Anderson, who retired in 1961, was an associate editor of *The Gerontologist* at the time of his death in 1966.

ODIN W. ANDERSON. Odin W. Anderson, who was born in Minneapolis in 1914, was attracted to the field of aging by Nathan Sinai (1894–1974), a professor of public health at the University of Michigan. Sinai hired Anderson to be his research assistant in 1942. Their first project relating to the elderly was a study of medical care for recipients of old-age assistance. Anderson was one of the first to show that nursing home care represented a major proportion of all care for the elderly. This was an unexpected finding, because few senior citizens were in nursing homes before 1945. The enactment of the Social Security Act in 1935, with its stipulation that old-age assistance recipients could not reside in almshouses, hastened the demise of that dreaded institution and the growth of private domiciliary residences for those too ill to care for themselves. Anderson's case study was noted in *Social Security Bulletin* and other scholarly journals, and provoked interest in the topic. See Odin W. Anderson, *Administration of Medical Care Problems and Issues: Based on an Analysis of Medical-Dental Care Programs for the Recipients of Old-Age Assistance in the State of Washington, 1941–1945* (University of Michigan, School of Public Health: Bureau of Public Health Economics Research), Series 2, 1947.

Anderson's major contribution to the field of aging is the five national surveys he conducted between 1956 and 1973 on the use of and expenditures for personal health services. The first and last panel studies, probably the best known, were done with his major collaborators. See Odin W. Anderson and Jacob Feldman, *Family Medical Costs and Voluntary Health Insurance: A Nationwide Survey* (New York: McGraw-Hill, 1956); and Ronald Andersen, *Two Decades of Health Services: Social Survey Trends in Use and Expenditures* (Cambridge, Mass.: Ballinger, 1976).

Anderson made his career as a medical sociologist, not a gerontologist. He was a founder and director of the Center for Health Administration at the University of Chicago, where he taught from 1962 to 1980. He was named in 1985 a Distinguished Health Services Researcher by the Association of Health Services Research. He is on the faculty of the Department of Sociology at the University of Wisconsin-Madison. He will retire in June 1995, but will maintain his office and individual directed study students. His retirement will hardly be fallow; in 1988, he was named one of Wisconsin's ten most admired senior citizens. The author or co-author of more than a dozen monographs and surveys, Anderson's best-known works are *Family Medical Costs and Voluntary Health Insurance* (New York: Blakiston Division, McGraw-Hill, 1956); *Elements of Health Insurance Today* (New York: Health Information Foundation, 1960); and *Medical Care Use in Sweden and the United States* (Chicago: Center for Health Administration Studies, 1970), none of which focuses much on aging.

Anderson merits inclusion in this volume because his empirical research took account of similarities in and differences between the consumption patterns of young and old and examined age-specific variations in expenditures. His careful analyses set high standards for gerontologically related studies in health services research. And his work had a practical impact in the policy arena. Anderson's surveys were often cited by his friend Wilbur Cohen* in drafting the landmark Medicare legislation of 1965.

REUBEN ANDRES. Reuben Andres was born in Dallas in 1923. He was a student at Southern Methodist University (1939–1941) and the College of Medicine at Baylor University (1941–1943), and earned his M.D. in 1944 from Southwestern Medical College. After military service Andres completed an internship in internal medicine at Gallinger Metropolitan Hospital in Washington and his residency from 1947 to 1950 at the Veterans Administration hospital in McKinney, Texas.

Andres joined the faculty of the Johns Hopkins University medical school in 1950, rising through the ranks. He was assistant chief of medicine at the Baltimore City Hospitals from 1958 to 1962, when he became assistant chief of the Gerontology Research Center at the National Institutes of Health. In 1976, Andres became clinical director of the National Institute on Aging. Early in his career, Andres contributed "Physiological Factors of Aging Significant to the Clinician" to the *Journal of the American Geriatrics Society,* 17 (1969): 274–77. There, he suggested that better subject selection and longitudinal-study techniques might correct medical students' misconceptions of the "biological pattern of life." In *Normal Human Aging: The Baltimore Longitudinal Study of Aging* (Washington, D.C.: Government Printing Office, 1984), Andres joined Nathan Shock* and others in presenting just such data. He offered specific research findings with Paul Costa and others on "hypertension, somatic complaints, and personality," with Virginia Elahi and associates on a longitudinal study of nutritional intake among men, a paper with John W. Rowe* among others on "the effect of age on creatinine clearance in men,'' and a paper with Shock and Jordan Tobin on "patterns of longitudinal changes in renal function."

Andres served as president of the Gerontological Society in 1981; that organization had honored him with its Kleemeier Award seven years earlier. In 1986 Andres received major awards from the American Geriatrics Society and the American Federation for Aging Research. The Allied-Signal Achievement award in aging was given to him that same year. The National Institutes of Health saluted his efforts in 1973 and 1978, and the Italian Society of Gerontology gave Andres its Enrico Greppi Prize in 1987.

TONI C. ANTONUCCI. Toni Claudette Antonucci was born in Brooklyn, New York in 1948. She majored in psychology at Hunter College and studied developmental psychology with Lillian E. Troll,* Robert Kastenbaum,* and Carolyn Shantz at Wayne State University. Antonucci was attracted to the field by Kastenbaum's "widespread intellectual curiosity that is both contagious and inspirational." Shantz and Troll proved to be important mentors, who were "supportive without being smothering." After spending six years in the Department of Psychology at Syracuse University, Antonucci came to the University of Michigan, Ann Arbor. Her primary appointment is in the Institute for Social Research (ISR); she is also an adjunct professor in psychology and a faculty associate at the Institute of Gerontology.

Antonucci's prolific works fall largely in the domain of life-span development, at the interstices of psychology and sociology. With her senior colleague Robert Kahn, she developed the notion of "Convoys over the Life Course: Attachment, Roles, and Social Support," in *Life-Span Development and Behavior, Vol. 3,* eds. Paul B. Baltes* and Orville Brim (New York: Academic Press, 1980). The notion of convoys provides a way to bridge macro- and micro-level analyses of patterns of affiliation, purposiveness, and reciprocal/non-reciprocal relationships over the life course. She is particularly interested in mapping hierarchies of social support networks, stipulating their effects on interpersonal efficacy and health. Earlier studies of social network characteristics have been extended over time in a series of articles focusing on gender differences in adult social relationships; see P. K. Adelmann, T. C. Antonucci, S. F. Crohan, and L. M. Coleman, "Empty-Nest, Cohort and Employment in the Well-Being of Midlife Women," *Sex Roles,* 20 (1989): 173–89. In conjunction with several ongoing ISR research projects charting the relationships among aging, health, and retirement, Antonucci has been exploring how social relations affect the health/well-being continuum.

With her husband James S. Jackson,* Antonucci has also been exploring possible racial and ethnic variations in social-support processes and mechanisms. "Although there is a convergence toward a resource, life-span model of ethnicity that transcends notions of traditional culture and assimilation, we noted the poor research and sparse empirical literature on the topic," the pair noted in a review article on "Cultural, Racial, and Ethnic Minority Influences on Aging" in the third edition of the *Handbook of Aging and the Social Sciences* (New York: Academic Press, 1990). Accordingly, Antonucci has tried to use a life-span framework to discover a mid-range theoretical construct that might organize whatever pertinent empirical data are available. Representative of this research thrust is J. Jackson and T. C. Antonucci, "Social Support, Interpersonal Efficacy, and Health," in *Handbook of Clinical Gerontology*, eds. L. L. Carstensen and B. A. Edelstein (New York: Pergamon Press, 1987), 291–311. With Kahn, Jackson, and other colleagues, such as Hiroko Akiyama, Antonucci has begun to compare social relationships among older people in the United States, Japan, and France.

Antonucci has been active in several organizations. In 1991 she chaired the Behavioral and Social Science Section of the Gerontological Society. She is a fellow of the American Psychological Association and American Psychological Society.

DAVID ARENBERG. David Arenberg has developed an impressive bibliography of work in over forty years of psychological research. He was Veterans Administration trainee from 1954 to 1956 before earning his Ph.D. from Duke University in 1960. Arenberg spent almost thirty years as a research psychologist, including twenty years as chief of the Cognition Section for the National Institute on Aging's Gerontology Research Center in Baltimore. He was an active officer of the American Psychological Association's Adult Development and Aging Division. He has also served as an editor of the *Journal of Gerontology* and consulting editor for *Educational Gerontology, Experimental Aging Research,* and *Psychology Aging.*

Arenberg's research has been primarily in cognition and aging, with a focus on reasoning in the elderly. Perhaps his most significant contributions have been the introduction of "poisoned food" problems for use with less educated subjects and informationally equivalent problems for use in longitudinal studies. See, for example, D. Arenberg, "Aging and Cognitive Processes" in *Changes with Age in Problems Solving,* eds. F. I. M. Craik and S. E. Trehub (New York: Plenum Press, 1982.)

According to Arenberg, research on reasoning tends to be focused on either "analytic" or "synthetic" processes. Therefore, he has designed problems that measure performance of each aspect separately. See D. Arenberg, "Cognitive Development in Adulthood: Progress in Cognitive Development Research" in *Analysis and Synthesis in Problem Solving and Aging,* eds. M. L. Howe and C. Brainerd (New York: Springer-Verlag, 1988).

Arenberg has collaborated primarily with Elizabeth Robertson-Tchabo, Leonard Giambra, Paul Costa, and Robert McCrae. He currently resides in Delray Beach, Florida, but continues to collaborate with his colleagues at the Gerontology Research Center.

ROBERT C. ATCHLEY. Robert C. Atchley was born in San Antonio in 1939. He moved to Ohio in 1952 and received his B.A. from Miami University in

1961. His strongest undergraduate influences were David T. Lewis, a demographer and civil rights activist whose inspiring undergraduate teaching and hardnosed approach to research attracted Atchley to an academic career, and W. Fred Cottrell, whose feedback systems theory and dedication to using social science ideas and data to influence social policy remained important intellectual tools for Atchley. While serving four years in the Marine Corps, Atchley pursued graduate work in sociology, demography, and social psychology at American University. In 1963 he took two courses in social gerontology from Clark Tibbitts,* a central figure in the development of social gerontology. Atchley's doctoral dissertation was on the impact of retirement on the self-concepts of women. Atchley returned to his alma mater, Miami University, in 1966, where he began a series of important studies on retirement and, along with Cottrell and Mildred M. Seltzer,* established the Scripps Gerontology Center, one of the first operational multidisciplinary gerontology centers in the United States.

Robert Atchley is probably best known for developing the first successful textbook in social gerontology, *The Social Forces in Later Life: An Introduction to Social Gerontology* (Belmont, Calif.: Wadsworth, 1972). Atchley integrated research findings about aging from a variety of disciplines such as biology, psychobiology, adult development, demography, sociology, economics, politics, and social welfare into a text that advanced undergraduates could understand. About a quarter of the book represented research that Atchley conducted to fill gaps in the research literature of the day. Now in its seventh edition and retitled *Social Forces and Aging,* the book remains an up-to-date prototype for organizing multidisciplinary materials in introductory social gerontology courses.

Atchley has also done considerable research on retirement. His first series of studies on individual adjustment to retirement found that retirement was a very positive transition and life stage for a large majority of retirees, contrary to the early gerontology literature, which had portrayed retirement as a negative life change. Atchley was among the first researchers to document that retirement had little effect on either physical or mental health. This work is summarized in his *The Sociology of Retirement* (Cambridge, Mass.: Schenkman, 1976). In an important article, "Retirement as a Social Institution," in the *Annual Review of Sociology* (1982), Atchley developed a feedback systems theory of the evolution of retirement in the United States. He also did comparative research on the relative influence of population aging and economic development on the development of social security-type public pension policy provisions throughout the world. See, for instance, R. Atchley, "Social Security-Type Retirement Policies: A Cross-National Study" in *Current Perspectives on Aging and the Life Cycle,* ed. Zena S. Blau* (New York: JAI Press, 1985).

Atchley is also well known for his development of a continuity theory of aging. Beginning with his "Retirement and Leisure Participation: Continuity or Crisis?" in *The Gerontologist* in 1971 and adding substantially to the theory in "A Continuity Theory of Normal Aging" in *The Gerontologist* in 1989, Atchley articulated a theory designed to explain the evolution of internal psychological structures and external lifestyles that people are predisposed to use as frames of reference in adapting to change.

In addition to Tibbitts and Cottrell, Atchley's closest associates have been his colleagues at Miami University, most notably Mildred M. Seltzer and Sheila J. (Miller) Atchley, and his students. Linda K. George's* praise of Atchley and the Scripps Gerontology Center that he has directed since 1974 is widely shared by his other students. Under his aegis, Miami has become one of the best, and arguably the most congenial, places to do graduate work in social gerontology, and Atchley developed a proposal for a doctoral program in social gerontology at Miami that is making its way through the approval process.

Atchley has also been active in professional organizations in aging. He served as president of the American Society on Aging from 1988 to 1990 and served on its board of directors for over a decade. He also held a number of offices and committee posts in the Gerontological Society of America and in the Association for Gerontology in Higher Education. He has served on the editorial boards of *The Gerontologist, Journal of Aging Studies, Generations, Aging Today,* and *Research on Aging,* and as founding editor of *Contemporary Gerontology: A Journal of Reviews and Critical Discourse.*

Atchley has been richly rewarded for his work in the field. In 1990, he received Miami University's highest award to a faculty member, the Benjamin Harrison Award. He has also received numerous awards from the Gerontological Society of America and the American Society on Aging.

JOSEPH C. AUB. Joseph Charles Aub was born in Cincinnati in 1890. He received his A.B. from Harvard College in 1911 and his M.D. from Harvard Medical School three years later. Aub completed his clinical training at Massachusetts General Hospital and then served as a physician there for the rest of his professional life. He also was on the staff of Peter Bent Brigham Hospital (1928–1942), and was physician-in-chief (1928–1943) and director of medical labs (1943–1956) at Collis P. Huntington Memorial Hospital of Harvard.

Aub served as an instructor of physiology at Harvard Medical School (1919), before rising through the ranks (assistant professor, 1920–1924; assistant professor of medicine, 1924–1928; associate professor, 1928–1943) and becoming department chair (1943–1956) and professor of research medicine (1948–1956). Much of his work focused on endocrinology, some on cancer. Aub retired in 1956.

In addition to his practice of medicine and teaching, Aub served on numerous advisory boards for the National Research Council. He was president of the Ella Sachs Plotz Foundation and sat on the board of the Worcester Foundation for Explorations in Biology, serving as its president from 1955–1959. Although he is better known for his work on cancer and endocrinology, Aub nonetheless served as president of the Gerontological Society in 1948.

Joseph Aub died in 1973.

B

JEANNE E. BADER. Jeanne Bader, born in 1943, earned her B.A. at the University of Delaware in 1965, where she majored in English and psychology. She took an M.A. in experimental psychology at the University of Vermont two years later. She spent five years at the Philadelphia Geriatric Center, working as a research psychologist. Bader earned her Ph.D. in 1979 at the University of California, San Francisco.

From 1981 to 1988, Bader directed the Center for Gerontology at the University of Oregon. After spending four years at the University of Minnesota, conducting the Minnesota Area Geriatric Education Center, Bader moved back west. Since 1992, she has directed the Gerontology Program at California State University, Long Beach, and she has directed its Center for Successful Aging.

During the last decade, Bader's activities have focused on beliefs and expectations regarding age and seniority as variables in higher education. This has been important in light of the 1994 elimination ("uncapping") of mandatory retirement for tenured faculty. She has produced two editions of the *Handbook of Research Abstracts on the "Uncapping" of Academic Mandatory Retirement* (Minneapolis, Minn.: University of Minnesota, 1989, 1990). In addition, she has conducted national research on this topic, published three refereed papers, and organized and staffed several conferences.

Her current work continues her interest in faculty seniority issues and includes research on older and retired gerontologists, geriatricians, and activities intended to foster greater collaboration and exchange among professionals in the fields of aging and disability.

Bader's teaching and networking skills, first at the University of Oregon, later

at the University of Minnesota, and now at California State University, Long
Beach, have influenced public and institutional policies. She has been a significant and creative networker, helping to define gerontology as a distinct field.
Bader has assumed several leadership roles in the Gerontological Society of
America since 1967, as well as in the formative years of the National Caucus
on the Black Aged and the Western Gerontological Society. She also has been
active in the Gray Panthers and Older Women's League.

She counts among her teachers and mentors M. Powell Lawton,* Carroll E.
Estes,* Robert Kane,* Nancy Eustis, Percy Tannenbaum, Maggie Kuhn,* and
Aaron Wildavsky.

GEORGE T. BAKER III. George T. Baker III was born in Waterbury, Connecticut, in 1940. After serving in the U.S. Naval Medical Corps (1958–1961),
he earned his baccalaureate degrees in zoology and chemistry from the University of Connecticut (1966). He earned his M.S. in biochemistry and physiology
from the University of Rhode Island, where he worked with George Trembley.
Under Morris Rockstein,* Baker won his Ph.D. in physiology and biophysics
from the School of Medicine at the University of Miami (1971).

Baker's interest in the field of aging initially was purely an intellectual one.
While working in 1965 as a research associate at the Cancer Research Institute,
under the direction of Olga Grengard, he recognized that the enzyme activity
measurements he was determining in animals in another research protocol context changed with adult age. He had to do a lesser number of experiments to
obtain statistical significance between various parameters under study. Baker
later became one of the first researchers to institute routine coextraction of biological materials as a standard experimental protocol in biological gerontology.
See his "Age-Related Activity Changes in Arginine Phosphokinase in the
Housefly, *Musca domestica L.,*" *Journal of Gerontology,* 30 (1975); 163–69.

Baker was one of the first biological scientists in modern times to understand
the concept of life-history strategy as a way of appreciating basic mechanisms
of aging and longevity. He was instrumental in reviving interest in the use of
Drosophila as a model system to study eucaryotic aging. See his essay on "Aging in *Drosophila*" in *CRC Handbook of Cell Biology of Aging,* ed. Vincent
Cristofalo* (Boca Raton, Fla.: CRC Series, 1985). At the same time, Baker has
long championed the importance of interspecies comparisons of age-related
changes to an understanding of basic mechanisms of biological aging processes.
As a close friend and supporter of Nathan W. Shock,* particularly in his retirement years, Baker reiterated his mentor's insistence on such comparative research. See N. W. Shock and G. T. Baker III, "Concepts in Aging Research,"
in *Potential for Nutritional Modulation of Aging Processes,* eds. D. Ingram, G.
T. Baker III, and N. W. Shock (Food and Nutrition Press, Washington, D.C.,
1991). Baker has also been active in promoting the development of bio-markers
of aging. See his essay with Richard Sprott (who oversees this area for National

Institute on Aging) on "Biomarkers of Aging," *Special Issues: Experimental Gerontology,* 23 (1988): 223–39.

Baker has been very active in establishing gerontology initiatives outside of the laboratory. He developed a gerontology institute at Drexel University, where he led a multidisciplinary team that published (with C. Krauser) the first *Catalog of Products and Services to Enhance the Independence of the Elderly* (Philadelphia: Drexel University Press, 1982). He then became director of the Center of Aging at the University of Maryland at College Park (1982–1986). During his tenure in College Park, approximately 400 students earned certificates of aging at the master's and doctoral levels. From 1985 until 1990, Baker served as founding president of the American Association for Advances in Health Care Research, an organization primarily consisting of marketing professionals with an interest in developing products and services for older individuals. Baker was particularly interested in disseminating bio-medical information as it relates to the problems of the elderly.

As a biologist who is interested in policy-relevant issues, Baker is keen to distinguish sharply between the processes of aging and the problems of the elderly in our society. He is an advocate of the development of intervention strategies to slow the processes of aging and reduce the incidence of age-associated diseases. See G. T. Baker III and G. M. Martin,* "Biological Aging and Longevity: Underlying Mechanisms and Intervention Strategies," *Journal of Aging and Physical Activity,* 2 (1994): 304–28. True to his scientific training, he believes that "only through our understanding of the basic mechanisms of aging processes will we in an efficacious manner alleviate the problems of the elderly. A balanced conceptual approach in allocation of resources is what must be advocated."

Since 1989, Baker has served as president of the Nathan W. and Margaret T. Shock Aging Research Foundation, which is dedicated to funding research to further our understanding of biological aging processes.

PAUL B. BALTES. Paul B. Baltes, who was born in Saarlouis, Germany, in 1939, earned his Ph.D. in psychology from the University of Saarland, Germany, in 1967. There he studied under Ernest E. Boesch, who earned his doctorate under Jean Piaget. Baltes became interested in aging-related research in the course of writing a doctoral dissertation on sequential models (cross-sectional and longitudinal sequences). Currently, he is a major figure in the Max Planck Institute for Human Development and Education in Berlin, one of the most prestigious research centers in the world. Baltes also taught at Penn State and West Virginia universities from 1968 to 1970. He counts his supervisors, Ernest Boesch and Gunnther Reinert, in addition to the German psychologists, and K. Warner Schaie,* Klaus F. Riegel,* O. G. Brim, and Matilda White Riley* among his role models. Margaret Baltes, John Nesselroade, and Sherry Willis* have been his major collaborators.

In Berlin, he currently works with a cohort of next-generation scientists such as Ulman Lindenberger, Jacqui Smith, and Ursula Staudinger. Among his earlier students and/or junior colleagues were Gisela Labouvie-Vief, Carol D. Ryff,* Steve Cornelius, Roger Dixon, Margie Lachman, Harvey Sterns, and Reinhold Kliegl. These biographical facts go some distance in explaining Baltes's pivotal role in the advancement of theory-building in the psychology of aging. Baltes is truly an international scholar, whose lifespan approach to developments in aging has had a significant impact on sociologists, historians, and clinicians, not just psychologists. This fact is evident in his honorary doctorates and election to several academies, including the American Academy of Arts and Sciences and the European Academy.

Baltes's initial publications took off from his dissertation. See, for instance, his "Longitudinal and Cross-Sectional Sequences in the Study of Aging and Generation Effects," in *Human Development, 11* (1968): 145–71, which by Social Science Citations standards became a classic. His recent publications represent major contributions to the theory and methodology of lifespan studies through his laboratory's research into the plasticity of intelligence and memory. He has explored opportunities for growth as well as limitations of the aging mind, such as the loss of capacity for basic memory. See, for instance, his "Theoretical Propositions of Life-Span Developmental Psychology: On the Dynamics Between Growth and Decline," in *Developmental Psychology, 23* (1987): 611–26. Like many other social scientists, Baltes also tried to formulate a rigorous and multifaceted conception of successful aging. Aware that some aspects of cognition declined while others improved with advancing aging, he proposed with Margaret Baltes a model of selective optimization with compensation. See *Successful Aging: Perspectives from the Behavioral Sciences,* eds. Paul B. Baltes and Margaret M. Baltes (Cambridge, England: Cambridge University Press, 1990).

More recently, Baltes and his colleagues (such as Jacqui Smith and Ursula Staudinger) at the Max Planck Institute have been connecting several lines of research into a programmatic, theory-driven empirical inquiry into the structure and dynamics of wisdom. Their model combines methods and concepts that are prevalent in cognitive psychology with those used in the study of knowledge systems. In an approach similar to the Cattell-Horn theory of crystallized/fluid intelligence, Baltes connects the knowledge-based "pragmatics" of intelligence with the knowledge-free "mechanics" of intelligence. Wisdom, which the Baltes group considers one of the prototypes of crystallized intelligence, reflects high expertise across five domains: (1) rich factual knowledge about life; (2) extensive procedural knowledge about ways of dealing with real-life problems; (3) lifespan contextualism; (4) relativism associated with variations in values and life priorities; and (5) an ability to recognize and manage uncertainty. See, for instance, Paul Baltes and Jacqui Smith, "The Psychology of Wisdom and its Ontogenesis," in *Wisdom: Its Nature, Origins, and Development,* ed. Robert J. Sternberg (Cambridge, England: Cambridge University Press, 1990), 87–120; see also his 1992 Kleemeier Award lecture for the Gerontological Society, published as "The Aging Mind: Potential and Limits," *The Gerontologist,* 33 (1993): 580–94.

With a large interdisciplinary team involving internal medicine, psychology, psychiatry, sociology and economics, Baltes has recently initiated a large-scale and extremely intensive study (fourteen sessions of observations) into advanced old age. The Berlin Aging Study involved a stratified random sample of 516 persons, ranging in age from seventy to 103 years. First summary results were published in a special issue of *Ageing and Society,* 13 (1993): 475–680.

CHARLES M. BARRESI. Sociologist Charles M. Barresi was born on December 20, 1928. He earned his graduate degrees (M.A., 1959; Ph.D., 1965), from the State University of New York at Buffalo, where he worked with Constance A. Yeracaris. Barresi did postdoctoral work at Miami University of Ohio, where he worked with Robert C. Atchley,* Fred Cottrell, Mildred M. Seltzer,* and Timothy Brubaker.

Barresi has taken the "life course perspective," and refined and developed it for the study of ethnic aging. The "life course" or biographical record of an individual, Barresi claimed, can be used to examine the timing of significant events such as marriage, child bearing and rearing, and retirement. Because the "proper" timing of such events is determined by cultural norms, Barresi finds this theoretical construct especially useful in explaining the social process of aging in general and the behavior of individuals bridging two sets of cultural norms. "It is most important when exploring the behavior of the migrant person who is in between two cultures, or the intergenerational relations between her or him and family members who are at different level in assimilating to the new culture," explains Barresi. His original work in this area appears in *Ethnic Dimensions of Aging* (New York: Springer Publishing, 1987), which he co-edited with Donald E. Gelfand.*

Emerging from this effort has been Barresi's concept of "ethnogerontology," elaborated in *Gerontology: Perspectives and Issues,* ed. Kenneth F. Ferraro* (New York: Springer, 1990). While it might be assumed that ethnogerontology is limited to the study of ethnic minorities, Barresi insists that it is essential to a proper understanding of groups that might be identified as "white ethnics," such as the Irish, Poles, and Italians. His most recent work, co-edited with Donald E. Stull, is *Ethnic Elderly and Long Term Care* (New York: Springer, 1993), and is a complete collection of information on ethnic elderly and long-term care. This book was selected as the Book of the Year by the *American Journal of Nursing* in 1994. Also in 1994, he edited and contributed to a monograph, *Health and Minority Elders: An Analysis of Applied Literature 1980–1990,* for the American Association of Retired Persons.

Barresi's interest in gerontology was sparked by work he did after joining the Department of Sociology at the University of Akron in 1966. Contracted to evaluate a U.S. Housing and Urban Development-sponsored workshop program on the elderly, Barresi eventually published two articles, one in *The Gerontol-*

ogist (1972), and one for *Industrial Gerontology* (1974). He has since published over thirty book chapters and journal articles. He is currently a professor emeritus and Life Fellow in the Institute for Life-Span Development and Gerontology at the University of Akron.

Barresi lives in Florida, where he is an adjunct professor in the Department of Gerontology, University of South Florida.

SCOTT A. BASS. After earning his B.A. from the University of Michigan in 1971, Scott Bass earned a combined doctorate in psychology and education in 1976 from his alma mater, where he worked with Elton McNeil. His conceptual work was further refined through an informal association with Seymour Sarason, "the father of community psychology," at Yale University. His interest in gerontology was sparked by Richard Rowland and Frank Manning of the Massachusetts Association of Older Americans, a statewide advocacy group.

While many gerontologists speak of the need to treat older people as valuable and productive members of society, Scott A. Bass has put this belief into practice.

Bass developed a comprehensive Gerontology Institute at the University of Massachusetts, Boston, that includes certificate, undergraduate, and graduate programs in gerontology. After building a coalition of academics and advocates, he negotiated the first Ph.D. program in gerontology and public policy at a public university. Particularly helpful in this venture was Frank Manning, a longtime leader of the Massachusetts Association of Older Americans. (The most prestigious chair in the program—the only chair directly established by the state legislature—is named for Manning.) More important, perhaps, the Institute engages older people as participants in the development of aging policy.

Along with Robert Morris,* Bass argues for the integration of the elderly as professionals and researchers in "The Elderly as Surplus People: Is There a Role in Higher Education?" *The Gerontologist,* 26 (1986): 12–18. Bass and Morris were founders in 1989 and co-editors of the *Journal of Aging and Social Policy.*

The two also collaborated on *Retirement Reconsidered* (New York: Springer, 1988), which established them as leaders in a movement that views older people as productive and valuable members of society. Bass has further refined the concept of "productive aging" through academic papers, publication, conferences, and research (sponsored by the Commonwealth Fund). A 1993 volume, *Achieving a Productive Aging Society* (Westport, Conn.: Auburn House Press, 1993), edited with Francis G. Caro* and Yung-Ping Chen,* examines the consequences of institutional norms and traditions on the role of the elderly in society. His most recent edited volume, *Aging and Active: Dimensions of Productive Engagement Among Older Americans* (New Haven, Conn.: Yale University Press, 1995), draws upon five years of Commonwealth Fund research and provides an analytical backdrop to the earlier conceptual work.

Through a Fulbright Research Scholarship, Bass is now exploring issues of work, role, and meaning in later life. The work has taken him to Japan, where he is studying the potential application of several innovative programs developed for older workers and retirees.

WALTER M. BEATTIE, JR. Walter M. Beattie, Jr. received his M.A. from the University of Chicago in sociology in 1950. From the start, Beattie's career and efforts were conducted mostly on his own, with little or no collaboration. Most of his teachers in the 1940s and early 1950s conceptualized aging as a problem or as "pathological." Most denigrated or avoided aging issues in teaching or research. This is not to say that there were no leaders in the field—Beattie was keenly aware at the time that there were experts in bio-medical specialties—but most were not interested in the social aspects of aging or in social policy. "Social research and studies were viewed as less rigorous and scientific" than bench science, Beattie recalls. "It was an uphill battle to reach out and get support and credibility."

Ollie A. Randall* became a continuing source of knowledge, support, and inspiration for more than a decade as gerontology and geriatrics programs began to be developed. With her assistance, Beattie became interested in the design and execution of action-research programs in long-term care. From 1953 to 1956, Beattie concentrated his efforts in Madison and Dane counties, Wisconsin; from 1959 to 1963, he worked in the metropolitan St. Louis area. These endeavors involved policymakers at the federal, state, and local levels; service providers in all related aspects of social, health, and environmental services; recipients of services; and research specialists. They participated in the formulation, design, and implementation of the action-research and in the design of relevant approaches to a community-based system of long-term care. Their emphasis was on identifying and matching individual social and psychological requirements to medical and health needs and resources on a continuing, long-term basis.

Beattie's primary intellectual contribution in this area was his emphasis on identifying the full range of individualized needs and in designing a community system of care responsive to such needs. "The concept of supportive environments—physical, psychological, and social—of the individual to promote maximum realization of potential self-determination throughout the life-span is essential," Beattie argued in "The Design of Supportive Environments for the Life-Span," *The Gerontologist,* 10 (1970): 190–93: "Central to social planning of the physical environment is the development of new conceptual frameworks which may serve as models for continuous experimentation." These efforts at community organization and planning research were carried out before the licensure of long-term care facilities had occurred. Because state and federal personnel were involved in these efforts, original legislation often reflected the ways analysts and lawmakers evaluated these grass-roots initiatives. See *Dane County Survey of Health Needs, Services, and Facilities for the Aging and Long-Term Patient* (Community Welfare Council of Madison, Wisconsin, 1956); and with

Jean Bullock, "Evaluating Services and Personnel in Facilities for the Aged," in *Geriatric Institutional Management,* eds. Morton H. Leeds* and Herbert Shore* (New York: G. P. Putnam's Sons, 1964).

The second area in which Beattie's contributions have been honored is education and teaching. He was a major figure in the design of an academic model for centers of multidisciplinary research, education, and practice in geriatrics and gerontology in higher education. In "Gerontology Curricula: Multidisciplinary Frameworks, Interdisciplinary Structures, and Disciplinary Depth," *The Gerontologist,* 14 (1974): 545–49, Beattie declared that program development had to be carried out in the context of changes in higher education itself; that the status of gerontology in higher education was as low as the status of older persons; that gerontologists had to make bridges to the humanities and scientific disciplines as well as a variety of professions; that planners had to get beyond the notion of aging as a "problem" in developing conceptual frameworks; that linkages that played creatively on the tensions between depth and breadth were key; that a critical mass of faculty was necessary; that students needed hands-on experience with the elderly; that the aged should be used as resources; that students be encouraged to design their own programs; and that policy issues be raised. This model was adopted by several North American universities, including Syracuse, which became Beattie's base of operations.

Especially during the 1960s and 1970s, Beattie traveled widely to develop curriculum materials and structure the training of leaders. He worked between 1963 and 1966 with the Chronic Diseases Section of the U.S. Public Health Service, particularly its chief, Austin Chinn, in the design and funding of a multidisciplinary gerontological curriculum project for the Gerontological Society. This resulted in several training publications. He also developed a series of workshops for training the trainers in New York, New Jersey, Delaware, Puerto Rico, and the Virgin Islands.

Beattie was a consultant, lecturer or visiting professor at fifty universities in the late 1960s through the mid-1970s. This led to the establishment of SAGE (the State Association of Gerontological Educators), now called the Society for Aging of New York. From 1972 to 1974, Beattie worked with the Gerontological Society's leadership and academicians to develop the Association for Gerontology in Higher Education (AGHE). That organization now gives an annual Walter Beattie award to a distinguished educator.

Beattie was also a pioneer in exploring the dimensions of minority aging. He conceived and developed a research protocol for the Ford Foundation in 1959, and published "The Aging Negro: Some Implications for Social Welfare Services," in *The Phylon: Review of Race and Culture,* 21 (1960): 131–35. This piece prompted the Urban League to establish a program on aging in the 1960s and to develop strategies for dealing with aging Blacks.

Finally, in the international arena, Beattie helped to formulate and conceptualize issues from a cross-cultural perspective. He served as a consultant on aging to the Center for Social Development and Humanitarian Affairs of the

United Nations (1972–1979). Beattie played a major role in writing the basic document for the United Nations' 1982 World Assembly on Aging, *Aging: the Humanitarian Issues.* He served on the executive committee of the board of directors of the International Center for Social Gerontology in Paris. This experience piqued his interest in differences in policy-relevant aging issues in lesser developed and advanced industrial cultures. See, for instance, his "Aging: A Framework of Characteristics and Considerations for Cooperative Efforts between Developing and Developed Regions of the World," in the U.S. Senate Special Committee on Aging's publication, *The Graying of Nations: Implications* (Washington, D.C.: Government Printing Office, 1978).

NEAL BELLOS. Neal Bellos earned his B.A. in general science in 1948, an M.A. in history from the University of Pennsylvania in 1950, and an M.S. in social work from Columbia University in 1958. After twelve years of community organizing in Dayton, Pittsburgh, and Cleveland, and as director of the antipoverty program in Louisville, Kentucky, Bellos joined the faculty of the Syracuse University School of Social Work in 1968. Walter M. Beattie, Jr.,* the dean of the school, first involved him in gerontology, appointing him as director of the school's Model Cities and Aging Project 1969–1972, funded by the U.S. Administration on Aging. That project developed a series of seven documents which were guidelines for the inclusion of elder concerns in model cities programs.

Bellos received his doctorate from Syracuse University in 1973, and joined the newly established All-University Gerontology Center as associate director for program development, becoming its director from 1980 to 1989. His primary contribution to the field originated in this development of the university's market-oriented professional programs involvement in gerontology education. These efforts culminated in the Syracuse Series in Gerontological Education, whose preparation was directed by Bellos in a number of Title IV grants from 1986 to 1989. The series published six volumes, designed to assist faculty in including gerontological content in advertising, industrial design, journalism, management, marketing, and retailing courses.

Bellos was president of the New York State Society for Aging in 1979 and of the Association for Gerontology in Higher Education from 1987 to 1988, and was a recipient of the Walter M. Beattie Jr. Award for Distinguished Service in Aging in 1986.

Now retired, he currently works on the images of age in science fiction, in developing multimedia computer-assisted distance education, and in teaching.

VERN L. BENGTSON. Vern L. Bengtson earned his B.A. in philosophy at North Park College in Chicago in 1963. Bengston claims that he had no idea what gerontology was, much less how to pronounce it, until he applied to the University of Chicago for graduate work. The only funding he was offered was a National Institutes of Health traineeship in gerontology. Opportunism aside,

Bengtson became convinced during the first quarter on the Midway that becoming a gerontologist was a shrewd professional move. He became part of a team that interviewed three-generation Black families in the Chicago slums. Bengtson saw continuities and changes in individuals and families with age. Having minored in history in college, the scope of macro-social change over decades and even centuries had always fascinated him. But as he thought more about the relationship between the micro- and macro-social levels, Bengtson developed an intellectual curiosity about the puzzle of continuity and change over time, in human lives and across birth cohorts. In many ways, Bengtson's entire career to date has been engaged in disentangling levels of units of analysis and developing concepts, to put them back together in a coherent manner.

During his graduate years, Bernice L. Neugarten* proved to be his most significant teacher. In Bengtson's words, Neugarten "intimidated me into becoming an empirical social scientist, and she taught me everything I know about clear writing and thinking. 'What's the intellectual plot line!,' she would scream in her pencilled margined comments on my drafts. [Neugarten] caused me to get through the Ph.D. program at Chicago in three and one-half years, thoroughly terrified lest she and the other faculty find out how dim my grasp of social science was." Bengtson earned his M.A. in 1965 and his Ph.D. in 1967.

Apparently, Neugarten's concern for methodological rigor paid off. Bengtson's first publication was a comment on cross-national research methods in aging, while the second presented data to demonstrate the differences between two occupations in patterns of retirement surveyed in six industrialized countries. See V. L. Bengtson and B. L. Neugarten, "Some Problems of Method in the Cross-National Study of Adjustment to Aging," in the *Proceedings of the Seventh International Congress of Gerontology* (Vienna: International Association of Gerontology, 1966); and B. L. Neugarten and V. L. Bengtson, "Cross-National Studies of Adulthood and Aging," in *Interdisciplinary Topics in Gerontology,* eds. Ethel Shanas* and J. Madge (Berlin: S. Karger, 1968).

James E. Birren,* who was building a gerontology program at the University of Southern California, recruited Bengtson to the faculty, where he has remained ever since. For Birren's mentoring, Bengtson has nothing but the utmost praise: "He helped make me what I am today, by inspiring confidence." In the five intellectual themes that characterize Bengtson's academic career can be seen the systematic development of ideas that became increasingly individuated (and extolled by peers) over time:

1. *The importance of comparative research on contrasting social contexts of aging.* Since his first year of graduate school, Bengtson has been intrigued by differences in age and aging reflected in different social contexts. He was fascinated by contrasts among social collectives in dealing with the universal phenomenon of aging, whether they be cross-national contrasts, contrasts between minorities and majorities, contrasts within ethnic groups, or contrasts between occupational groups. One line of research under this rubric concerned aging in American minority populations. Bengston and a team of his students expanded

contrasts among Black, Mexican-American, and Anglo respondents in patterns of family relationships, awareness of plenitude, attitudes toward death and dimensions of well-being.

See, for instance, V. L. Bengtson, "Cultural and Occupational Differences in Level of Present Role Activity in Retirement," in *Adjustment to Retirement,* eds. Robert J. Havighurst* et al. (Utvecht: Van Gorkum, 1969); S. Luebeck and V. L. Bengtson, "Measures for Relational Propositions," *Sociology and Social Research,* 58 (1973): 45–56; V. L. Bengtson, "Comparative Perspectives on the Microsociology of Politics and Aging," in *Justice and the Older Americans,* ed. M.A.Y. Rifai (Lexington, Va.: D. C. Heath, 1977); and Pauline K. Regan and V. L. Bengtson, *Aging among Blacks, Mexican-Americans, and Whites: Development, Procedures and Results of the Community Survey* (Washington, D.C.: Report to the National Science Foundation, 1977).

2. *Generations and their role in social continuity and change.* Once again, this intellectual interest stems from Bengtson's graduate school experiences. Neugarten required him to read several of Karl Mannheim's essays on the "problems of generations." This aroused his interest in cohorts as well as in the difference between cohort and family relationships with the passage of time. In 1970, Bengtson developed a survey to compare and contrast three generations. This longitudinal study now spans nearly three decades, enabling Bengtson to study continuities and changes in family relationships as members age.

Three ideas stand out among the findings that have emerged and been reconfirmed over the decades. First, the term "generations" spans at least three distinct conceptual and empirical scientific domains; researchers must be clear about what they mean when they use this term. Second, the "generation gap" is neither as deep nor as specific as many observers have suggested. Third, cohort effects and family intergenerational transmission effects are quite different. See, for instance, an early essay that remains frequently cited, V. L. Bengtson and J. A. Kuypers, "Generational Differences and the 'Developmental Stake,'" *Aging and Human Development,* 2 (1971): 249–60; V. L. Bengtson and K. D. Black, "Intergenerational Relations and Continuity in Socialization," in *Life-Span Developmental Psychology and Socialization,* eds. Paul B. Baltes* and K. Warner Schaie* (New York: Academic Press, 1973); and V. L. Bengtson, "The 'Generation Gap': A Review and Typology of Social-Psychological Perspectives," *Youth and Society,* 2 (1970): 7–32.

3. *Family relationships and old age across the life course.* Greatly influenced by the work of Reuben Hill, Bengtson has made several contributions here. First, building on his essay with Kuypers, Bengtson has advanced the "generational stake hypothesis," the idea that each generation distorts its perceptions of the others, and its own relationship with them. The distortion is always more positive down the generational line, that is, from father to son, and more negative from son to father. There are, nonetheless, high and stable degrees of affect between parents and children across the life course. The solidarity that inheres in family relationships in fact can be conceptualized across at least six distinct

domains, which can be reduced to three overarching dimensions. By analyzing and synthesizing parts and the whole, Bengtson has underscored the dubious interplay between family solidarity and psychological well-being. Finally, challenging contemporary wisdom, Bengtson acknowledges that the grandparent-grandchild relationship is usually cordial, but of relatively little importance to either party.

For some of the major pieces that have come out of this research, see V. L. Bengtson, "Generation and Family Effects in Value Socialization," *American Sociological Review*, 40 (1975): 358–71; A. C. Acock and V. L. Bengtson, "Socialization and Attribution Processes: Actual versus Perceived Similarity between Parents and Children," *Journal of Marriage and the Family*, 42 (1980): 501–15; Lillian Troll and V. L. Bengtson, "Generations in the Family," in *Theories about the Family*, ed. W. Burr, R. Hill and I. Nye (New York: Free Press, 1979); and Judith R. Treas and V. L. Bengtson, "Family in Later Years," in *Handbook on Marriage and the Family*, ed. Marvin G. Sussman* and S. Steinmetz (New York: Plenum, 1986).

4. *The crucial importance of theory and theory-development to research in social gerontology.* In this area, his intellectual partnership with James Birren becomes more evident. "I would like to be remembered," he wrote for his volume, "to be remembered as a scholar who developed intellectual bridges: between stages of the life course, between macro- and micro-levels of analysis, between behaviors and attitudes in the analysis of aging." Bengtson has been a major force at the Andrus Gerontology Center's Andrew Norman Institute in the creation of ideas. With Birren, he edited *Emergent Theories of Aging* (New York: Springer Publishing, 1988). In an essay on "Sociological Theories of Aging: Current Perspectives and Future Directions" with Patricia Passuth, he stressed the importance of assessing current theoretical perspectives as well as future prospects: "While the study of aging has drawn upon sociological theories in general, it has lagged behind in its theoretical development." Enthusiastic about richly contextualized analyses of the aging process, Bengtson has been a major force in emphasizing life-course perspectives as an emerging paradigm of gerontology. Among the conceptual nubs that emerge from his work have been notions about the "social-breakdown syndrome" and the "double-jeopardy versus age as a leveler hypothesis."

5. *"Generational equity" and the action of "justice between generations."* Bengtson chose to commemorate his year as president of the Gerontological Society by staging a conference at the University of Southern California to explore whether

something new seems to have happened in the latter decades of the twentieth century. Traditional problems of generational relations have been altered by phenomena of worldwide population aging—in which average life expectancy has almost doubled in the Western world during the past century, and the 'normal' balance of generational support has tilted toward the upper end of the life cycle. . . . Once accused of viewing all older people as marginal and poor, journalists now exaggerate elders' power in the voting booth and chide them as 'greedy geezers.'

See V. L. Bengtson and W. Andrew Achenbaum, eds., *The Changing Contract across Generations* (New York: A. de Gruyter, 1993).

Despite his prolific outpouring, Bengtson takes special pride in his contributions as a teacher—a disseminator of existing knowledge, a mentor, and an intellectual midwife. His teaching has been recognized several times at USC. In addition to be awarded a chair of the American Sociological Association's Section on Aging, he has also been a president of the Gerontological Society. Bengtson was twice awarded the Reuben Hill Award for outstanding research and theory on the family by the National Council of Family Relations. He has also received a MERIT award from the National Institute on Aging.

RUTH BENNETT. Ruth Bennett was born in New York in 1933. She graduated *magna cum laude* from Brooklyn College, City University of New York, where she was elected to Sigma Xi and Phi Beta Kappa. Bennett served as a research assistant in Cornell Medical School's Comprehensive Care and Teaching Program from 1953 to 1956. In 1958, she began a twenty-year affiliation with the Jewish Home and Hospital for the Aged as a research associate in sociology. While working as a research scientist, doing gerontological research for Biometrics Research of the New York State Office of Mental Health (1957–1990), Bennett earned her Ph.D. in 1962 from Columbia University.

Bennett was first attracted to research on aging by one of her teachers, Joseph Zubin. Her first published paper (with N. Tee), in *Social Problems* (1959–1960): 226–32, dealt with "social isolation and difficulties in social interaction in residents of a home for the aged." It is also worth noting that Bennett published a paper on "the aged recluse" with Frederic Zeman, a luminary at the Jewish Home, in 1960. These two articles signaled a research interest that would last more than three decades. In the mid-1960s, sometimes with one of her associates (such as Lucille Nahemow), Bennett published papers on the social and mental adjustments of nursing-home residents. She was one of the first to introduce Frying Goffman's conception of institutional totality to the nursing home field. In "Psychopathology and Deviance: Treatment or Intervention?" (in *Psychopathology: Contributions from the Biological, Behavioral, and Social Sciences,* eds. Muriel Hammer, Kurt Salzinger, and Samuel Sutton (New York: Wiley-Inter-Science Publications, 1972), 175–90), Bennett (with E. Sanchez) contributed to an interdisciplinary approach to the fields of psychopathology and deviance as experienced by the aged.

Bennett is probably best known for work in three areas:

1. *Social isolation in the aged.* Of major concern has been the detection of an isolate, identifying different types of isolates, assessing the consequences of isolation, determining which types of isolates need help and can benefit from

help, and determining what sorts of help they need. In New York and London, Bennett has explored the negative impact of social isolation on the aged, which seems to reduce their ability to adjust. Isolation among the elderly does not seem to correlate with age, sex, mental status, or education. It is not synonymous with mental disorder, though it may result in some behavior patterns associated with mental disorder such as poor social adjustment and cognitive functioning. The effects of isolation are sometimes reversible, through interventions such as resocialization programs and the use of services.

Bennett's critical contribution has been to establish a typology for social isolation. She distinguishes between lifelong (voluntary) isolates and late-life (involuntary) ones, early isolates and non-isolates. For more on this subject, see R. Bennett, ed., *Aging, Isolation, and Resocialization* (New York: Van Nostrand Reinhold, 1980); and M. Aronson, R. Bennett, and Barry Gurland, eds., *The Acting Out Elderly,* (New York: Haworth, 1983).

2. *Long-term care.* In the face of the bias against institutions and in favor of community-based care, Bennett has tried to "counter the polemics so rampant in the 1960s and later" with systematic, objective evaluations of facilities in terms of their environment and in terms of their outcomes and impacts on patients and other groups. "When aged individuals are institutionalized, it is often assumed that they will remain there until their death and that any social interaction in which they participate will be so limited that it is of no consequence," Bennett noted in an early paper in this area ("The Meaning of Institutional Life," *The Gerontologist,* 3 (1963): 117–25). "What is ignored is the fact that, depending on the role it plays in society, each institution develops a specific way of life to which inmates are socialized and expected to adjust."

Thus, Bennett's work in this area was an extension of her realization that the institutionalization of the aged meant the need to adjust to a new lifestyle, which is difficult for isolates. Nursing home life and other alternatives are described in a trio of books she edited with Barry Gurland: *Coordinated Service Delivery Systems for the Elderly: New Approaches for Care and Referral* (New York: Haworth, 1984); *Handbook of Innovative Programs for the Impaired Elderly* (New York: Haworth, 1984); and *Continuing Care Retirement Communities* (New York: Haworth, 1984).

3. *Attitudes toward aging.* Her early work in this area, such as in R. Bennett, "Attitudes in the United States Aged: A Critical Examination of Recent Literature and Implications for Future Research" (in *The Psychology of Adult Development and Aging,* eds. Carl Eisdorfer and M. Powell Lawton* (Washington, D.C.: American Psychological Association, 1973), 575–98), assayed to distinguish behavior from attitudes. Her later work deals with how family members tend to view the elderly, especially those who are demented. See, for instance, R. Bennett, "Family Burden and Dementing Illnesses," in *Advances in Neurology,* eds. R. Mayeux and W. Rosen (New York: Raven, 1983), 239–51.

In addition to her research, Bennett helped form an interdisciplinary graduate program in Gerontology at Columbia University, first in its Teachers College

(1968) and then at the School of Public Health. Since 1979, she has been deputy director of the Columbia University Center for Geriatrics and Gerontology. Six years later, Bennett became director of graduate education in the Division of Geriatrics and Gerontology in Columbia's School of Public Health. She has also been a professor of clinical public health in that unit since 1989.

Bennett has served on several study sections for the Administration on Aging, the National Institutes of Health, and U.S. Public Health Services. In 1984, she received the Northeastern Gerontological Society's Ollie Randall Award and the New York State Association of Gerontological Educator's Walter Beattie Award. She also has participated in many advisory committees related to New York City, New York State, national and international activities in aging.

FELIX M. BERARDO. Felix M. Berardo was born in Waterbury, Connecticut, in 1934. He earned his B.A. and Phi Beta Kappa key at the University of Connecticut and his Ph.D. four years later at Florida State University.

His research and teaching agenda span the fields of family sociology and social gerontology. Berardo counts Meyer Nimkoff and F. Ivan Nye—with whom he did course work during his doctoral program—as his mentors in family sociology. But as a gerontologist, he names his colleague Gordon F. Streib* as a mentor.

After spending four years at Washington State University as an assistant professor of sociology and assistant rural sociologist, in 1969 Berardo joined the sociology faculty at the University of Florida, where he has remained. He chaired the department from 1985 to 1991.

The sociology of death and widowhood has been Berardo's primary area of interest. An early piece on widowhood, "Widowhood Status in the United States: Perspective on a Neglected Aspect of the Family Life-Cycle," appeared in *The Family Coordinator: Journal of Education, Counseling, and Service,* 17 (July 1968): 191–203. It remains widely cited.

Survivorship, broadly defined, constitutes a secondary research agenda for Berardo. Here, he focuses on life preservation, including issues of risk-taking as they relate to health and longevity. He has written several articles on the subject for a special issue of the journal *Death Studies,* including "Social Networks and Life Preservation," 9:1 (1985), 37–50. He also edited a special issue on "Middle and Late Transitions" for the *Annals* of the American Academy of Political and Social Sciences (1982).

In branching out, he has begun to examine transitions in life by focusing with colleagues on "age-discrepant" marriage. Although Berardo has worked with a variety of collaborators, Hernan Vera has been his primary collaborator in this field. See Hernan Vera, Felix M. Berardo, and Joseph Vandiver, "Age Irrelevancy in Society: The Test of Mate Selection," *Journal of Aging Studies,* 14:1 (1991):81–96.

Berardo has served a number of editorships, including two terms as editor of the *Journal of Marriage and the Family* (1976–1981), and as associate editor for *Death Studies,* the *International Journal of Sociology of the Family, The Family Coordinator,* and the *Journal of Marriage and the Family.* He taught one of the first graduate-level seminars on death and dying, and teaches a highly regarded undergraduate course on the sociology of death and survivorship. He also teaches a variety of courses on the sociology of the family. For his contributions in this area, Berardo received the Arthur Peterson Award in Death Education.

Berardo is the former chairman of the Department of Sociology at the University of Florida. He has just completed a book on the general topic of survivor education, *Living is Risky: Staying Alive in Spite of Ourselves.* It examines a wide range of factors that shape the quality and length of our lives.

RICHARD W. BESDINE. Richard W. Besdine has devoted his career in academic medicine to the well-being of older persons. He attended Haverford College and earned his M.D. from the University of Pennsylvania in 1965. His grandfather, Samuel Bronstein, was the first person to interest him in doing work in geriatrics.

For more than two decades, Besdine has developed and managed educational, research, and clinical programs on aging. He has built recruitment and training programs for future leaders in geriatrics, and designed programs to meet educational needs in geriatrics for primary health care professionals. After developing a solid grounding in clinical care of older persons across the spectrum of community, hospitals, and nursing homes, including a Royal Society of Medicine Fellowship to train in Scotland with Sir W. Ferguson Anderson (the first chaired professor of geriatrics in Europe), he returned to the Harvard faculty and established an academic career of teaching, research, administration, public policy and international affairs in geriatrics. Besdine is listed in both editions of *Best Doctors in America* for internal medicine and geriatrics.

Besdine is director of the Travelers Center on Aging and Travelers Professor of Geriatrics and Gerontology at the University of Connecticut Health Center's (UCHC) School of Medicine. He is professor of internal medicine, of community medicine and health care, and of family medicine, and is chief of the Division of Geriatrics in the Department of Medicine. As director of the School of Medicine's Geriatrics Fellowship Program and the University's Geriatric Education Center, he exerts major influence on geriatrics education and clinical care in the university and the region. As director of the recently endowed Travelers Research Institute on Health Promotion and Aging, he oversees studies of interventions for prolonging vitality in older persons.

Prior to coming to Connecticut, Besdine was on the Harvard Medical School faculty for fifteen years. During that time, he and John W. Rowe* developed Harvard's Division on Aging; Besdine was responsible for its large academic fellowship training program in geriatric medicine, one of the first in the nation.

At UCHC, he chairs the Research Advisory Committee, charged with advising the CEO on research and with the distribution of $3.3 million annually in research funds to faculty in grants competitions. He also chairs the committee evaluating the institution's research infrastructure, and the committee to explore institutional options to increase competitiveness in clinical and research programs. He has served on committees restructuring the medical school curriculum, and interviews applicants to the medical school nearly weekly. In the area of health policy, he has served as a panelist on the elderly on the President's Commission on Mental Health, as a consultant to the National Institute on Aging, on the National Institute on Aging's Task Force on Reversible Dementia in the Elderly, and on two NIH Consensus Development Panels. He has also given congressional testimony in multiple areas related to geriatrics care, research and education. On a HCFA-supported health promotion demonstration project with Blue Cross/Blue Shield of Massachusetts, he was the major clinical adviser. He has served on numerous scientific review panels and study sections for the federal government and private foundations. He serves on the board of directors for the American Federation for Aging Research and for the Hospital for Special Care, and on the Scientific Advisory Board of the Alliance for Aging Research and the Brookdale Foundation.

Besdine is co-editor of the textbook *Geriatric Medicine,* and author of more than ninety publications, chiefly in geriatrics and gerontology. He has chaired two Western delegations to research conferences on aging in the Far East. He serves on numerous journal editorial boards and is a Fellow of the American College of Physicians, the Gerontological Society of America, and the American Geriatrics Society. His national reputation for leadership in geriatrics was recognized with the American Geriatrics Society's 1991 Milo D. Leavitt Award for eminence in geriatric education. He is board-certified in internal medicine, geriatrics, and infectious disease.

ROBERT H. BINSTOCK. Robert H. Binstock was born in New Orleans in 1935. He graduated with honors in government from Harvard College in 1956, where he studied with Sanford Lokoff. After spending a year as a Harvard College/ University of Chicago Law School Scholar, Binstock returned to Harvard to pursue his Ph.D. From 1959 to 1960, he was a Ford Foundation Fellow in metropolitan studies. A specialist in urban politics, Binstock produced through the Joint Center for Urban Studies of the Massachusetts Institute of Technology and Harvard University two reports on politics: the first on Worcester, Massachusetts (1960), and the second on Manchester, New Hampshire (1961). This work culminated in his dissertation, "Ethnic Politics and Reform Ideal" (1965), under the direction of Edward C. Banfield.

Binstock was first attracted to research on aging by Robert Morris,* then at Brandeis University, who hired him in 1963 to be a research associate on a Ford Foundation Project in Community Organization for the Elderly. Through this connection, Binstock met Ollie A. Randall.* The issue that impressed Binstock most was that existing programs for the elderly and the social welfare literature treated the population as if it were a homogeneous age group. Binstock thought this a mistake, and he has spent much of his subsequent career explaining the significance of the error. Binstock was also struck by the ways that efforts of professional social workers to help older Americans were hampered by their sparse knowledge of micro- and macro-politics. Binstock recognized the potential for career possibilities if he were to augment the research and educational opportunities available to professionals. As an initial step, he co-wrote with Robert Morris his first monograph, *Feasible Planning for Social Change* (New York: Columbia University Press, 1966).

Having committed himself to a career in aging, Binstock tried to convey (in a fashion that went beyond civic textbooks, "Beltway" generalization, or journalistic conventional wisdom) the complexities of politics as they apply to the political behavior of older persons and age-based organizations. He also has explained major issues in policies on aging to people inside and outside the field. He related this specific focus to mainstream political science in five editions of a textbook co-written with Peter Woll of Brandeis University, *America's Political System*. The first four editions were published by Random House (1972–1984), the last by McGraw-Hill (1991).

Four themes emerged from this effort. First, Binstock underscores and explains the fact that the enormous growth of American policies on aging, while helping many older persons, was doing little for those among the older population who were most severely deprived—and would probably do little to help them in the future without drastic changes in policies. Second, he uses empirical evidence to indicate that older persons do not behave in a homogeneous fashion politically, and that the agenda of old-age-based organizations are rarely focused on helping the most deprived elderly. Third, Binstock calls attention to the likelihood that policies on aging and the political behavior of old-age-based organizations may engender a political backlash against the elderly, with possibly dire consequences. Finally, he suggests policy reforms that would move away from age-categorical programs and focus on injustices and on needs to be found among all age groups in American society.

One of his most cited publications dealing with these themes was R. H. Binstock, "Interest Group Liberalism and the Politics of Aging," *The Gerontologist*, 12 (1972): 265–80. This article, applying Theodore Lowi's seminal theoretical critique of American interest-group liberalism to the field of aging, was the first to undertake a critical analysis of the politics of aging-based organizations. It demonstrated that such organizations were not essentially motivated to advocate for the disadvantaged elderly. It pointed out that older persons are not homogeneous politically, and why that is so. And it concluded that while the aged had their fair share of power in the American political system, that power was not being used to enhance the situations of the most severely disadvantaged aged.

The themes in this early article have been analytically and empirically developed in a number of subsequent publications, documenting the voting behavior of older persons, analyzing the interest groups, pointing up the plight of the disadvantaged elderly and explaining why the extant patterns of politics in the field of aging would be unlikely to help them, and recommending policy changes that might be politically feasible for ameliorating conditions among the disadvantaged. See R. H. Binstock, "National Policies and the Vulnerable Aged: Present, Emerging, and Proposed," in *The Vulnerable Aged: People, Services, and Policies,* ed. Zev Harel (New York: Springer, 1990), 235–47; R. H. Binstock, "Older Voters and the 1992 Presidential Election," *The Gerontologist,* 32 (1992): 601–606; R. H. Binstock, "Changing Criteria in Old-Age Programs: The Introduction of Economic States and Need for Services," *The Gerontologist,* 34 (1994): 726–30; and R. H. Binstock and C. L. Day, "Aging and Politics," in *The Handbook of Aging and the Social Sciences,* eds. R. H. Binstock and L. K. George* (San Diego: Academic Press, in press).

Another line of contributions has focused specifically on analyzing the Older Americans Act, dealing with the political and policy dilemmas posed by its broad mission and the scant resources and authority available for implementing it, as well as recommending policy changes for improving the Act's mission and effectiveness. These efforts began with a thirty-eight-page blueprint, *Planning, Background Paper for the 1971 White House Conference on Aging.* They have continued through the succeeding two decades in such publications as R. H. Binstock, Carolyn Cherington, and Peter Woll, "Federalism and 'Leadership-Planning': Predictors of Variance in State Behavior," *The Gerontologist,* 14 (1974): 114–21; R. H. Binstock, Jill Grigsby,* and Thomas D. Leavitt, *An Analysis of "Targeting" Policy Options Under Title III of the Older Americans Act,* Working Paper No. 16 of the National Aging Policy Center on Income Maintenance (Brandeis University, 1983); R. H. Binstock, "Title III of the Older Americans Act: An Analysis and Proposal for the 1987 Reauthorization," *The Gerontologist,* 27 (1987): 259–65; and R. H. Binstock, "From the Great Society to the Aging Society: 25 Years of the Older Americans Act," *Generations,* 15 (1991): 11–18.

A more recent line of work has focused on health policy and biomedical ethics, including three new co-edited books: R. H. Binstock and Stephen G. Post, eds., *Too Old for Health Care? Controversies in Medicine, Law, Economics and Ethics* (Baltimore: Johns Hopkins University Press, 1991); R. H. Binstock, Stephen G. Post, and Peter J. Whitehouse, eds., *Dementia and Aging: Ethics, Values, and Policy Choices* (Baltimore: Johns Hopkins University Press, 1992); and R. H. Binstock, Leighton E. Cluff, and Otto von Mering, eds., *The Future of Long-Term Care: Social and Policy Issues* (Baltimore: Johns Hopkins University Press, in press). A chapter in the first debunks the economic, political, and clinical assumptions and reasoning in proposals for rationing health care for older people; see Dennis W. Jahnigen and R. H. Binstock, "Economic and Clinical Realities: Health Care for Elderly People," pp. 13–43. A chapter in the second analyzes the politics of expanding public reimbursement for the care of patients suffering dementia and other chronically ill and disabled persons; see R. H. Binstock and Thomas H. Murray, "The Politics of Developing Appro-

34   ROBERT H. BINSTOCK

priate Care for Dementia," pp. 153–70. A chapter in the third analyzes political
prospects for the enactment of federal long-term care insurance in the wake of
President Clinton's failed health care reform proposal; see "The Politics of
Enacting Long-Term Care Insurance." In addition, Binstock has offered general
analyses of health care policy and aging, for example, R. H. Binstock, "Health
Care of the Aging: Trends, Dilemmas, and Prospects for the Year 2000," in
Aging 2000: Our Health Care Destiny, eds. Charles M. Gaitz* and Thaddeus
Samorajski (New York: Springer-Verlag, 1985), 3–15; R. H. Binstock, "Health
Care Costs Around the World: Is Aging a Fiscal 'Black Hole'?" *Generations,*
17 (1993): 37–42; R. H. Binstock, "Older People and Health Care Reform,"
American Behavioral Scientist, 36 (1993): 823–40; R. H. Binstock, Dennis W.
Jahnigen, and Stephen G. Post, "Exploring the Future of Health Care for Older
People," in *Aging and the Quality of Life,* eds. Ronald P. Abeles,* Helen C.
Gift, and Marcia G. Ory* (New York: Springer, 1994), 350–66. More specific
contributions have focused on issues of rehabilitation, aging, and ethics. See R.
H. Binstock, "Aging and Rehabilitation: The Birth of a Social Movement?" in
Aging and Rehabilitation: Advances in the State of the Art, eds. S. J. Brody*
and G. Ruff (New York: Springer Publishing, 1986), 349–56; R. H. Binstock,
"Rehabilitation and the Elderly: Economic and Political Issues," in *New Issues
in Stroke,* eds. Ruth Dunkle and J. Schmidley (New York: Springer Publishing,
1987), 186–200; and R. H. Binstock, "Allocation of Resources to Rehabilitation: Intellectual and Political Challenges," in *Aging and Rehabilitation, Vol. 2*
eds. Stanley Brody and L. G. Pawlson (New York: Springer Publishing, 1990),
315–32. On ethics in recent years, see R. H. Binstock, "The Clinton Proposal
and Old-Age-Based Rationing: A Plea for Informed Public Debate," *Journal of
Aging and Social Policy,* 6 (1994): 167–77; R. H. Binstock, "Long-Term Care
for Older People: Moral and Political Challenges of Access," in *Ethics: Critical
Issues for Today's Health Professionals,* eds. John F. Monagle and David C.
Thomas (Rockville, Md.: Aspen Publishers, 1994), 158–67; R. H. Binstock,
"Old-Age-Based Rationing: From Rhetoric to Risk?" *Generations,* in press;
R. H. Binstock and Roger C. Klein, "Health Care for the Aged in the United
States: Jewish Perspectives on Ethical and Moral Dilemmas," in *Jewish Aged:
People and Services,* eds. Zev Harel, David Biegel, and David Gutman* (New
York: Springer Publishing, in press).

From this prolific outpouring of ideas and words, probably Binstock's most
significant contribution has been to show how "compassionate ageism," expressed through decades of programs benefiting older people in the United
States, led to the emergence of the older person as scapegoat for a variety of
problems that began to confront American society in the 1970s and continued
through the 1990s, and laid the foundation for issues of so-called intergenerational equity. This line of analysis began in the mid-1970s, when Binstock suggested that the most likely political implication of population aging would not
be enhanced political power for older persons, but a strong political backlash
against an artificially homogenized group termed "the elderly," because of the

enormous cost implications of policies on aging. See "The Aging as a Political Force: Images and resources," in *Aging: A Challenge to Science and Social Policy—Volume II, Medicine and Social Science,* eds. A. J. J. Gilmore, A. Svanborg,* M. Marois, W. M. Beattie,* and J. Piotrowski (New York: Oxford University Press, 1981), 390–96.

In his 1982 Kent Lecture to the Gerontological Society of America, "The Aged as Scapegoat" (*The Gerontologist,* 23 (1983): 136–43), Binstock characterized ageism as "the attribution of the same characteristics, status, and just deserts to a heterogeneous group that has been artificially homogenized, packaged, labeled, and marketed as 'the aged.' " This enabled him to distinguish between previous definitions (such as Robert Butler's) of ageism as a prejudicial construct employed against older persons, and the compassionate ageism that had undergirded the creation of an "old age welfare state." Binstock argued that compassionate ageism had laid the groundwork for a reversal of stereotypes, in which older persons were becoming portrayed as prosperous, politically powerful, and an unsustainable burden for American society—and being made the scapegoat for a variety of problems in America.

This theme was elaborated in 1985 in "The Oldest Old: A Fresh Perspective or Compassionate Ageism Revisited?," *Milbank Memorial Fund Quarterly/ Health and Society,* 63 (1985): 420–51, in which Binstock presciently argued that the identification of the "oldest-old" (persons aged 85 years and older) as a special group might lead to a reconstruction of compassionate ageism on a higher old-age ground and feed into pernicious constructs of intergenerational equity. Binstock anticipated the old-age-based health care rationing proposals of Daniel Callahan and others, warning that "if the issues of health care allocations continue to be framed as tradeoffs between age groups, it does not take much imagination to envision that a stereotyped group termed the 'oldest old' will be assembled in the front row of the trading block" (433). This line of reasoning was extended most recently in R. H. Binstock, "The Oldest Old and 'Intergenerational Equity'," in *The Oldest Old,* eds. Richard Suzman, David Willis, and Kenneth Manton (New York: Oxford University Press, 1992), 394–417; R. H. Binstock, "Another Form of 'Elderly Bashing'," *Journal of Health Politics, Policy, and Law,* 17 (1992): 269–72; R. H. Binstock, "Transcending Intergenerational Equity," in *Economic Security, Intergenerational Justice: A Look at North America,* eds. Theodore R. Marmor, Timothy M. Smeeding, and Vernon L. Greene (Washington, D.C.: Urban Institute Press, 1994), 155–85.

In addition to generating his own contributions to the field, Binstock has generously enabled other scholars to add to the literature. He edited four editions of the *Handbook of Aging and the Social Sciences,* which have served as major sources for ideas, research agenda, and up-to-date literature in the field. His co-editor on the first two editions was Ethel Shanas; Linda K. George co-edited the third and fourth. As a major figure in Brandeis University's aging center in the 1970s and early 1980s, Binstock directed the graduate training of some of the field's rising stars. In recent years he has served as a mentor for those interested in aging-policy issues from this base at Case Western Reserve University, where he has served as a professor of aging, health, and society.

Binstock has also performed many professional duties. He served as executive director of a White House Task Force on Aging for President Lyndon B. Johnson (1967–1968), which made thirty-three policy recommendations, many of which were subsequently enacted as law—among them, the major components of the Employee Retirement Income Security Act of 1974. He has been active in the Gerontological Society. As the founding chairman of its Public Policy Committee (1968–1970), Binstock facilitated, for the first time, invitations for members of the GSA to testify at congressional hearings and thereby represent the organization's position on public policies. As the society's president (1975–1976), he put the organization on a stable financial footing, through reorganization of financial accounting, financial management, and policies for automatic reconsideration of dues increases. Through appointments and providing budgets to committees, Binstock was able to revitalize what then was a relatively moribund committee structure in GSA. And by arranging for the opening program of the annual meeting to be an official hearing of the U.S. Senate, with Senator Charles Percy of Illinois presiding (an unprecedented practice at that time), on "Medicine and Aging: An Assessment of Opportunities and Neglect," Binstock was able to give the members of the organization a solid sense that it was important in the public policy world. He is currently chairman of the Gerontological Health Section of the American Public Health Association (as of Fall 1995).

One gets a sense of Binstock's contributions from the following testimonial, offered by the National Association of State Units on Aging, which honored him at its twenty-fifth anniversary:

We honor Bob today because:

- he has continually challenged us to "break set" in how we conceptualize and operate the state service and advocacy system;
- he continues to offer new and provocative conceptual models and practical solutions for the design and management of aging policies and programs;
- we have always deeply appreciated his extraordinary understanding of the political environment within which state agencies must work, and his sincere commitment to help us improve how we serve the older citizens of our states;
- he has served individual states as a "devil's advocate," to critique policy options, regulatory issues, and legislative proposals;
- lastly, we honor Bob because he exemplifies the very best of how the academic community and state aging networks can and should work together for the betterment of older Americans.

JAMES E. BIRREN. James E. Birren was born in Chicago in 1918. After attending Wright Junior College, he earned his B.Ed. from Chicago State University in 1941. He then earned his M.A. from Northwestern University before becoming a test constructor for the U.S. Army and then, as an officer in the U.S. Naval Reserve, a research psychologist in the Naval Medical Research Institute (1943–1945) and head of the institute's Psychology and Statistics Facility (1945–1946). In this latter capacity Birren collaborated with biological scientists on measuring fatigue. This work then inspired his dissertation work on seasickness; he earned his Ph.D. from Northwestern in 1947.

From the start of his career, he recalled in a 1987 interview, Birren enjoyed investigating how "biological and environmental factors modulated behavioral expressions of physiological mechanisms." Birren would spend his entire academic career investigating "big" problems that enabled him to cut across disciplinary domains as he explored how human biological and psychological responses to social and environmental contests changed over time.

Birren began his research career in federal laboratories and scientific centers. He was a research fellow with the U.S. Public Health Service from 1946 to 1947, and then spent four years as a research psychologist in the National Heart Institute's gerontology unit, which was headed by Nathan W. Shock.* (His wife Betty, whom he married in 1942, helped Shock compile the first edition of his definitive *Classified Bibliography on Gerontology and Geriatrics.*) During the 1950–1951 academic year, Birren was a postdoctoral fellow at the University of Chicago. He extended his stay in Chicago for an additional two years, becoming an assistant professor of anatomy. During this period he formed lifelong friendships with Robert J. Havighurst,* Bernice L. Neugarten,* and other members of the Committee on Human Development. In the early 1960s, Birren returned to the Midway to teach one course per year as a visiting professor of human development and psychology.

In 1953 he returned to Bethesda, where he served as chief of the section on aging at the National Institute of Mental Health. When federal research programs on aging were consolidated and transferred to the newly established National Institute of Child Health and Human Development, Birren served as the first director of the Aging Program. Despite increasing administrative responsibilities, Birren maintained an active lab. He considered his time spent with Alan T. Welford* at Cambridge University during a sabbatical in 1960–1961 especially helpful.

Birren made his reputation publishing studies that documented how the functioning of the nervous system changed with age. Among his most important collaborators in this period were Jack Botwinick* and Klaus Riegel.* See two back-to-back essays that he published with Botwinick on "Age Difference in Finger, Jaw, and Foot Reaction Time to Auditory Stimuli" and "Speed of Response as a Function of Perceptual Difficulty and Age," *Journal of Gerontology,* 10 (1955): 429–36. Birren served as editor of the *Journal of Gerontology* from 1956 to 1963, imposing the same rigorous scientific standards for presentation of data that was evidenced in his own research.) See also his ''Psychophysio-logical Aspects of Aging'' in *Duke University Council on Aging* (1959): 157–73; and a summary paper, with K. F. Riegel and P. F. Morrison, ''Age Differences in Response Speed as a Function of Controlled Variations of Stimulus Conditions: Evidence of a General Speed Factor,'' *Gerontologia,* 6 (1962): 1–18.

Perhaps the most important volumes with which Birren was involved during this period became the basis for the various *Handbooks* that he was to edit throughout his career. In 1955 he began, with Robert N. Butler,* among others, a project that focused on interrelations between cerebral physiological changes, psychological capacities, and psychiatric symptoms expressed with advancing age. This culminated in the production of *Human Aging I: A Biological and Behavioral Study* (Bethesda, Md.: National Institute of Mental Health, 1961). In addition to co-writing an introductory and two concluding chapters, Birren also analyzed ''interrelations of mental and perceptual tests given to healthy elderly men.'' He and his research team examined thirty-two variables, many taken from the Wechsler Adult Intelligence Scale, to determine the influence of health status. The investigators found that while age was more important in speed measures, health was more important in verbal measures. With Wilma Donahue,* Ernest W. Burgess,* and other social scientists, Birren also helped to compile a trilogy of collections of essays; his own volume, *Handbook of Aging and the Individual,* was published by the University of Chicago Press in 1959. In introductory remarks he noted that

> research on aging is undergoing a metamorphosis into an experimental field, and as facts about aging increase, more and more attention will be given to method and theory, not only to manage and systematize the increasing data base but also to save time in devising more efficient experiments. The essential ingredient is an investigator who is aware of the problems of the field and is alert for new or different methods for their solution.

In 1964, the University of Southern California (USC) began to recruit Birren to head its new aging center. University president Norman Topping counted his success in luring Birren to Los Angeles as the second most important appointment of his tenure—after recruiting John McCay to be the football coach. Part of the enticement was the promise of solid funding. In February 1964 USC signed a contract with the Rossmoor Corporation so that ''research concerning the problems of retirement and aging may be conducted in Rossmoor's and the public's behalf by the University . . . in an efficient and integrated manner, for the ultimate benefit of retired and elderly persons throughout the United States and the World.'' Rossmoor, which had designed retirement communities called ''Leisure Worlds,'' promised to give USC a $50,000 advance and then contribute $50 for every unit sold in southern California. The arrangement was potentially worth millions of dollars.

The deal with Rossmoor, however, did not work out as planned. Although President Topping had promised him support for the first three years, Birren sought financial support through training grants from the U.S. Public Health Service Training grants. The funds enabled him to attract first-rate graduate students and promising young faculty such as Vern Bengtson.* In 1967, Birren sponsored his first Summer Institute for Study in Gerontology and with seed money from the National Institute of Mental Health conducted workshops for professionals. Committed to multidisciplinarity, Birren encouraged his colleagues and students to conduct research projects in biology, psychology, sociology, economics, and urban studies. "Right now planning for the aging is done without fundamental understanding of the meaning of aging biologically, psychologically, and socially," he wrote in 1966.

In addition to building his center at USC, Birren was emerging as a major spokesman for research on the psychology of aging. See, for instance, his entry on "Aging: Psychological Aspects," in the *International Encyclopedia of the Social Sciences,* ed. David L. Sills (New York: Crowell, Collier and Macmillan, 1968); J. E. Birren, "A Developmental View of Aging," in *Developmental Psychology: An Introduction* (New York: CRM Books, 1970); and J. E. Birren, "Toward an Experimental Psychology of Aging," *American Psychologist,* 25 (1970): 124–35. Birren also continued his research at the interstices of biological and behavioral domains. See his "Age and Decision Strategies," in *Decision Making and Age,* eds. A. T. Welford and J. E. Birren (Berlin: Karger, 1969); L. H. Hicks and J. E. Birren, "Aging, Brain Damage, and Psychomotor Slowing," *Psychological Bulletin,* 74 (1970): 377–96.

Birren also became a major spokesman for gerontological training. With Robert W. Kleemeier,* he wrote the lead essay, "Society and the Study of Aging" for *Graduate Education in Aging within the Social Sciences,* eds. Rose E. Kushner and Marion E. Bunch* (Ann Arbor: University of Michigan Press, 1967). He and J. L. Moore looked at "Doctoral Training in Gerontology: An Analysis of Dissertations on Problems in Institutions of Higher Learning in the United States, 1934–1969," *Journal of Gerontology,* 26 (1971): 249–57, updating the study with "A Bibliography of Doctoral Dissertations on Aging from American Institutions of Higher Learning, 1969–1971," *Journal of Gerontology,* 27 (1972): 399–402. For the 1971 White House Conference on Aging, Birren, Dianne Woodruff (a former graduate student), and K. J. Gribbin prepared *Training: Background.* With Woodruff, he prepared "Academic and Professional Training in the Psychology of Aging" for *The Psychology of Adult Development and Aging,* eds. Carl Eisdorfer and M. Powell Lawton* (Washington, D.C.: American Psychological Association, 1973).

In 1968 the American Association of Retired Persons (AARP) approached Birren about the possibility of erecting a facility at USC to honor its founder, Ethel Percy Andrus, who had been a principal at a high school near University

Park. Prize-winning architect Edward Durell Stone was commissioned to erect a 55,000-square-foot building, complete with wet labs, multipurpose rooms, and a courtyard. The setting was fitting proof of Birren's extraordinary leadership. According to the author's analysis, USC's net return on its $7.6 million investment exceeded $22 million in research-generated overhead, tuition, and gifts between 1965 and 1980. During those first fifteen years, Birren and his faculty supervised ninety-five doctoral dissertations. During its first five years, the Leonard Davis School of Gerontology, a branch of the Andrus Center, graduated 214 individuals, a third of whom earned certificates or bachelor's degrees.

During the 1970s Birren secured his position as one of the nation's preeminent gerontologists. In 1976 and 1977, under his editorship, three handbooks of aging were commissioned: *The Handbook of the Biology of Aging, The Handbook of Psychology and Aging,* and *The Handbook of Aging and the Social Sciences.* "It is expected that investigators will use these books as the basic systematic reference works on aging, resulting in the stimulation and planning of needed research," Birren wrote in the series Foreword. "A decision was made, therefore, to develop a multidisciplinary project, the purpose of which was to organize, evaluate, and interpret research data, concepts, theories, and issues on the biological, psychological, and social aspects of aging." These volumes were updated in 1985 and 1900; the fourth editions were due in 1995. With each edition Birren became more insistent in urging his colleagues to reevaluate the way they defined key issues. In the 1990 *Handbook of the Psychology of Aging,* for instance, he proposed that "dynamic terms be introduced, such as *senescing* to refer to the biological processes of aging, *eldering* to refer to the social processes of aging, and *geronting* to refer to the psychological processes of aging." Note that even these three terms hew to the tripartite disciplinary division that Birren has advocated all along—with perspectives from the humanities strategically injected into gerontologic analysis.

Although Birren no longer ran his own lab, he continued to explore new areas of research in gero-psychology. With Vivian Clayton,* for instance, he explored "The Development of Wisdom across the Life Span: A Reexamination of an Ancient Topic," *Life Span Development and Behavior,* 3 (1980): 103–35. With another student, William Cunningham, he continued to write about "Age Changes in the Factor Structure of Intellectual Abilities in Adulthood and Old Age," *Educational and Psychological Measurement,* 40 (1980): 271–90. He also wrote about mental health issues and the relationship between well-being and aging: "The field of health psychology is burgeoning and needs co-opting by the concerns of aging," he wrote in *The Course of Later Life,* eds. Vern L. Bengtson* and K. Warner Schaie,* a Springer volume published in his honor in 1989. And then, in words he might have written in the 1940s, he added, "The well-being of the organism is perhaps best expressed by the capacity of the organism to adapt and change in relation to environmental demands." See also his essay with V. L. Renner, "Concepts and Criteria of Mental Health and Aging," *American Journal of Orthopsychiatry,* 51 (1981): 242–54.

Birren also tried to reach larger audiences by writing textbooks and editing collections that would appeal to a wide range of readers. Two of his more successful ventures were *Developmental Psychology,* with D. Kinney, K. Warner Schaie, and Diane Woodruff (Boston: Houghton Mifflin, 1981); and *Aging: Scientific Perspectives and Social Issues* with Woodruff (Berkeley: Brooks-Cole, 1983), which went through several editions. At USC he began to offer courses on autobiographies.

Birren was also a prime mover in the Carnegie Corporation's Aging Society project, which issued *Our Aging Society,* edited by Alan Pifer and Lydia Bronte. Birren's contribution, "The Process of Aging," (New York: W. W. Norton, 1986) offers a succinct, balanced overview of various explanations of the causes of aging, highlighting theories about the hardening of arteries, digestive putrification, endocrinal functions, and the connection between immunity and aging. With his colleague Vern Bengtson, Birren tried to extend disciplinary boundaries, particularly through seminars held at the Andrew Norman Research Institute in the Andrus Center. Their *Emergent Theories of Aging* (New York: Springer Publishing, 1988) offered "an attempt by researchers to begin to address the data-rich but theory-poor state of current research on aging, and to encourage cross-disciplinary interchange that focuses on theory development in aging."

After retiring as dean of the Leonard Davis School of Gerontology, director of the Andrew Norman Institute for Advanced Study in Gerontology and Geriatrics, and executive director of the Andrus Gerontology Center, Birren served as a Brookdale Distinguished Scholar. He also helped launch the Boren Center for Gerontological Research at the University of California, Los Angeles, serving as director and adjunct professor of medicine/gerontology. Looking back "on events during the formative years of my career," Birren affirmed his long-standing belief "that the problems of aging are in most cases not like the lock-and-key problems of many areas (e.g., poliomyelitis and immunization), in which there is one single solution. They become transformed over time and as our standards and expectations rise, even as the topics seem to remain the same." With his friends Gary M. Kenyon* (a Canadian philosopher) and Johannes J. F. Schroots (a Dutch gerontologist), Birren edited *Metaphors of Aging in Science and the Humanities* (New York: Springer Publishing, 1991). Birren and Jackie Lanum noted in their contribution to the volume, "Metaphors of Psychology and Aging," that "a scientific metaphor is the implicit thought structure or underlying root concept a scientist uses in the pursuit of research and scientific explanation. A new metaphor, like an invention, is seeing a connection where none has been seen before."

Birren has been honored often during his career. He received an honorary doctorate from the University of Goteborg in 1983. The Association for Gerontology in Higher Education bestowed upon him the Distinguished Educator Award the same year. In 1978 Birren received the Distinguished Contribution Award from the American Psychological Association's Division on Adult Development and Aging. Earlier in his career, the University of Michigan saluted him as one of the American Pioneers in Aging (1972). He served as president of the Gerontological Society in 1961–1962; he also was president of the Western Gerontological Society, which became the American Society on Aging, and the Division on Adult Development and Aging of the American Psychological Association. Birren, who was a senior advisor to the 1995 White House Conference on Aging, currently serves as a member of the World Health Organization's Expert Advisory Panel on Health and Elderly Persons. It is not surprising, given his governmental, foundation, and university connections, that Birren has served on countless review boards. He also has volunteered his services in Los Angeles.

ZENA SMITH BLAU. Zena Smith Blau was born 1922 in New York, and reared in a radical Yiddish family and community in Detroit. She attended Detroit's Wayne State University (A.B., 1943; M.S.W., 1946). She was invited by Edward Suchman, John Dean, Milton Barron, and Gordon Streib* at Cornell University to join them as a research fellow, which was her first taste of research on the aging. She was trained as a sociologist by Paul F. Lazarfeld and Robert K. Merton; the latter directed her 1957 dissertation at Columbia. "To interest him in aging, I presented a proposal delineating a novel sociological perspective on old age, which aroused his interest and support," Blau says. Her topic focused on how people's status changed in old age.

A long time Chicago resident, Blau taught at the University of Illinois's Medical Center in Chicago (1958–1965), was a lecturer at the University of Chicago (1967–1969), and a Northwestern University associate professor from 1969 to 1974. Since 1976 she has been a professor of sociology at the University of Houston, and served as chair of the department from 1976 to 1979.

Her widely cited article, "Structural Constraints on Friendships in Old Age," *American Sociological Review,* 26 (1961): 426–36, provided evidence that the effects of widowhood and retirement on older people's friendships are not uniform but are governed by the prevalence of each type of exit among their age, sex, and social class peers. An exit that places an individual in a minority position among age peers interferes with friendship opportunities. But when an exit becomes prevalent among age peers, the individual who retains that role exhibits less friendship participation.

Blau's 1973 book, *Old Age in a Changing Society* (New York: Franklin Watts), developed the concept of "role exit." She proposed that "roleless statuses," such as widowhood among women and retirement among men, distinguished old age from earlier stages of life. "Each signifies exit from a core social role that had provided structure, meaning and purpose to individuals," she argues. In addition, the late stage of life has no "cultural script" to follow, so that friendship participation and other optional roles take on great significance. This book has become a classic in the literature on social gerontology.

Blau collaborated with Rose Goldsen in the design of the Kips-Bay interview

carried out in New York City and was aided by Jessie Cohen in the analysis of
the Elmira and Kips-Bay data sets. She was co-principal investigator with Richard Stephens of Aging in Texas, supported by the Texas Department of Human
Resources (1976–1978). A second edition, *Aging in a Changing Society,* incorporating new findings from the Texas study, was published in 1981 (New York:
Franklin Watts). Her book, *Black Children/White Children: Competence,
Socialization and Social Structure* (New York: Free Press-Macmillan), was also
published in 1981.

   She is the series editor of ''Current Perspectives on Aging and the Life Cycle,'' and editor of *Work, Retirement, and Social Policy,* Vol. 1 (Greenwich,
Conn.: JAI Press, 1985). Three subsequent volumes with guest editors focus on
Family Relations (1987); *Personal History over the Life Course* (1989); and
Delinquency and Drift over the Life Course (1995). Her most recent publication
is ''Social Structure, Socialization Processes and School Competence of Black
and White Children'' in *The Question of Discrimination: Racial Inequality in
the U.S. Labor Market,* eds. Steven Shulman and William Darity, Jr. (Middle-
town, Conn.: Wesleyan University Press, 1989).

DAN G. BLAZER. Dan German Blazer was born in Nashville in 1944. He
earned his A.B. from Vanderbilt in 1965. After attending the Harding Graduate
School of Religion in Memphis, where he worked toward an M.A. with studies
in cross-cultural religion, Blazer decided to go to medical school; he received
his M.D. from the University of Tennessee in 1969. Blazer became a resident
in psychiatry in 1973, after completing his internship and spending two years
as medical director of the Christian Mobile Clinic in Cameroon. Except for a
year as a fellow in the Department of Psychiatry at Montefiore Hospital in the
Bronx, Blazer has remained in Durham, North Carolina.

   Blazer was first attracted to work in gerontology by colleagues in the Duke
University Medical Center. George Maddox* and Dorothea Leishton interested
him in epidemiology and social factors in aging, and Ewald W. Busse* introduced him to geriatric psychiatry. Maddox and Busse remain his role models.
From 1976 to 1981, Blazer was associate director for programs at Duke's Center
for the Study of Aging and Human Development. For the next four years he
headed the university's Division of Social and Community Psychiatry. From
1985 to 1990, Blazer was director of the Affective Disorders Program in the
Department of Psychiatry, and was head of the Division of Geriatric Psychiatry
from 1988 to 1990. From 1990 until 1992, he served as interim chair of psychiatry. Blazer now serves as dean of medical education.

   In the late 1970s, Blazer undertook graduate training in Chapel Hill. He
earned an M.P.H. in epidemiology in 1979, and his Ph.D. in epidemiology from
the University of North Carolina a year later, where he was greatly influenced
by Berton Kaplan. Blazer has held an adjunct appointment as professor in the
Department of Epidemiology at UNC since 1986.

   He has done extensive work in the study of depression in late life. Three of his early, influential studies were "The Epidemiology of Late Life Depression," which appeared in the *Journal of the American Geriatrics Society,* 30 (1982): 587–92; and, with L. Hyer, "Depressive Symptoms: Impact and Problems in Long Term Care Facilities," *International Journal of Behavioral Geriatrics,* 1 (1982): 33–44; and "Impact of Late-Life Depression on the Social Network," *American Journal of Psychiatry,* 140 (1983): 162–66. In "The Epidemiology of Depression in an Elderly Community Population," *The Gerontologist,* 27 (1987): 281–287, an article with Linda K. George* (one of his primary collaborators) and Dana Hughes, Blazer screened over 1,300 adults over age sixty living in communities for depressive symptomatology. Among the 27 percent who reported depressive symptoms were older people who also suffered problems in other psychiatric areas assessed, which suggested that the categories set forth in the standard instrumental (then DSM-III) did not capture the true nature of late-life depression.

Blazer considers his major aging-related contributions to be documenting the lower prevalence of major depression in the elderly, as compared with other stages of the life cycle; and second, documenting the impact of impaired social support upon mortality among older adults, especially those perceived to have inadequate support. He has summarized much of his work to date in "Epidemiology of Depression: Prevalence and Incidence," in *Principles and Practice of Geriatric Psychiatry,* eds. John R. M. Copeland, Mohammed T. Abou-Saleh, and Dan G. Blazer (New York: John Wiley, 1994). Comparing his own studies with other researchers' findings, he concluded that 1 percent to 3 percent of all older people suffer from major depression, but perhaps even more important, another 15 percent "experience clinically significant symptoms not captured by the diagnosis of major depression." Cautious in interpreting data, Blazer is careful not to extrapolate longitudinal trends from cross-sectional patterns designed in different ways.

A fellow of six professional organizations and member of five others, Blazer has served on the editorial boards of the leading geriatric and gerontologic journals. He was associate editor of the *Journal of Gerontology: Medical Sciences* from 1988 to 1993. He has served as president of the Psychiatric Research Society and of the American Geriatrics Society. Blazer received the Distinguished Service Award from his alma mater's School of Public Health in 1989 and the Jack Weinberg Award in Geriatric Psychiatry from the American Psychiatric Association in 1992. In 1990 he was appointed J. P. Gibbons Distinguished Professor of Psychiatry at Duke.

JUNE E. BLUM. June E. Blum has had broad experience in clinical psychology. She began her career as a school psychologist. She earned a master's degree from Columbia University in 1950, a doctorate from St. John's University in 1969, and completed an eight-year postdoctoral psychoanalytic program in New York at the Postgraduate Center for Mental Health in 1976. Currently in private practice, she is clinical assistant professor of psychology in psychiatry at Cornell

University Medical College. She is also assistant attending psychologist at New York Hospital, a post she has held since 1977.

Blum's interest in gerontology began as a participant in the 20-year follow-up study of the aging twins originally begun by Kallman and Lissy Jarvik.* The research results led her to develop strong, positive views on aging, notably that older adults are not in a static monolithic group. Rather, they are in a developmental period—"elderhood"—that is more heterogeneous than any of the earlier periods. As a result, her work has focused on establishing clinical geropsychology as a force for adding *life* to the extended lifespan.

In 1977, Blum published a curriculum for clinical gerontology in *Geropsychology: A Model of Training and Clinical Services,* ed. W. D. Gentry (Cambridge, Mass.: Ballinger). In 1980, her paper, "Psychotherapy with the Elderly: A Holistic Approach," was published in the *Annual Review of Gerontology and Geriatrics,* Vol. 1, 204–34.

Her study and practice continue to refute Freud's early position that older adults (age forty and above) could not profit from psychotherapy. In fact, a major portion of Blum's professional career has been devoted to the positive effect of therapeutic intervention in the later years.

HERMAN T. BLUMENTHAL. Herman T. "Butch" Blumenthal's interest in aging was evident in the early 1930s in his master's thesis at the University of Pennsylvania. There, he worked with L. V. Heilbrunn on his studies of calcium deposition, a common aging phenomenon. In 1935, he went to Washington University to work in the laboratory of Leo Loeb, an eminent parasitologist who was professor and chairman of the Department of Pathology.

Although Loeb never joined the Gerontological Society, he was the first person on the Washington campus doing gerontologic research, though not on aspects of human aging. Loeb also encouraged his colleague, anatomist Edmund Vincent Cowdry,* to study senescence. Blumenthal earned his Ph.D. under Loeb in 1938 and then, with help from Cowdry, who had just published his *Problems of Ageing* (Baltimore: Williams and Wilkins, 1939; 2nd ed., 1942), earned his M.D. four years later.

Blumenthal has maintained a research appointment at Washington University for more than half a century. Marion Bunche recruited him to teach biology when trying to establish a first-rate Psychology Department. He collaborated with Albert Lansing (whom he first met in Heilbrunn's lab) on the calcification of vascular tissues. With Dr. Y. Hirata, a research fellow from Japan, he studied autoimmune phenomena associated with diabetes in the 1950s. For nearly four decades, he has worked with Dr. B. N. Premachandra on aging phenomena that occur in the endocrine system. It should be noted that much of Blumenthal's time and energy after 1962 were focused on his Medical Diagnostic Laboratory, which grew to gross $2 million before being bought out. Profits from this venture underwrote Blumenthal's gerontologic research.

As a pathologist, Blumenthal's major interest has been the origins of diseases in the elderly. Blumenthal readily acknowledges that his view—that the aging-disease dichotomy is false—is a minority position among researchers on aging. It is a position, however, that he has stressed tenaciously. See, for instance, his efforts in revising the second edition of Cowdrv's *Arteriosclerosis* (Springfield, Ill.: C. C. Thomas, 1967); H. T. Blumenthal, "Aging: Biologic or Pathologic," *Hospital Practice,* 13 (1978): 127–42; and, with B. N. Premachandra, "Bridging the Aging-Disease Dichotomy. I: The Amyloidosis Model," *Perspectives in Biology and Medicine,* 33 (1990): 402–20. It is significant that Van Nostrand Reinhold chose to publish and market Blumenthal's edited collection, *Handbook of the Diseases of Aging* (1983), separately from the first and second editions of the trilogy of *Handbooks of Aging* assembled by James E. Birren.*

To Blumenthal, aging is a "pathobiological entity." Without any sense of being illogical, Blumenthal's definition of aging gives him a distinctive spin on gerontologic research. He lauds efforts by Robert Butler* and T. Franklin Williams to promote research on Alzheimer's, but he deplores the politics of National Institute in Aging (NIA) study sections. In addition, Blumenthal has long been dismayed by the "artificial" separation of the Gerontological Society's biological and medical sections. Realizing that he probably will not effect a restructuring that will merge the two sections, he has instead tried to promote closer communication between clinicians and bench scientists concerning the pathological and biological processes that occur in aging.

Blumenthal has published broadly and widely. His over 200 research papers, reviews, and book chapters have applied an aging perspective to issues in endocrinology, cancer, vascular disease, and neurobiology. Like many biogerontologists, Blumenthal drew a distinction between intrinsic and extrinsic factors, but he went on to argue that if environmental risk factors were eliminated, there would still be disease derived from the intrinsic aging phenomena. Lately, he also has been writing on the future of health care planning in terms of population aging. This latter interest stems from his appointment to the Department of Community Medicine at St. Louis University School of Medicine, in addition to being a research professor in gerontology at Washington University. He is particularly interested in chronic diseases in patients with dementia and cardiovascular disease not associated with risk factors. Hence, it is not surprising that the subtitle of his forthcoming book is "Reflections on the Intrinsic Origins of Aging-Dependent Diseases." His concept has received increasing support in England and from such luminaries in the United States as Hubert Warner.

EDWARD L. BORTZ. Edward Leroy Bortz was born in Greensburg, Pennsylvania, in 1896. After attending Pennsylvania State College, he graduated from Harvard in 1919 and received his M.D. degree from Harvard Medical School four years later. Bortz did graduate work in pathology at the universities of Vienna and Berlin.

After completing an internship at Lackenau Hospital in suburban Philadelphia

(1923–1925) and some specialized research at the Mayo Clinic and the University of Illinois, Bortz joined the faculty of the School of Medicine at the University of Pennsylvania, serving as an associate professor of medicine from 1932 until his retirement. He was also chief of medical services (1932–1961) at Lackenau Hospital, and then senior consultant in medicine until his death.

Bortz was active in civic affairs. A president of the American Geriatrics Society (1960–1961), he won the Society's Gold Medal in 1960. Bortz served as an adviser to the 1961 White House Conference on Aging and was honored by the International Association on Aging for his writings on nutrition, metabolism, and aging. In addition to editing the *Encyclopedia of Medicine, Surgery and Specialties,* he also wrote *Creative Aging* (1963). He published "Retirement and the Individual" in the *Journal of the American Geriatrics Society,* 16 (1968): 1–15. There, he stressed the positive challenges of retirement as well as the threats of disuse through excessive leisure. He recommended ways to engage in preventive geriatrics and pre-retirement counseling.

Edward Bortz died in 1970.

WALTER M. BORTZ II. Walter M. Bortz II earned his B.A. from Williams College in 1951 and his M.D. four years later from the University of Pennsylvania School of Medicine. He was first attracted to research on aging by his father, who has also been his primary role model, mentor, and teacher. Edward L. Bortz* was one of the pioneers of geriatrics in the United States in the 1940s. The Bortz father-son pair represents one of the few truly generational partnerships in the gerontological community.

Walter Bortz has spent much of his career at the Palo Alto Medical Clinic, where he has been elaborating the distinctions among aging, disease, and disuse. See, for instance, his "Redefining Human Aging," *Journal of the American Geriatrics Society,* 37 (1987): 1092–96; and an earlier article, *Journal of the American Medical Association,* 248 (1982): 1203–09. To the extent that he differentiates between aging and disease, his work echoes ideas enunciated by his father and by another of Walter Bortz's teachers and mentors, Nathan W. Shock.* More than his elders, however, Walter Bortz from the start of his career has stressed the proposition that most of today's norms are actually artifacts of our inactive status. See his early articles, "The Disuse Syndrome," *Western Journal of Medicine,* 141 (1984): 64–78; and "Physical Exercise as an Evolutionary Function," *Journal of Human Evolution,* 14 (1985): 145–56. Lately, he has recast the thesis, arguing that aging is a thermophysical event. See "Aging as Entropy," *Experimental Gerontology,* 21 (1986): 321–28.

Walter Bortz's clinical observations have informed his assessment of current medical-care practices in the United States. He asserts, for instance, that precious health care resources should be allocated according to function rather than to age. See W. Bortz, "The Trajectory of Dying: Functional Status in the Last Year of Life," *Journal of the American Geriatrics Society,* 38 (1990): 140–50. He has elaborated this argument for lay audiences in W. Bortz, *We Live Too*

Short to Die Too Long (New York: Bantam Books, 1991). In this line of reasoning, one sees the influence of his conversations with Stanford University health care economist Victor Fuchs and social psychologist and reformer John Gardner.

Walter Bortz has played an active role in the American Geriatrics Society. In addition to the public policy issues noted above, Bortz is convinced that geriatric medicine is the job of nearly all physicians, "not the exclusive province of an elite cadre of internists." Hence, he was active in establishing a common geriatrics exam for internal medicine and family practice.

JACK BOTWINICK. Jack Botwinick was born in Brooklyn, New York, in 1923. After serving in the U.S. Army in World War II, he returned to Brooklyn College, where he earned his B.A. in 1946 and completed all course work toward an M.A. in psychology. He then joined James E. Birren* at the Gerontology Laboratory of the National Heart Institute in Baltimore (which later became the Gerontology Center of the National Institute of Aging). During this period, he completed his thesis for the M.A. degree awarded by Brooklyn College in 1950.

Botwinick left the Gerontology Laboratory to continue graduate studies at New York University, receiving his Ph.D. in 1953. In 1955 he joined the staff of the Laboratory of Psychology of the National Institute of Mental Health, again working with James E. Birren. Much of his research was in cognition and psychomotor function. Eight years later, in 1963, Botwinick accepted an appointment as associate professor (later, professor) at the Gerontology Center and Department of Psychiatry of Duke University Medical School. It was here that he wrote his first text, *Cognitive Processes in Maturity and Old Age* (New York: Springer, 1967). At that time, the published literature of behavioral aging was hardly more than disparate, scattered reports in a wide variety of journals. Botwinick's book provided an organization and integration of this scattered literature and elucidated methodological research problems seen in many of the studies. He also provided theoretical structure to this basically empirical literature when possible.

In 1969, Botwinick moved on to what was to be his final work station. He became professor of psychology at Washington University in St. Louis. He continued his research in aging, taught undergraduate and graduate classes, and guided graduate students in his role of director of the Aging and Development Program. He published *Aging and Behavior* in 1973 (New York: Springer), revised it in 1978 and again in 1984. The latter revision was extensive, effectively constituting a new book. *Aging and Behavior* has been used as a text in several universities and became a much used secondary research source.

His next book was co-written with Martha Storandt, *Memory, Related Functions and Age* (Springfield, Ill.: C. C. Thomas, 1974). This book reported an extensive series of studies of a wide variety of behavioral functions as they relate to age. The authors attempted to determine the relationship among these functions and to see whether they could be described by just a few organizing themes. His next book, *We Are Aging,* published in 1981 by Springer, was designed for a less technically advanced audience. This book was translated into Japanese.

Botwinick's vita includes over 100 published studies in refereed journals and his efforts on behalf of gerontological research extended beyond his own laboratory. He was a major participant in establishing the Geriatric Research, Education and Clinical Center (GRECC) of the St. Louis Veterans Administration, and the Alzheimer Disease Research Center of the Washington University School of Medicine under Leonard Berg's direction. Botwinick was appointed professor of neurology (psychology) in 1982 and co-director of clinical research in the Alzheimer Center in 1985.

Botwinick is past president of the Behavioral and Social Sciences Section of the Gerontological Society of America (GSA). He is also past president of Division 20 (Adult Development) of the American Psychological Association (APA). He served on the Council of Representatives of the APA. Botwinick is a recipient of several honors, including the Distinguished Contribution Award from Division 20 of the APA (1979) and the Kleemeier (1979) and Brookdale (1984) awards of the GSA.

Botwinick retired in 1988.

CYRIL F. BRICKFIELD. Cyril F. Brickfield was born in Brooklyn, New York, in 1919. After serving as a major in the Air Force during World War II, he earned his LL.B. from Fordham University in 1948. Brickfield spent the next two years as a law clerk to the chief judge of the New York State Court of Appeals. While serving as council to the U.S. House of Representatives Judiciary Committee (1951–1961), he earned his LL.M. (1953) and S.J.D. (1957) from George Washington University. He wrote several reports, including *Problems Relating to a Federal Constitutional Convention* (Washington, D.C.: Government Printing Office, 1957). Brickfield was general counsel for the Commonwealth of Virginia from 1961 to 1963.

Brickfield served in a number of key positions with the Veterans Administration from 1961 to 1967. He was appointed general counsel and thereafter became chief benefits director, in which post he supervised veterans' housing, education, disability compensation, and pension programs. He was then named deputy administrator, with jurisdiction over 183,000 employees and 173 hospitals and a yearly budget of $14 billion.

Brickfield's affiliation with the American Association for Retired Persons began in the 1960s; he served as its executive director from 1967 to 1969. In private practice from 1969 to 1977, he returned to AARP as its executive director from 1977 to 1987. During this decade the organization became the most powerful organization in the so-called "gray lobby." Under his leadership, AARP grew from 1 million to more than 28 million members. The association is now, according to the *Los Angeles Times,* "a major force in American life." After stepping down from the top position, Brickfield became an honorary pres-

50   JOSEPH H. BRITTON

ident of AARP, a trustee of the organization's Investments Trust, and a special counsel.

In addition to his work at AARP, Brickfield served as president of the National Senior Citizens Law Center (1977–1979) and, since 1981, has been president of the Corporation for Older Americans. Brickfield was a U.S. delegate to the 1982 U.N. World Assembly on Aging. He headed the Leadership Conference of Aging Organizations in 1980, 1983, and 1986. He also co-wrote, with Gerald D. Facciani, "Can We Repair the Cracks in the Social Security System?" *Association Management,* 34 (September 1982): 58–62.

JOSEPH H. BRITTON. Joseph H. Britton earned his bachelor's degree in biology, psychology, and education from Albion College, and a master's and Ph.D. in human development from the University of Chicago, completing his formal education in 1949.

His philosophy of gerontology has always stressed its interdisciplinary nature. "Gerontology belongs to academic disciplines and professions wherever individuals wish to cultivate it," Britton believes. That philosophy was nurtured by Robert J. Havighurst* and the Committee on Human Development at the University of Chicago. It is expounded in J. H. Britton, "Multidisciplinary Programs in Gerontology," *Gerontology in Higher Education: Perspectives and Issues,* eds. Mildred M. Seltzer,* Harvey Sterns, and Tom Hickey* (Belmont, Calif.: Wadsworth, 1978).

Britton was appointed assistant professor of psychology at Pennsylvania State University in 1949. There he brought together various faculty interested in aging education and research. In persuading Penn State President Milton Eisenhower to formalize the group, Britton conceived the Committee for the Study of Adulthood. This small, cross-campus mechanism was used to promote gerontology. Over the years Britton made Penn State a major gerontological education and research center.

The growth of gerontology at Penn State parallels Britton's career because of his ability to infuse a lifespan developmental perspective into various disciplines and professions. He served as chairman of the Gerontology Center and chairman of the Department of Individual and Family Studies. He also served as acting dean of the College of Health and Human Development and as acting director of the Institute for the Study of Human Development. His national impact is measured in his service on the 1956 Inter-University Council, during which he encouraged the development and publication of a series of three *Handbooks on Aging.* He served as president of the Division of Adult Development and Aging of the American Psychological Association (1968–1969), chairman of the Psychological and Social Sciences Section, and vice president of the Gerontological Society of America (1967–1968).

Britton's work at Penn State was interrupted on two occasions. In 1963/64 he was a Fullbright Professor in Finland at the University of Jyväskylä and received visiting appointments in Wales, Scotland, and Germany during that

time. In 1971 he was a visiting professor in gerontology at the University of
Southern California. Data collected in Finland resulted in several published
cross-cultural comparisons of children's perception of moral and emotional behavior and the behavior of their parents.

His book, co-written with his wife, Jean Oppenheimer Britton, on *Personality
Changes in Aging: A Longitudinal Study of Community Residents* (New York:
Springer, 1972), was an important early contribution to the understanding of
personality changes and aging. His publications report research on such subjects
as retirement attitudes and adjustment of teachers and university faculty and
alumni, the rural elderly, survivorship, and young people's perception of aging.

ELAINE M. BRODY. Elaine M. Brody was born in New York in 1922. She
earned her M.S.W., specializing in psychiatric work with children, at the University of Pittsburgh. She spent more than three decades of her career at the
Philadelphia Geriatric Center, which she originally chose because it was a part-
time job close to home. There she worked closely with Bernard Liebowitz, M.
Powell Lawton,* Morton H. Kleban,* and Arthur Waldman. At the time of her
retirement, she was the center's associate director of research, and arguably
gerontology's best-known student of caregiving across generational lines. For
many years, she had also been director of the center's Department of Human
Services.

Brody focused largely on the demographic, psychological, social, and political
conditions of "women in the middle," those middle-generation women who
have responsibilities for their aging parents and often for jobs and growing
children. She found that three-fifths of all women who were overburdened felt
guilty about not doing enough for their mothers; an even greater percentage
bemoaned the decline in filial responsibility. Brody claimed, however, that guilt
had nothing to do with the current realities or conditions in the past. Thanks to
increased longevity, we now live more and more often in four-generation families, with fewer adult children to shoulder the care of the increasing number of
dependent or impaired elderly, who would have been dead in earlier times.
Although women bear the brunt of the responsibility, parent care affects the
entire family. To ease the burden, especially in a society in which women are
also increasingly expecting and expected to be gainfully employed, Brody advocated in-home services, changes in nursing homes (such as those by the Philadelphia Geriatric Center), and government-financed long-term care insurance.

Brody's best-known scholarly contribution was her 1984 Kent Lecture before
the Gerontological Society (she was president of the organization three years
earlier), which was published as "Parent Care as a Normative Family Stress,"
in *The Gerontologist*, 25 (1985): 19–29. There, she referred at length to findings
reported at a 1963 symposium sponsored by Duke University and the Gerontological Society, as well as the research by fellow gerontologists such as Ethel
Shanas.* She reported for the first time that many women had to quit their jobs
to take care of elderly parents. Brody was careful not to dichotomize public vs.

private dimensions or the realms of dependence and independence, since they were really operating along a continuum. She also stressed that for many women, parent care was not a single, time-limited episode. "The strains families experience are not completely preventable or remediable," Brody concluded, but "knowledge, properly used, can do much to prevent families from reaching the limits of endurance and can help us as a society to meet our collective filial responsibilities."

A past president of the Gerontological Society of America, Brody received an honorary doctorate, D.Sc., from the Medical College of Pennsylvania in April 1987 and has been elected a Distinguished Scholar of the National Academies of Practice. Among other awards she has received are the 1985 Brookdale Award of the Gerontological Society of America, the 1983 Donald P. Kent Award of the Gerontological Society of America, and the 1982 Distinguished Alumni Award of the University of Pittsburgh School of Social Work. Brody was selected a Woman of the Year, by *Ms. Magazine* in January 1986. She has served on the editorial boards of many professional journals and on review committees at the National Institute of Mental Health, the Administration on Aging, and a number of foundations. She was a member of the Congressional Advisory Panel on Alzheimer's Disease. Her publications include six books, many book chapters, and over 200 journal articles. She has directed fifteen federally financed research studies on subjects such as individualized treatment of the mentally impaired aged; mental and physical health practices of older people; the dependent elderly; women's changing roles; women, work, and care of the aged; and parent care, sibling relationships, and mental health.

For more, see Lindsy Van Gelder's sketch of Brody in the January 1986 issue of *MS, 47ff.*

HAROLD BRODY. Harold Brody was born in Cleveland, Ohio, in 1923. After army service from 1942 to 1946, he earned his B.S. in 1947 at Western Reserve University and his Ph.D. in anatomy from the University of Minnesota six years later. From 1950 to 1954, Brody served as assistant professor of anatomy at the University of North Dakota. While in the Department of Anatomy at the State University of New York at Buffalo, Brody earned an M.D. in 1961.

After 1964 Brody spent most of his career in Buffalo. He became a professor in the Department of Anatomy in 1963 and served as chairman of the Department of Anatomical Sciences from 1971 to 1992. From 1956 to 1960, he was associate director of the Project for Medical Education. In the late 1960s he was dean for student affairs in the medical school, leaving that position for the anatomy chairmanship. Brody served as acting director of SUNY-Buffalo's Multidisciplinary Center for the Study of Aging from 1977 to 1980. Over the course of his career, Brody held visiting professorships at the universities of Toronto, Winnipeg, and Kentucky, and returned frequently to the departments of neurology and anatomy at the University of Copenhagen, where he had been a Fulbright Fellow in 1963.

Brody was especially interested in conducting quantitative and morphological studies of aging in the central nervous system. One of his first articles, now identified as a classic study of nervous system gerontology, was the "Organization of Cerebral Cortex: A Study of Aging in the Human Cerebral Cortex," *Journal of Comparative Neurology,* 102: (1956): 511–56. See also his "Structural Changes in the Aging Nervous System," in *Interdisciplinary Topics in Gerontology,* ed. Herman Blumenthal (Basel: S. Kargel, 1970). He also investigated early postnatal changes in the nervous system, the presence of mercury in the human brain, and the effects of stress upon the hypothalamus. See, for instance, his contribution with C. A. Glomski and S. K. K. Pillay, "Distribution and Concentration of Mercury in Autopsy Specimens of Human Brain," *Nature,* 232 (1972): 200–201, as well as several articles with one of his principal collaborators, N. Vijayashankar: "A Study of Aging in Human Abducens Nucleus," *Journal of Comparative Neurology,* 173 (1977): 433–37; and H. Brody, "A Quantitative Study of the Pigmented Neurons in the Nuclei Coeruleus and Subcoeruleus in Man as Related to Aging," *Journal of Neuropathology and Experimental Neurology,* 38 (1979): 490–97. Much of his early work in this area is summarized in his *Clinical, Morphological, and Neurochemical Aspects of Aging in the Central Nervous System* (New York: Raven Press, 1975), which Brody edited with D. Harman and J. M. Oray.

Among Brody's contributions to anatomy has been the development of neuroanatomical techniques. See, for instance, his article, with J. E. Wirth, on "A Staining and Plastic Embedding Technique for Macroscopic Brain Sections," *Anatomical Record,* 127 (1957): 65-14. By measuring changes in the deposition of pigments in nerve cells of the human cerebral cortex and inferior olive, Brody was able to trace development with aging. See, for instance, H. Brody, "The Deposition of Aging Pigment in the Human Cerebral Cortex," *Journal of Gerontology,* 15 (1960): 258–61; and with R. Monagle, "The Effects of Age upon the Main Nucleus of the Inferior Olive in the Human," *Journal of Comparative Neurology,* 155 (1974): 61–66; with N. Vijayashankar, "Cell Loss in Aging Brain," in *Aging Brain and Senile Dementia,* eds. K. Nandy and A. Sherwin (New York: Plenum Press, 1977); H. Brody, "Neuronal Loss," in *Biological Mechanisms in Aging,* ed. R. T. Schimke (Bethesda, Md.: Department of Health and Human Services, 1981), pp. 563–66; H. Brody, "Comments on Neuron Numbers and Dendritic Extent in Aging and Alzheimer's Disease," *Neurobiology of Aging,* 8 (1987): 566; and H. Brody, "The Aging Brain," *Acta Neurologica Scandinavica,* 85 (1992): 40–44. Most recently has been his contribution, "Structural Changes in the Aging Brain," in *Principles and Practice of Geriatric Psychiatry,* eds. J. R. M. Copeland, M. T. Abore-Saleh and D. G. Blazer* (New York: Wiley, 1994).

Brody has been active in the Gerontological Society. He served as president from 1974 to 1975. He was editor of the Biological Sciences Section of the *Journal of Gerontology* from 1973 to 1975, before serving as editor-in-chief of the entire journal for the next five years. In this capacity, as well as his chairmanship of the Society's Publications Committee (1984–1987), Brody made special efforts to increase the range of disciplinary perspectives in the pool of scientific contributors. Brody was also active in planning the meetings of the International Association of Gerontology in Kiev and in Tokyo in the 1970s. From 1975 to 1979, he served as a founding member of the National Advisory Council of the National Institute on Aging.

In addition to his service on national and international boards, Brody, with his wife Anne, has been active in developing health care and social services in western New York. Brody, for instance, has served on the board of directors for Legal Services for the Elderly, the Western New York Alzheimer's Disease Society, Meals on Wheels, and on the advisory committee of Adult Day Services for the town of Amherst.

STANLEY J. BRODY. Stanley J. "Steve" Brody was born in New York City in 1918. He earned his B.S. from Columbia University in 1936 and completed his law degree there three years later, where he was greatly influenced by Herbert Wechsler. In 1941, Brody earned his M.S.W. from the University of Pittsburgh's School of Applied Science, where he worked with Marion Hathaway. Brody's career before entering the field of aging was quite varied but focused on social and health policy. He served as a legislative analyst for the Social Security Board's Bureau of Public Assistance, where he served with his primary mentor, Wilbur J. Cohen.* He was executive secretary of the Bronx Council for Social Welfare, an officer of the Philadelphia Community Chest, and editor of *Washington Bulletin,* published by the Social Legislation Information Service Inc.

In the 1950s, Brody continued his activities in rethinking health care and welfare programs in the public sector. He served as chairman of the Pennsylvania Commission on Mental Health and as a member of the State Welfare Board. He was appointed to the President's Committee on Juvenile Delinquency and Youth Crime in 1960. He was executive secretary of the State and Local Welfare Commission for the Commonwealth of Pennsylvania (1961–1962), for which he published *A Reallocation of Public Welfare Responsibilities* (1963), emphasizing care and continuity of care. Brody then served as executive director of the Governor's Hospital Study Commission (1962–1965). In that capacity, he edited four volumes dealing with hospital costs, utilization, operations, and construction.

From 1964 to 1969, he served as regional director and deputy secretary for the metropolitan Philadelphia area of the Commonwealth of Pennsylvania's Department of Public Welfare. It was in this capacity that Brody first became sensitive to the needs of the elderly. As an administrator of multiple programs, he became aware of how much the elderly were at risk. His first aging-related article, "The Aged, Their Families and The Law," was published with his wife, Elaine M. Brody,* in *Womens Law Journal,* 53:3 (1967): 686ff.

In 1969, Brody left state government and became associate professor and

Community Medicine Commonwealth Fellow in the Fels Center of Government Wharton School, and associate director of the Regional Medical Plan at the University of Pennsylvania. Over the next twenty years, until his retirement, he held a number of appointments in the schools of business, medicine, and social work. He became professor of rehabilitation medicine in psychiatry in 1976, and of health care services. He chaired the Graduate Group in Social Gerontology (1978–1986). Perhaps his most important responsibility was directing the National Center for Rehabilitation of Elderly Disabled Individuals, a consortium underwritten by the National Institute on Aging, the Administration on Aging, National Institute of Mental Health, and the National Institute of Disability and Rehabilitation Research. Brody made more than 150 presentations at annual meetings of the American Hospital Association, Gerontological Society, and nursing home associations. He argued that rehabilitation is a valid intervention for the elderly. See, for instance, his "Is Rehabilitation a Legitimate Intervention for the Elderly?" in *Aging 2000,* ed. Charles M. Gaitz* et al. (New York: Springer, 1985), as well as his collection of essays with G. E. Ruff, *Aging and Rehabilitation: Advances in the State of the Art* (New York: Springer, 1986) and *Aging and Rehabilitation II* (New York: Springer, 1990), edited with L. G. Paulson.

Brody was instrumental in the 1980s in arguing that long-term care was an insurable risk. See his "Chronically Disabled Elderly's Long-Term Care Needs are not a Bottomless Pit," *American Hospital Association News,* 37 (September 21, 1987): 4; and S. J. Brody and J. S. Magel, "Long-Term Care: The Long and Short of It," in *Caring for the Elderly: Reshaping Health Policy,* ed. Carl Eisdorfer (Baltimore: Johns Hopkins University Press, 1989). In his 1986 Kent lecture to the Gerontological Society, published as "Strategic Planning: The Catastrophic Approach" (*The Gerontologist,* 27 (1987): 131–38), Brody noted that, having addressed the elderly's need for income maintenance and acute medical care, the time had come to deal with continuity of care. He stressed that a measurement of need for long-term care that he had proposed in the 1970s—Activities of Daily Living (ADL)—be used as a criterion, since survey data suggested that roughly 30 percent of the U.S. elderly population required functional assistance. He made more than a dozen major testimony presentations to Congress, culminating with a series before the U.S. Senate Finance and House Ways and Means committees on ADL as a criterion for the need for long-term care. Congress adopted this instrument in the short-lived Catastropic Coverage Act of 1988, and it has continued as an eligibility criterion. The field of rehabilitation accepted the elderly as appropriate for service because of the efforts of the Center for Rehabilitation for the Elderly. Brody became emeritus professor of rehabilitation medicine in psychiatry and health care services at the University of Pennsylvania in 1970. His most recent article, "A Responsible Citizen's Analysis of the Clinton Health Proposal," *The Gerontologist,* 35:5 (1994): 586–89, was a continuation of a lifelong interest and commitment to health and social legislation.

HERMAN BROTMAN. Herman Brotman was born in 1909. His career in the federal government began in the 1930s, when he did background research for the staff that designed the 1935 Social Security Act. During World War II, he served in Austria. Brotman remained in Europe to help with reconstructing the war-torn countries; upon his return to the United States in 1952, he won the Army's Meritorious Civilian Award.

Brotman joined the Special Staff on Aging in the Office of the Secretary of Health, Education, and Welfare. There, he worked on special studies and helped to draft the legislation known as the Older Americans Act (1965). When the Administration on Aging was established, Brotman joined the staff. Eventually he became chief of the Data Analysis Division and, later, special assistant to the Commissioner on Aging. Brotman produced a series of statistical studies and publications for students and practitioners in the field.

After retiring in 1973, Brotman served as a consultant to both the Senate and House committees on aging. For a number of years he produced "Every Tenth American," a statistical overview of the demographic and socioeconomic status of older people that prefaced the annual report, *Developments on Aging,* of the Senate Special Committee on Aging. (This report has been expanded over the years; the American Association of Retired Persons now issues it as *Aging America: Trends and Projections.*)

Brotman was the first recipient of the Gerontological Society's Donald Kent Award in 1973. Three years laters, upon his death, George Mason University established the Herman B. Brotman Fund for Gerontology Students.

VICTORIA E. BUMAGIN. Victoria E. Bumagin, born in 1923, received her B.A. from Brooklyn College in 1945. She received her M.S.S.W. from Columbia in 1969. Her subsequent practice has been based on the concept that family ties usually bind their members to be available to each other when need arises, and that their responses cross generational lines in both directions. She believes that "family relationships are based on reciprocity, mutuality, and interdependence at all ages." She has found that while service trends might recast discrete services for the elderly into a respite framework intended to ease family stress, national family policy directions must reflect a high degree of family involvement. To offer professionals and families understanding and guidance for such involvement, she co-wrote *Aging Is a Family Affair* (New York: T. Y. Crowell, 1979) and *Helping the Aging Family* (New York: Springer, 1990).

With this framework, Bumagin has contributed to the development of gerontological social work that builds on family systems theory and the concept of multidisciplinary service provision. In a practice based on a psycho-dynamic view of human behavior, she assesses, evaluates, and relies on the principle of minimal intervention to strengthen family interactions and coping strategies. She is a pioneer of "case management," giving the elderly continuing opportunity to live independently and preserve self-determination. Her thinking on service systems is abstracted in V. Bumagin, "Integrated Social Services for the Aged in England and the United States," *Aging International,* 6 (1979). Her comparative work between the United States and England is based on practical work in England during the early 1970s. Having become familiar with the pros and cons of the British "cradle-to-grave" approach to welfare, Bumagin became intrigued by the questions of intergenerational equity posed by the commitment to universal access to services. Expanding on this experience, in 1990–1991 Bumagin was involved in a study of the then Soviet social and health service delivery system through the Institute of Gerontology, Kiev, Ukraine.

Her current practice includes teaching, training, consultation, and individual and family treatment. Montay College in Chicago awarded Victoria Bumagin an honorary L.H.D. in 1993.

MARION E. BUNCH. Marion Estel Bunch was born in Rochester, Kentucky in 1902. He earned his A.B. at the University of Kentucky in 1925, his M.A. at Washington University in 1926, and his Ph.D. in psychology from the University of Chicago in 1934. Except for a year (1948–1949) serving as a professor of psychology at the University of Illinois, Bunch spent his entire academic career at Washington University in St. Louis.

Bunch's research focused on the psychology of learning, human and animal memory, and the experimental study of emotions. Thanks to his association with Robert W. Kleemeier,* however, Bunch became involved in two gerontologically related projects. First, with Rose E. Kushner, he edited *Graduate Education in Aging Within the Social Sciences* (Ann Arbor, Mich.: Division of Gerontology, 1967). With Helen Flint, he contributed a chapter to that volume on "strategies for educational administration and support for doctoral education in social gerontology." Second, following Kleemeier's untimely death, Bunch helped organize with Paul M. Paillat a colloquium on "Interdisciplinary Topics in Gerontology." Supported by the National Institute of Child Health and Human Development, the project followed up a 1966 symposium in Austria. The report of the proceedings, *Age, Work and Automation* (New York: S. Karger, 1970), dealt with medical, psychological, social, and economic aspects of the aged; special attention was placed on those between the ages of sixty and sixty-five who were in good health.

ERNEST W. BURGESS. Ernest Watson Burgess was born in Tilbury, Ontario, in 1886. He earned his A.B. at Kingfisher College in 1908, and his Ph.D. in sociology at the University of Chicago five years later. After teaching at the universities of Toledo, Kansas, and Ohio State, Burgess joined the sociology faculty of the University of Chicago in 1916. He became a full professor in 1927. From 1946 until his retirement, he chaired the department.

In the early stages of his career, Burgess became well known for his work in family studies and urban sociology. He edited *The Urban Community* (Chicago: University of Chicago Press, 1926); with Herbert Blumer, *Personality and the*

Social Group (Chicago: University of Chicago Press, 1929), and *The Human Side of Social Planning* (Chicago: University of Chicago Press, 1935). With his colleague Robert Park, Burgess wrote several landmark texts, including *Introduction to the Science of Sociology* (Chicago: University of Chicago Press, 1921) and, four years later, *The City.* With Leonard Cottrell, Jr., he wrote *Predicting Success or Failure in Marriage* (Chicago: University of Chicago Press, 1939). He also wrote *The American Family: The Problems of Family Relations Facing American Youth;* and *The Family, From Institution to Companionship.*

Burgess's interest in research on aging began in the 1940s, when he chaired a Social Science Research Committee survey of social-scientific inquiries in gerontology. With his colleague Robert J. Havighurst,* Burgess made work on late adulthood and aging a component of the research and teaching mission of the University of Chicago's Committee on Human Development. With Ruth Shonle Cavan and others, Burgess prepared the research instruments that were set forth in *Personal Adjustment in Old Age* (Chicago: University of Chicago Press, 1949). With Sidney Spector, he prepared *The States and Their Older Citizens* (Chicago: University of Chicago Press, 1955), which became a classic analysis of public policy initiatives in aging at the state level.

Burgess is probably best remembered in gerontology for his work with the Inter-University Training Institute in Social Gerontology, in Bethesda, Maryland, which was supported by the National Institute of Mental Health. In addition to serving on the project's executive committee, Burgess edited *Aging in Western Societies: A Survey of Social Gerontology* (Chicago: University of Chicago Press, 1960). Burgess focused on the economic, societal, and cultural dimensions of demographic aging, older people's problems, and social action for their welfare in France, Italy, the Netherlands, Sweden, the United Kingdom, and West Germany. He hoped that the analysis would be useful to U.S. policymakers and citizens engaged in the 1961 White House Conference on Aging.

Burgess died in 1966.

RICHARD V. BURKHAUSER. Richard V. Burkhauser was born December 27, 1945. He received his B.A. in economics from St. Vincent College in 1967, his M.A. in economics from Rutgers University in 1969, and his Ph. D. in economics from the University of Chicago in 1976. Burkhauser was one of the first economists to consider social policy questions from a life-cycle perspective. During his training at Chicago, Burkhauser was attracted to gerontology by Bernice L. Neugarten,* who sparked his appreciation for multidisciplinary research. Neugarten's National Science Foundation (NSF) sponsored graduate seminar in 1974–1975 led Burkhauser to think of Social Security and employer pensions as assets whose value changed over time.

In subsequent research with Joseph Quinn, Burkhauser's pension asset model was used to examine the influences of mandatory retirement and Social Security benefit rules on work. They argued that mandatory retirement rules have far less impact on retirement decisions than do changes in pensions and Social Security benefit rules. Burkhauser, Quinn, and Daniel Meyers co-wrote the 1990 volume *Passing the Torch: The Influence of Economic Incentives on Work and Retirement* (Kalamazoo, Mich.: W.E. Upjohn Institute for Employment Policy), which summarizes their research and that of others in the field.

Burkhauser was among the first to use "life-course" or duration analysis to examine how the economic well-being of the elderly changes over time. See, for example his work with Karen Holden and David Feaster, "Incidence, Timing and Events Associated with Poverty: A Dynamic View of Poverty in Retirement," *Journal of Gerontology,* 43 (March 1988): 46–52. This work led to a long collaboration with Greg Duncan and Richard Hauser on the relative economic well-being of women and men in the United States and Germany. They found that women are at greater risk because of a failure of social policy to adjust to changes in family structure. See, for example, "Sharing Prosperity across the Age Distribution: A Comparison of the United States and Germany in the 1980s," *The Gerontologist,* 34 (April 1994): 150–60.

Most recently, Burkhauser has been evaluating the influence of government policy, including the Americans with Disabilities Act, on people with disabilities. He is currently a professor of economics and the associate director for the Aging Studies Program, Center for Policy Research, Syracuse University.

LYNDA C. BURTON. Lynda C. Burton earned a B.A. from Pennsylvania State University in 1960, an M.L.A. in 1972 from the Johns Hopkins University Evening College, and her Sc.D. at the Hopkins School of Hygiene and Public Health in 1991. She has remained at Hopkins as an instructor teaching courses such as "Perspectives on Aging: Introduction to Gerontology," "Health Promotion and Disease Prevention Among the Elderly," and "Health Care Systems for Aging Populations."

Burton's most important gerontological work to date has been a demonstration and evaluation of preventive services for Medicare beneficiaries. This work was done at Hopkins, one of five sites carrying out the Health Care Financing Administration-funded study. The principal investigator at Hopkins was Pearl S. German, Sc.D. In the randomized trial, the group offered free preventive services (N = 2,105) and a modest health benefit with no negative cost impact, as compared with the controls (N = 2,090). See P. S. German and L. C. Burton, "Does Adding a Benefit for Preventive Services for Older Persons Have an Impact on Utilization and Costs Under Medicare?" *American Journal of Public Health,* a February 1995 publication.

Burton has also published research findings on the treatment of nursing-home elderly. Her primary collaborator in this work has been German, and funding came from the National Institute on Aging. In a study presented to the 1990 meeting of the Gerontological Society of America, Burton correlated the use of physical restraint with the diagnosis of mental illnesses. Predictors of restraint included inability to transfer, a combination of limitations to activities of daily living, and cognitive impairment. See L. C. Burton, P. S. German, Barry W.

Rovner, and Larry J. Brant, "Mental Illness and the Use of Restraints in Nursing Homes," *The Gerontologist*, 32 (1992): 164–70.

The team raised the possibility in a follow-up study that restraint could contribute to cognitive impairment. Restraint use alone and in combination with neuroleptic use was associated with poor cognition in a sample of 437 nursing home residents—particularly in residents who had moderate or no cognitive impairment at admission. See P. S. German and L. C. Burton, "Physical Restraint Use and Cognitive Decline Among Nursing Home Residents," *Journal of the American Geriatrics Society*, 40 (August 1992): 811–16.

EWALD W. BUSSE. Ewald W. Busse was born in St. Louis in 1917, earned his B.A. degree at Westminster College, which awarded him the Sc.D. degree in 1960, and received his M.D. from Washington University in St. Louis in 1942. His psychiatric training was at the University of Colorado Medical Center.

Busse joined the Duke University faculty as chairman of the Department of Psychiatry in 1953, a position he held for twenty-one years. Between 1974 and 1982 he served as dean of medical and allied health education and associate provost. In 1965 he was named J.P. Gibbons Professor of Psychiatry. He held numerous positions within the Medical Center, including chief of staff. He became professor emeritus in 1987. He was president and chief executive officer of the North Carolina Institute of Medicine from 1987 to 1994. He has served as president of the American Psychiatric Association, the American Geriatrics Society, the Gerontological Society of America, the American Association of Departments of Psychiatry, the Southern Psychiatric Association, the Southeastern Medical-Dental Society, and the International Association of Gerontology. Busse is a member of the Academy of Sciences-Institute of Medicine and was director of the American Board of Psychiatry and Neurology for eight years.

Busse held the position of founding director of the Duke University Center for the Study of Aging and Human Development from 1957 to 1970. He has received numerous research and professional awards, including the Edward B. Alien Award, 1967; the Strecker Award, 1967; the Kleemeier Award, 1968; the Menninger Award, 1971; the Modern Medicine Award, 1971; the Freeman Award, 1978; the Thewlis Award, 1979; the Brookdale Award, 1982; the Sandoz Award, 1983; the Weinberg Memorial Award, 1983; the Alumni Achievement Award (Westminster College), 1984; a Commendation for Leadership, Commitment, and Dedication to Service on behalf of Aging Veterans, 1985; the Warren Williams Assembly Speaker's Award (APA), 1987; Distinguished Service Award (APA), 1988; the Distinguished Alumni Award (Washington University, St. Louis), 1992; the President's Medallion for Gerontological Research (International Association of Gerontology, Budapest), 1993; and the Pioneer Award from the Governor's Commission on Reduction of Infant Mortality. He was also recognized for Contribution to Gerontology in Latin America by the Latin American Committee of Gerontology in 1993.

Busse was honored in 1985 with the dedication of the E. W. Busse Building for gerontology at Duke University. An international research award was established in 1990 honoring Busse, and the North Carolina Department of Human Resources established the Ewald W. Busse Award in 1990.

Busse was a member of the President's Biomedical Research Panel from 1976 to 1981 and was made a fellow of the American Association for the Advancement of Science in 1981. He chaired for four years the Geriatrics and Gerontology Advisory Committee of the Veterans Administration and served for six years as a member of the Special Medical Advisory Group. He is a member of the jury for the International Sandoz Prize for Gerontological Research and has served as chairman of the jury. He has been on the DHR Advisory Committee on Home and Community Care since 1989. He is listed in *Who's Who in America* and *Who's Who in Frontier Science and Technology*.

Author and co-author of more than 250 scientific articles, Busse has edited several books, including: *Behavior and Adoption in Late Life; Mental Illness in Later Life; The Handbook of Geriatric Psychiatry; The Duke Longitudinal Studies of Normal Aging 1955–1980; Aging—The Universal Human Experience* (1987); and *Geriatric Psychiatry* (1989).

ROBERT N. BUTLER. *Note:* Robert N. Butler's biography is longer than most entries for two reasons. First, his career has been unusually rich and rewarding. Second, Butler was prompted by our questionnaire to trace in considerable detail his professional and personal growth. Because we feel this is an important narrative, we have done minimal editing.

Robert N. Butler received his B.A. from Columbia University in 1949, where he was greatly influenced by political scientist Dean Lawrence Chamberlain, biologist Charles Dawson, and chemist Charles Van Doering. Butler earned his M.D. from Columbia's College of Physicians and Surgeons four years later. His interest in aging dates to his internship, when he was struck by the high average age of his patients. This on-rounds impression did not jibe with his medical school experience, in which not much attention had been given to older persons. Butler began to ground himself in the literature by reading articles by Alexis Carrel on his experiments at Rockefeller University in the 1920s, by Clive McCay on prolonging rats' lives by restricting their caloric intake, by Anton Carlson* on physiology, by Henry Simms on biology of aging, and by Albert Szent-Gyorgi on muscle physiology. This wide-ranging curiosity was to serve Butler well in a career that has traversed many intellectual domains and enabled him to interact with politicians, policymakers, and experts from many disciplines and domains.

Butler's interest in aging was further stimulated at the Langley Porter Clinic by Drs. Karl Bowman and Alexander Simon,* the chairman and vice chairman, respectively, of the Department of Psychiatry at the University of California, both of whom had an interest in aging. Butler did studies on the first tranquilizers, chlorpromazine and reserpine. When he joined the Laboratory of Clinical

Science at the National Institute of Mental Health under the leadership of the "father" of U.S. neuroscience, Dr. Seymour Kety, he had the opportunity, as a principal investigator, to explore central nervous system functioning in older people, utilizing the Kety-Schmidt method of measurement. He was a principal investigator of the interdisciplinary Human Aging Study, which extended over eleven years and, along with the studies at Duke University, became a model for research on healthy older persons living in the community.

Among other things, the findings by Butler and his colleagues that senility was not an inevitable consequence of aging *per se* but rather the result of various diseases was derived directly from the Human Aging Study. They found that cerebral physiological variables do not decline as a function of age *per se* but of disease. This work was amply confirmed in the 1980s by the more precise technique of positron emission tomography. The interdisciplinary nature of the Human Aging Study also became an important model for later investigations of human senescence, such as Nathan Shock's Baltimore Longitudinal Study on Aging. The work is described in James E. Birren,* Robert N. Butler, Samuel Greenhouse, Louis Sokoloff and Marian Radke Yarrow, *Human Aging 1: A Biological and Behavioral Study* (Bethesda, Md.: National Institute on Mental Health, 1963). *Human Aging 2* was edited by D. Granick and J. Paterson in 1971. Butler's own interpretation of the Human Aging Studies is contained in the paper, "The Facade of Chronological Age," *American Journal of Psychiatry,* 119 (1963): 721–28, which expressed forcefully the idea that much that is attributed to aging is in fact due to physical disease, personality, and social economic circumstances:

> We have found evidence to suggest that many manifestations heretofore associated with aging *per se* reflect instead, medical illness, personality variables, and social-cultural effects. It is hoped that future research may further disentangle the contributions of disease, social losses, and pre-existent personality so that we may know more clearly what changes should be regarded as age specific. If we can move behind the facade of chronological aging, we open up the possibility of modification through both prevention and treatment.

Prior to the publication of the books and various papers related to the Human Aging Study, Butler began to investigate the applicability of intensive psychotherapy to older persons, including hospital in-patients. He wrote about the major adverse "counter-transference" attitudes of mental health professionals toward older persons and the fact that older persons benefit from psychotherapy in "Intensive Psychotherapy for the Hospitalized Aged," *Geriatrics,* 15 (1960): 644–53. Butler set up perhaps the first experimental hospital in-patient psychotherapy unit for older persons at Chestnut Lodge, Maryland, in 1958.

Impressed by the extraordinary importance of reminiscence, which at that time was regarded as primarily pathological and not as having possible therapeutic value, Butler wrote "Life Review: An Interpretation of Reminiscence in the Aged," *Psychiatry,* 26 (1963): 655–76. The concept has been widely studied and translated into a therapeutic approach, "life review therapy," which Butler wrote about with Myrna I. Lewis* in *Geriatrics,* 29 (1974): 165–69. The therapy is often used in nursing homes, homes for the aging, and hospitals by nurses as well as by social workers, psychologists, psychiatrists, and other therapists.

Butler also emphasized the importance of comprehensive psychiatric evaluation of the aged, including an experimental study of older people's reactions to their mirror images. See "Life Review," *Geriatrics,* 18 (1963): 220–32. Throughout his professional career, Butler was struck by the negativism toward older persons that comes from medicine, psychiatry, and the other mental health professions, as well as the public at large. He wrote about the minimal extent to which older persons were provided psychiatric evaluation and treatment and about adverse nursing home conditions and direct abuses. Social worker Phyllis Brostoff and Butler described the "battered old person's syndrome," now called "elder abuse," for the first time in the gerontologic literature; see *Aging and Human Development,* 3 (1972): 319–22.

In 1968 in "Ageism," Butler proposed the word "ageism" as a counterpart of sexism and racism, reflecting the extent to which discrimination is based on age (*The Gerontologist,* 9 (1969): 243–46). He noted that the term could apply to prejudice from older persons toward the young as well as from younger persons toward the old. To Butler, the stereotypes and prejudice encapsulated in ageism paralleled those embedded in racism or sexism. Much of Butler's work has been concerned with overcoming prejudices based on age, and the word *"ageism"* has entered everyday language in the *Oxford English Dictionary.*

Butler fought the "deinstitutionalization" movement within American psychiatry nationally and in Washington, D.C., in both the professional and public arena (as did Alvin Goldfarb and Jack Weinberg*). He regarded the concept of community care for the chronically mentally ill as valuable but limited, especially since funds had not been made available to provide such care. Moreover, improvements to mental hospitals were sacrificed. The result was the re-creation of the conditions over 100 years before that prompted Dorothea Lynde Dix to lead the struggle to create state asylums. (Now, perhaps one-third of the homeless are mentally ill persons who should be in protective settings.) The motivation for the movement was primarily financial—state governments wanted to save money. The movement also falsely assumed that "senile dementia" was a social problem, not a neuropsychiatric condition.

In 1972, Myrna I. Lewis and Butler wrote what he believes was the first comprehensive textbook of the psychiatry of old age in the United States. This book is now in its fourth edition (*Aging and Mental Health: Positive Psychosocial Approaches,* Columbus, Ohio: Merrill, 1991). Thus, along with Alvin Goldfarb, Jack Weinberg, and a few others, Butler helped to found the field of geriatric psychiatry.

In 1975, Butler published *Why Survive? Being Old in America* (New York: Harper and Row), which was awarded the Pulitzer Prize a year later. This work provided a portrait of old age in America and offered policy solutions. It included a major critique of deinstitutionalization, the commercial nursing home industry, medicine, psychiatry, and other professional fields in meeting the needs of older persons. It encouraged passage of the Age Discrimination in Employment Act and the end of mandatory retirement. It called for a National Institute of Gerontology. *Why Survive?* was the stimulus for the Pulitzer Prize-winning play, *The Gin Game.*

The first stage of Butler's career was dominated by concern about negativism toward aging. Thus, his basic biomedical research (the Human Aging Studies), his attention to the psychiatric aspects of aging (evaluation and treatment), his portrait of the social treatment of old age (*Why Survive?*) and, with Myrna I. Lewis, his writings about mental health and one of the most profound forms of ageism, negativism toward the sexuality of older persons (*Sex After 60,* which appeared in 1976), all illustrate his basic goal of exposing prejudice and introducing medical, psychiatric, social, and economic interventions into the aging process.

In 1976, Butler became the founding director of the National Institute on Aging (NIA) of the National Institutes of Health. There, he endeavored to establish a wide range of priorities, from the basic biology of aging to social and behavioral studies, concluding that the successful historic development of the National Institutes of Health was due to what he called "the health politics of anguish." Butler identified Alzheimer's Disease and related dementias as a major NIA priority. NIH Director Donald Fredrickson, Arthur M. Flemming,* and Congressman Claude Pepper served as key political mentors. Butler intended to make dementia, specifically Alzheimer's Disease, a national priority and a household word, but he did not intend for the institute to become as unbalanced in favor of Alzheimer's Disease research as it has become. Rather, Butler called for the study of fourteen major topics including basic biology, pharmacology, prevention, nutrition, the impact of retirement, and bereavement. Today, he favors greater financial support from the NIA of studies for the dementias, including Alzheimer's Disease and multi-infarct dementia, but believes it is vitally important to expand the aging agenda as he originally formulated it. For this reason, Butler worked to gain the support of the Commonwealth Fund and Pew Memorial Trust to sponsor the National Academy of Sciences Institute of Medicine National Agenda for Research on Aging (*Extending Life, Enhancing Life,* 1991). It might be time, he suggests, to rename the NIA the "National Institute on Aging and Longevity Science."

Butler compiled an impressive record during his tenure as director of NIA. He:

- stimulated the development of academic geriatrics by sponsoring, for example, the Geriatric Medicine Academic Award and the NIA Teaching Nursing Home Award;

- forced the addition of women to the Baltimore Longitudinal Study on Aging at NIA's Gerontology Research Center in 1976 (among other changes);

- pressured the Food and Drug Administration to emphasize aging in drug evaluation in animal and human studies and to improve labeling for consumers;

- made an epidemiologist the associate director of an NIH Institute (NIA) for the first time in order to develop population studies on special topics, such as "the last days of life" and clinical trials, the Systolic Hypertension of the Elderly Program as well as epidemiological studies in East Boston, New Haven, and Iowa;

- created the Interagency Committee on Aging to advance aging issues and research throughout the federal government;

- worked with the Bureau of Census, National Center of Health Statistics, Social Security Administration, Department of Labor, and other statistics-gathering elements of government to achieve disaggregation of age-related data;

- instigated and organized the contribution regarding old age for Healthy People, the Surgeon General's Report on Health Promotion and Disease Prevention;

- participated in developing a symposium, Cancer and Aging, with Congressman Pepper and Drs. Arthur Upton and Vincent DeVita, directors of the National Cancer Institute. Butler and DeVita phased out age limits on treatment protocols and urged use of full dosages in the combined chemotherapy study of breast cancer in post-menopausal women. Throught this project, Butler emphasized the basic biological aging predisposition to cancer. He held out the possibility that cancer essentially might be considered "failed aging," and asked whether there are "geronto genes" that are anti-oncogenes;

- developed programs and wrote on the protection of voluntary research subjects in aging and with Alzheimer's Disease;

- stimulated study of *Mammalian Models For Research on Aging* (1981) at the Institute of Laboratory Animal Resources, National Academy of Sciences;

- helped establish the Biomarker study led by the NIA and the National Center for Toxicological Research;

- led research planning in aging—*Our Future Selves* (Bethesda, Md., 1978) and *Toward an Independent Old Age* (Bethesda, Md., 1982), and participated actively in developing the National Agenda for Research on Aging's *Extending Life, Enhancing Life* (Bethesda, Md., 1991) as well as the NIH Women's Health Research Agenda 1992;

- helped stimulate Travelers Company Foundation Awards to medical students as well as the Travelers Center on Geriatrics. Butler also helped persuade the Merck Company as well as the Commonwealth, John A. Hartford, and Greenwall Foundations to support geriatrics;

- promoted nationwide interest in aging research and the health problems of older persons;

- worked with Jane Shure in developing "Age Pages," which gave succinct, straightforward information about various manifestations and diseases associated with aging.

The National Institute on Aging is a research organization, but Butler also wished to influence medical education. At the National Institute on Aging in 1976–1977, he arranged to bring key national figures interested in geriatrics to Bethesda to discuss the development of geriatrics in American medical education. Butler also wrote a paper conceptualizing the "teaching nursing home" to indicate the importance of moving away from the preoccupation with acute ailments in hospitals to chronic illness and nursing home care. See "The Teaching Nursing Home," *Journal of the American Medical Association,* 245 (1981): 1435–37.

In 1982, Butler left the NIA and founded the first department of geriatrics in an American medical school at the Mount Sinai School of Medicine in New York, which he hoped would influence medical education at large. To change stereotypes, he established the Healthy Elderly Program at the 92nd Street YMCA for medical students' rotation. Butler argued that pediatrics is made attractive to medical students in part because of the "well baby clinics." If they saw only children with Down syndrome and cancer they might be turned off to pediatrics; so, too, if students see only older persons with dementia and terminal illness, they may not find the field attractive.

Butler believed that just as teaching hospitals were important standard setters for American hospitals, education and research in nursing homes associated with medical schools would help bring about new standards of care, supplementing regulations and their enforcement. He presented the case for geriatrics before the American Board of Internal Medicine and later before the American Board of Neurology and Psychiatry in special meetings. Along with the work of others, his efforts helped lead to the decisions of these boards as well as the American Academy of Family Practice to offer examinations for "a certificate of added competence in geriatrics" (see R. N. Butler, "Developments in New Disciplines of Relevance to the ABIM; Geriatrics in American Board of Internal Medicine," *Summer Conference Report,* Carmel Valley, California, 1984). Butler has emphasized maintaining or integrating geriatrics within all primary care and specialty medicine and developing academic and consultative geriatrics, but not creating a new practice specialty *per se.*

During and since his tenure as director of the National Institute on Aging, Butler encouraged international studies on individual and population aging and longevity so that through collaboration we may learn from one another. He actively participated in the World Health Organization as an adviser. Butler serves as American member of the Board of the United Nations International Institute on Aging, and was founding co-director of the International Leadership Center on Longevity and Society (U.S.-Japan).

In 1982, Butler chaired a Salzburg Seminar in Austria, where he chose to highlight "productive aging"—the mobilization of the continuing contributions of older people to their families, the community, and to the nation at large through paid or unpaid work. Nearly two decades earlier, Butler had done studies of creativity in the middle and later years (see "Studies of Creative People and the Creative Process after Middle Life" in *Psychodynamic Studies on Aging: Creativity, Reminiscing and Dying*, ed. S. Levin (Washington, D.C.: Universities Press, 1967)). He had written about "Successful Aging" in the *Journal of the American Geriatrics Society*, 22 (1974): 529–35. In 1976, his chapter on "middle age" was the first in a major American psychiatric textbook (*Comprehensive Textbook of Psychiatry*, Baltimore, Md.: Alfred M. Freedman, 1975). Its premise was simply that it will be valuable for individuals and for society alike if older persons continue to contribute throughout life. As in the earlier Human Aging Studies, Butler and his colleagues found evidence that goals and structure in people's lives were related to better adaptation and survival. Two books, *Productive Aging* (1985) and *The Promise of Productive Aging* (New York: Springer Publications, 1990), expound on this premise. See also "The Relation of Extended Life to Extended Employment," *Milbank Memorial Fund Quarterly*, 61 (1983): 420–29. With the rise of "new ageism," exemplified by the epithet, "Greedy Geezer," Butler views "productive aging," the notion that older persons continue to contribute to our national life, as a useful political strategy as well as sound practice.

Butler's other interests defy neat categorization, so they will be noted in chronological order. He has, for instance, a long-term interest in the protection of experimental subjects in research. See *Archives of General Psychiatry*, 8 (1963): 139–41. For more on the privileged communication and confidentiality of research subjects, see also, R. N. Butler, "Protection of Elderly Research Subjects," *Clinical Research*, 28 (1980): 35; and R. N. Butler, "Guidelines Addressing the Ethical and Legal Issues for Research in Alzheimer's Disease," *Journal of the American Geriatric Society*, 32 (1984): 531–36.

In 1965, Butler founded the Forum for Professionals and Executives in Washington, D.C., which is similar to the Institute of Retired Professionals, New School for Social Research, New York (founded in 1962). He also advised in the creation of the Fromm Institute of Lifetime Learning, San Francisco. As director of the NIA, Butler worked in the late 1970s to change the Federal Aviation Agency's over-60 rule for pilots.

With Bernice L. Neugarten, he conceptualized the need for long-term human development studies. His article on the "psychiatry of the life cycle" appeared in *Aging in Modern Society* (Washington, D.C.: American Psychological Association, 1968). Although he never wrote a paper with Neugarten, she has been a key collaborator for decades.

Myrna I. Lewis and he endeavored to expand the interest of the women's movement in the field of aging; see Myrna I. Lewis, "Why Is Women's Lib Ignoring Older Women," *Aging and Human Development,* 3 (1972): 223–31. He sought to emphasize the key importance of older women's issues.

In 1978, Butler proposed the founding of the American Association of Geriatric Psychiatry and the APA Commission on Service, Training and Research on Aging at the annual meeting of the APA. See *World Journal of Psychosynthesis,* 12 (1980): 22–26.

Butler has also headed several significant blue-ribbon panels. From 1985 to 1991, he chaired the Commonwealth Fund Commission on Elderly People Living Alone, which established the special vulnerability of the group to poverty and institutionalization. Nearly 100 reports were produced. A special program was established within the American Association of Retired Persons to continue the work.

He also chaired the National Advisory Committee for the multi-foundation-sponsored Living At Home Program, which supported twenty program sites throughout the United States. The program's purpose was to demonstrate methods of coordinating community resources to help older patients remain in their homes as long as possible. Since 1985, Butler has chaired the Brookdale Foundation's National Fellowship Program in Geriatrics, dedicated to the support of promising leaders in the field.

Butler also helped found the Alzheimer's Disease Association, the American Federation for Aging Research, and the U.S-.Japan International Leadership Center on Longevity and Society. He testified in court as an expert in favor of funding by the Buck Foundation (created by the late Beryl H. Buck in Marin County, California) for the Buck Center for Research in Aging. This testimony required confirmation of the legal concept cy-pres ("so near"), which honors to every degree possible the wishes of the testator, and was a landmark case in philanthropy.

In 1994 he became a member of the Advisory Committee of *Project on Death in America* (Open Study Institute of George Soros) to help transform the care of the dying.

C

EVAN CALKINS. Evan Calkins was born in Newton, Massachusetts, in 1920. He earned his M.D. from Harvard Medical School in 1945. Calkins considers his chief mentor to be Walter Bauer, M.D., Jackson Professor of Medicine at Harvard and chief of medical services at Massachusetts General Hospital. Bauer opened Calkins's eyes to the fascination of long-term illness. Calkins became particularly interested in crippling rheumatic diseases; he wanted to work with patients in defeating the ravages of disease and in mustering the strength and determination to survive, and possibly surmount, the limitation and burden of illness. "This balance between the 'human element' of illness, and the disease itself," wrote Calkins, "has proved to be the focal point for my medical practice and my teaching."

Calkins is the author of more than eighty-five scientific publications and thirty-two book chapters, and has co-edited three books, including *The Practice of Geriatrics* (Philadelphia: W. B. Saunders Publications, 1986, 1991). Perhaps his most important scientific contribution was the elucidation, with Dr. Allen Cohen, that amyloid, previously thought to be an amorphous hyaline material, was actually composed of characteristic and definable fibrils. This discovery, aided by the use of electron microscopy, opened the way for understanding the diverse nature of the amyloid proteins and the clinical syndromes that accompany their deposition.

Calkins's major contributions to gerontology and geriatrics, however, are to be found not in the laboratory, but in creating networks for the advancement of research on aging and medical training in geriatrics. As the first chairman of medicine at the University of Buffalo, after it was incorporated into the State

University of New York system, Calkins realized that he had the opportunity to create a true university department from what had previously been a divided, parochial, and insecure department. During his seventeen-year tenure as chairman, Calkins devoted considerable effort to attracting and retaining able physicians to academic medicine. He also was keen to foster ties with health care facilities in western New York. Building on the notion of "resource exchange" developed by Yale organizational psychologist Seymour Sarason, Calkins developed what he called a "model community-wide university-linkage network." The network brought together scholars, practitioners, and private citizens from a seven-country region to coordinate continuing education in the field. So successful was the venture that the Bureau of Health Professions of the U.S. Public Health Service in 1978 designated Buffalo, along with Harvard, Michigan, and the University of Southern California, as one of the nation's prototypical "geriatric education centers."

Calkins also took advantage of the close proximity of a Veterans Administration hospital to the medical school to provide geriatric clinical services. By 1985, Calkins was overseeing a Hospital Based Home Care Program, Geriatric Evaluation and Medical Rehabilitation unit, Nursing Home unit, and two long-term-care wards—together totaling 140 in-patients and eighty home-care patients. The unit also served three community-based nursing homes, with an additional 225 patients. See E. Calkins, "Aging on the Inside," *Transactions of the American Clinical and Climatological Association,* 97 (1985): 175–82. When the Veterans Administration established a fellowship program, Buffalo qualified for support in the second round.

For his efforts at institution-building, Evan Calkins received the 1986 Milo D. Leavitt award from the American Geriatrics Society.

RUTH CAMPBELL. Ruth Campbell has been a senior social worker and director of the Psycho-Social Program of the Turner Geriatric Clinic at the University of Michigan since 1977.

An English major (Temple University, 1960), she first became attracted to the field of aging in 1962, when, expecting to work with teen gangs, she was asked to work with a group of senior citizens—African-Americans, Puerto Ricans, and immigrant whites—who were living in East Harlem, New York. Over the next decade she worked (with interruptions for child-rearing) as a group worker at the Casita Maria-Carver Community Center in New York. In 1973, she was program director of the Day Care Center for the Elderly at the Montefiore Community Center in the Bronx. In the course of graduate training at the University of Michigan, where she earned her M.S.W. in 1976, Campbell continued to focus on adults. She engaged in group and individual counseling in field work at Michigan's Milan Federal Correctional Institute and at the University of Michigan Medical Center's pilot geriatric arthritis program.

As team social worker from the inception of a multidisciplinary health team at the Turner Geriatric Center, a University of Michigan-based geriatric outpatient clinic, Campbell was instrumental in developing an innovative psychosocial program for a large out-patient population. She received funding from the U.S. Administration on Aging from 1978 to 1980 for a model project on "peer support," which consisted of health education workshops, small support groups, and peer counseling. Campbell stressed the importance of involving peer counselors in designing programs for older people and for fostering collaboration between staff and volunteers in an article she wrote with Barbara Chenoweth, "Health Education as a Basis for Social Support," *The Gerontologist,* 21 (1981): 619–27; and in her book, *Peer Supports for Older Adults* (Ann Arbor, Mich.: Institute of Gerontology, 1981). Working with Katherine Supiano, Campbell has also been enthusiastic in encouraging elderly people in the community and nursing homes to write about their feelings and experiences. See her article, "Writing Groups for the Elderly," in *Individual Change Through Small Groups,* eds. Paul Glasser et al. (New York: Free Press, 1985), 546–59.

Campbell shares with her husband, political scientist John Creighton Campbell, a love for Japan. She has won two Fulbrights and a Japan Foundation Fellowship to do research on care-giving and social services. In 1994 she received an Abe fellowship from the Social Science Research Council to write a book, *Japan's Aging Society: At Home and in the Community.* One of her major themes has been the role that Japanese women play in providing transgenerational care. Among her publications in this area is an article (with two of her collaborators, Hiroko Akiyama and Toni C. Antonucci*), "Rules of Support Exchange among Two Generations of Japanese Women," in *Growing Old in Different Societies,* ed. Jay Sokolovsky* (Westport, Conn.: Greenwood Press, 1991).

WALTER B. CANNON. Walter Bradford Cannon was born in Wisconsin in 1871. A member of the Harvard Class of 1896, he began to contribute to physiology as a first-year medical student: With the aid of primitive X-ray apparatus, he watched pearl buttons pass through the esophagus of a dog as a way to study the motor activity of the alimentary tract. A few weeks later, he repeated the experiment to demonstrate the nature of diglutition in a goose at the American Physiological Society.

After completing his M.D., Cannon joined the Harvard Medical School faculty. Among his landmark publications were *The Mechanical Factors of Digestion* (Cambridge, Mass.: Harvard University Press, 1911); *Bodily Changes in Pain, Hunger, Fear and Rage* (Cambridge, Mass.: Harvard University Press, 1915; rev. 1929), which reflected his collaborations with Pavlov; and eight editions of a *Laboratory Course in Physiology* (Cambridge, Mass.: Harvard University Press). In 1932, he explicated his understanding of homeostasis and the role of autonomic systems in regulating bodily functions in *The Wisdom of the Body* (Cambridge, Mass.: Harvard University Press). Although he never won a Nobel Prize, Cannon was highly regarded as a scientist. His autobiographical account, *The Way of an Investigator* (Cambridge, Mass.: Harvard University

Press) published in 1945, the year of his death, attests to the keenness of his scientific acumen and his generosity of spirit.

At a symposium at the State University of New York Downstate Medical Center at the centennial of his birth, Chandler McC. Brooks, Kiyomi Koizumi, and James O. Pinkston noted (published in *The Life and Contributions of Walter Bradford Cannon, 1871–1945* (1975)) that

> he was one of the first to use X-rays, but no one considered him to be a radiologist. He made major discoveries in the field of gastroenterology, but he was not considered to be a gastroenterologist. He contributed as much to our knowledge of the autonomic nervous system as has any man, but he was not thought of as a neurophysiologist. In much of his work on transmitters he employed drugs to facilitate and drugs to block chemical actions, yet he was not a pharmacologist. Certainly he did much research relative to the function of the endocrine glands, but he is not considered to have been an endocrinologist. His work on emotional expression has been of great importance to psychologists and behaviorists, yet he was not classified as either. His studies of homeostasis, reactions to stress, the means used by the body to maintain required balances as well as his studies of traumatic shock qualify him to be considered a physician of major attainment. He was always considered to be a physiologist, no other title would suffice. (pp. xx–xxi)

In none of the memorial exercises or biographical accounts has any attention been paid to Cannon's contributions to gerontology, yet his work on homeostasis was expanded and refined by some research on aging. In his William Henry Welch lectures, published in the *Journal of Mt. Sinai Hospital*, 5 (1939): 587–606, Cannon spoke at length about homeostasis in senescence. And in a revision of his *Wisdom of the Body* (New York: W. W. Norton, 1939), he added a chapter on changes in regulatory capacities with advancing age, which reflected his exposure to research ideas discussed at the 1937 Woods Hole conference on aging. He also contributed a chapter on the "ageing of homeostatic mechanisms" in the second edition of *Problems of Ageing*, ed. Edmund Vincent Cowdry (Baltimore: Williams and Wilkins, 1942). Cannon also trained two early presidents of the Gerontological Society, Joseph C. Aub* and Roy Hoskins. Thus, while Cannon cannot be characterized as a gerontologist, his interdisciplinary turn of mind, especially his desire to establish homeostasis as a gerontologic metaphor, surely makes Walter Bradford Cannon a forefather of the emerging field.

MARJORIE H. CANTOR. Marjorie H. Cantor received her B.A. *cum laude* in economics from Hunter College in 1943, where she was elected to Phi Beta Kappa. She then did graduate work in economics at Harvard before joining the

National War Labor Board (1943–1945) as an economist. In 1964, she earned an M.A. in psychology from Columbia University's Teachers College.

After the war, Cantor worked on a variety of projects. From 1949 to 1951, she was assistant research director of a study of migrant farm labor in New York State sponsored by the Florida Lasker Foundation and New York Consumer's League. During the next two years she was a field interviewer for Cornell Medical School's "Midtown Study of Mental Health." From 1953 to 1964, she was a research associate in the program department of Girl Scouts, U.S.A. From 1965 to 1967, she directed research for the Phoenix Project in the West Side Urban Renewal Area.

Cantor's academic career resumed in 1965, when she became a lecturer on social welfare research in Columbia University's School of Social Work and directed its Vista Research Project. From 1967 to 1968, she served as a research consultant for a pre-retirement training program at Fordham University, and then spent the following year as a senior fellow at the Metropolitan Applied Research Center.

Cantor received on-the-job training in gerontology as director of research, planning, and evaluation for the New York City Department for the Aging. Each year, with M. Mayer, she produced *Facts for Action* (New York City Department for the Aging). The pair also published several monographs, including *The Elderly in the Rental Markets of New York City* (1969); *The Health Crisis for Older New Yorkers* (1972); and *Dial a Ride: The New York City Experience* (1975), through the department. She also gave testimony and wrote papers for federal units concerned with the elderly. See, for instance, her 1970 report for the Administration on Aging, *Elderly Ridership and Reduced Transit Fares,* which reported that senior-citizen ridership increased 26 percent during the first ten months of the program. Her report on health care of older New Yorkers, which appeared in a 1973 U.S. Senate Special Committee on Aging report, *Barriers to Health Care for Older Americans,* inspired reforms.

In 1977, Cantor became director of research and faculty development at Fordham University's Brookdale Center on Aging. From 1978 to 1988, she served as Brookdale Professor of Gerontology in the Graduate School of Social Service, when she became a university professor and Brookdale Distinguished Scholar. Cantor has been associate director of the Third Age Center at Fordham since 1978, and she has directed the Brookdale Research Institute on Aging as well as Fordham's doctoral training program in research on aging since 1986.

Cantor's publications have focused on the diversity of informal and family support systems across ethnic, racial, and geographic lines. Her essay with M. Mayer, "Health and the Inner City Elderly," *The Gerontologist,* 16 (1976); her contribution, "Effect of Ethnicity on Life Styles of the Inner City Elderly," in *Community Planning for an Aging Society,* ed. M. Powell Lawton,* Robert Newcomer,* and Tom Byerts (New York: McGraw-Hill, 1976); as well as "Life Space and the Urban Elderly," in *The Later Years,* ed. Richard Kalish (Monterey, Calif.: Brooks/Cole, 1977) all attest to her perspective. Her subsequent writings increasingly focused on the health care and social service needs of minorities and women in the inner city and the resiliency (or lack thereof) in family networks. See, for instance, her "Strain among Caregivers," *The Gerontologist,* 23 (December 1983); "Social Care: Family and Community Support Systems," in the *Annals of the American Academy of Political and Social Science,* 503 (May 1989): 99–112; and "Families and Caregiving in an Aging Society," *Generations,* 18 (1992): 67–70. Through the Third Age Center, Cantor (with K. Brook and J. Mellor) wrote one of the first monographs on *Growing Old in Suburbia* (New York: Columbia University Press, 1986).

Cantor has served on many prestigious foundation, New York City, state, and federal advisory panels. She was a 1981 delegate to the White House Conference on Aging and representative to the World Assembly on Aging a year later. She has been active in the Gerontological Society since 1974, serving as president from 1983 to 1984. Her Kent Award lecture was published as "Family and Community: Changing Roles in an Aging Society," in *The Gerontologist,* 31 (June 1991): 337–46.

ANTON J. CARLSON. Anton Julius Carlson was born in Svarteborg, Sweden, in 1875. He became a naturalized U.S. citizen in 1896. Carlson earned his B.A. (1898) and A.M. (1899) from Augustana College, in Illinois, which honored him with an LL.D. in 1923. He earned his Ph.D. from Stanford in 1902. After spending the 1903–1904 academic year at the Carnegie Institution in Washington, D.C., Carlson joined the faculty of the University of Chicago. There he rose quickly through the ranks: In addition to chairing the Department of Physiology (1916–1940), he served as Frank P. Nixon Professor from 1929 until his retirement.

Carlson is primarily known for his research in the comparative physiology of the circulatory system. He studied the rate of conduction of nerve impulses and the nature of the heart beat. He did work on the physiology of the thyroid and parathyroid, the sensory nervous system, and the alimentary tract. He was interested in lymph formation and salivary secretion. Among his best-known books were *Machinery of the Body* (Chicago: University of Chicago Press, 5th edn., 1961); and *Control of Hunger in Health and Disease* (Chicago: University of Chicago Press, 1919). The latter book stressed the "biological, medical, and economic importance" of work in the fields of clinical medicine and comparative physiology.

As a member of the National Research Council and past president of the Federation of Societies for Experimental Biology and incoming head of the Union of American Biologists (1940–1943), Carlson was well connected with those who advised the Macy Foundation in studying senescence. His contribution to Edmund Vincent Cowdry's* *Problems of Ageing* (Baltimore: Williams and Wilkins, 1939), "The Thyroid, Pancreatic Islets, Parathyroids, Adrenals, Thymus and Pituitary," focused on how increases and decreases in hormone production affect the aging process. Loath to give functional interpretations to differences in structural findings, his essay underscored how little was truly known about endocrinological mechanisms. Accordingly, he paid particular attention to the instability of the "nervous machinery," but could not determine whether changes were due to hereditary or environmental influences.

A president of the American Association for the Advancement of Science and a founder and early president of the Gerontological Society, Carlson died in 1956.

FRANCIS G. CARO. Francis G. Caro was born in 1936. He graduated *summa cum laude* from Marquette University in 1958 and earned his Ph.D. in sociology from the University of Minnesota four years later. His interest in aging dates to 1963, when two of his mentors, Arnold Rose and Warren Peterson, enlisted him to assist with a project of the Midwest Council for Social Research on Aging while he was serving as a research associate at Community Studies Inc. in Kansas City. Then came a series of short appointments as a research associate with Community Progress Inc. in New Haven (1964–1965); as an assistant professor of sociology and anthropology at Marquette (1965–1967); and as assistant director for program evaluation in the Institute for Behavioral Science, University of Colorado (1967–1970). During this period he edited *Readings in Evaluation Research* (New York: Russell Sage Foundation, 1971), a widely used resource for the teaching of evaluation research.

In 1970, Caro was appointed an assistant professor of social research at Brandeis's Florence Heller Graduate School for Advanced Studies in Social Welfare and associate director of its Levinson Gerontological Policy Institute. For four years, he helped to shape what was then the nation's premier center for research on the political economy of aging. In 1974 Caro became director of research at the Community Service Society of New York, a position he held for fourteen years. Here, his work included research and demonstration projects concerned with community care of functionally disabled populations. See, for instance, F. G. Caro, *Family Care of the Elderly: Public Initiatives and Private Obligations* (Lexington, Mass.: Lexington Books, 1981), and F. G. Caro, *Quality Impact of Home Care for the Elderly* (New York: Haworth Press, 1988). He also held an adjunct appointment in the Department of Public Administration at Baruch College during most of this period.

In 1988, Caro became director of the Research Division and a professor of gerontology at the University of Massachusetts-Boston. There, he rejoined his eminent Brandeis mentor, Robert Morris,* with whom he had done some of his most creative work in the field of aging.

In the early 1970s, Morris and Caro developed the Personal Care Organization, a conceptual service-delivery model for provision of comprehensive home care services to the functionally disabled elderly that had a capitated framework calibrated according to the severity of functional disability. Although the academic formulation of Personal Care Organization remains buried in 1971 and 1973 Levinson Institute working papers, the working model itself was widely circulated, stimulating the development of several state-level case-managed home care demonstrations. The idea also influenced the development of several social health-maintenance-organization demonstrations in New England.

From this work, Caro sought to measure the immediate behavioral effects of home care for the elderly, especially those whose functional disabilities cause problems in coping with daily tasks. He introduced the concept of "quality of circumstances" to measure the immediate experiences and capacities of older people in such domains as shelter, household supplies, and eating. The focus of Caro's index parallels the content of Activities of Daily Living (ADL) and Instrumental Activities of Daily Living (IADL) scales. The construct has the potential for evaluation research not only in community-based long-term care programs but also in establishing a framework for performance-based home care services.

At the Gerontology Institute of the University of Massachusetts-Boston, Caro now focuses largely on evaluation research involving senior citizens. In addition to his interest in home care programs, he has been studying retraining and volunteer opportunities for older people.

NEENA LANE CHAPPELL. Neena Lane Chappell was born in Toronto in 1948. She earned her B.A. from Carleton University in Ottawa in 1970 and her M.A. from McMaster University in Hamilton, Ontario, in 1973. It was during the master's program that an attraction to gerontology arose from her interest in thanatology. Chappell considered the elderly people she knew to be wise. They possessed an abundance of life experiences (and a capacity to interpret those experiences) that she felt was heightened by their proximity to death. Thus, for her M.A. thesis she explored "future time perspective among the institutional elderly and a phenomenological interpretation of senility." Her Ph.D. thesis, under the direction of Frank Jones, focused on "work, commitment to work and self-identity among women." During her years at McMaster University, she had professors (none of whom were gerontologists) who reinforced and nurtured both her fascination with the promise of science and her intense interest in social issues.

Chappell's academic career to date has been spent largely at the University of Manitoba. It was here that she met individuals in the community who were committed to the value of scientific research for helping to solve problems associated with gerontology. While writing her dissertation, she was a research associate in the Department of Social and Preventive Medicine. In 1982, Chappell became founding director of the university's Centre on Aging. She became a full professor in the Department of Sociology and in the Department of Community Health Sciences six years later. In this capacity, she has worked closely with Betty Havens,* then Provincial Gerontologist and Assistant Deputy Minister of Continuing Care Programs in the Province of Manitoba. Chappell admires Havens for "her steadfast commitment to program improvement for seniors and for her belief in the value of scientific research to solve practical problems.'' The application of scientific thinking to relevant community questions has characterized Chappell's own endeavors in gerontology.

The publication dates and titles of Chappell's first three books—*Aging and Health Care: A Social Perspective* (Holt, Rineholt and Winston of Canada, 1986); *Aging and Ethnicity: Toward an Interface* (Toronto: Butterworths, 1987); and *Social Support and Aging in Canada* (1992)—suggest the energy with which she applies scientific rigor to a wide range of social issues. Whether dealing with the receipt of care from family and friends, the utilization of the formal health care system, or the interface between public and private networks, Chappell pays particular attention to differences in living arrangements, to variations in race and ethnicity, and to the significance of gender roles in giving and receiving care. Some of the findings challenge conventional gerontological wisdom. For instance, in ''Living Arrangements and Sources of Caregiving,'' which appeared in the *Journal of Gerontology: Social Sciences,* 46 (1991): S1–S8, Chappell and associates argued that living with someone (not necessarily one's spouse) was the most important predictor of informal care among the elderly. Some of her articles are state-of-the-art reviews, such as ''Home Care Research: What Does It Tell Us,'' *The Gerontologist,* 34 (1994): 116–20; and some focus on applied research with rigor, such as ''Gerontological Research in the '90's: Strengths, Weaknesses and Contributions to Policy,'' *Canadian Journal on Aging* (1995).

More than some gerontologists, Chappell has tried to combine scientific rigor with relevant and timely research questions. She understands that ''care'' is a broad concept, with dimensions that do not neatly conform to scholarly typologies. Much of her work thus probes the boundaries of self-care, informal care, and formal care. She recently moved to Canada's retirement community to be the first director of the Centre on Aging at the University of Victoria. That center is being built on the twin foundations of scientific excellence and applied community relevance.

YUNG-PING (BING) CHEN. Yung-Ping Chen was born in 1928. He earned his Ph.D. at the University of Washington in 1960. At the suggestion of his adviser, James K. Hall, a professor of public finance, Bing focused on Social Security financing for his dissertation. This project sparked his interest in gerontology.

Social Security financing has remained a primary interest. His introductory textbook, *Social Security in a Changing Society* (1980; rev. edn., 1983) is well respected, notably for the often unorthodox approach that Chen takes to esoteric topics. Indeed, Chen has often played an important role in policy debates by being a maverick. In 1976, when lawmakers and the public decried the ''burden'' of rising Social Security costs, Chen wrote a paper on ''Total Dependency Burden and Social Security Solvency,'' published by the New York-based Industrial Relations Research Association, in which he argued that experts must factor in young-age dependency along with old-age dependency in calculating societal costs and benefits. Viewed this way, the "crisis" was less dire than pundits declared: The total dependency ratio of young and old vis-à-vis the working population had peaked in the 1960s and would not attain those levels for the foreseeable future. Five years later, as the debate over Social Security benefits escalated, Chen was the first to call attention to "the growth of fringe benefits" in assessing the solvency of Social Security in a November 1981 article in the *Monthly Labor Review.* This became a key to the taxation of pension benefits for higher-income recipients under the 1983 Social Security Amendments.

Chen's work on home-equity conversion further illustrates one way that technical analyses can contribute practical solutions to some of the problems that elderly Americans face. To resolve the dilemma of aged men and women who are income-poor and house-rich, Chen made the case for a voluntary conversion of home equity into annuity income, based on the total income concept (that is, current income plus annuitized income from net worth including home equity). Chen first presented the idea at the University of Wisconsin in 1963 in "Property Tax Burden on Aged Homeowners and Income Potential of Their Houses." With support from the U.S. Department of Housing and Urban Development, Chen refined the idea, elaborating his full argument in his *Unlocking Home Equity for the Elderly* (Cambridge, Mass.: Ballinger, 1980). Dr. Robert N. Butler,* director of the National Institute on Aging, praised the notion, which has been adopted in some regions of the country.

Chen has been working on other aspects of the economic status of the aged since 1963, when he published an article on the elderly's tax burdens. He served as a technical consultant to the 1971 and 1981 White House Conferences on Aging. After serving as director of research at the Boettiger Institute in Bryn Mawr, Pennsylvania, Chen became in 1988 the first Frank J. Manning Eminent Scholar's Chair in Gerontology at the University of Massachusetts-Boston. Lately, to deal with the health care crisis, Chen has been suggesting a trade in which older people would exchange some pension in return for basic long-term care protection. He first presented this idea to the Advisory Council on Social Security in 1990.

AUSTIN B. CHINN. Austin B. Chinn, born in 1908, earned his M.D. from the University School of Medicine. He moved to Cleveland in 1932 to train at University Hospital. After serving in the military during World War II, he returned to Cleveland and joined the medical faculty at Western Reserve University. He was a faculty member for sixteen years, and was eventually appointed associate dean.

In 1952, Chinn became Medical Director of the Benjamin Rose Hospital. There he initiated a program in which a multidisciplinary staff of physicians and allied health professionals developed comprehensive treatment and rehabilitation of chronic diseases of the aged. Within five years a research program, which included basic as well as clinical research, was started.

In 1962 he became the first chief of the Gerontology Branch of the Division of Chronic Services of the U.S. Public Health Service. There Chinn focused on developing a curriculum in applied gerontology which eventually resulted in a standard geriatric textbook, *Clinical Aspects of Aging*.

Dr. Chinn moved to Los Angeles in 1967 as professor of medicine and director of the Rehabilitation Research and Training Center of Southern California. He died in 1989.

DAVID A. CHIRIBOGA. Born in Boston in 1941, David A. Chiriboga received his B.A. from Boston University in 1964. There, Dr. Freda Rebelsky in the Department of Psychology encouraged him to delve into the literature on gerontology. Chiriboga was particularly struck by an article by Robert N. Butler,* then a psychiatrist practicing in Washington, D.C., which noted that the most mentally healthy older people self-identified as being middle-aged rather than aged. He was also intrigued by the research by Tuckerman and Lorge, which demonstrated that older people could learn a new language just as well as younger college students. Early on, Chiriboga became interested in what promoted and impeded adult development in later years.

Chiriboga did his graduate studies under the Committee on Human Development at the University of Chicago, where he worked principally under Bernice L. Neugarten.* In 1965, he conducted content analyses of in-depth transcribed protocols of the Middle Adult Life Project and trial research on an inquiry into self-actualization among middle-aged males. For three years Chiriboga worked closely with Neugarten and Robert Havighurst* (both of whom became his role models) on their Cross-National Project. From 1968 to 1972, he worked on his dissertation, "The Nature and Effects of Relocation in the Aged," in which he first began to explore how the aged adapted and survived under conditions of stress, a topic that still dominates much of his scholarly interest.

In 1969, Chiriboga moved to the University of California, San Francisco, to work with Marjorie Fiske (Lowenthal),* who was to become one of his principal mentors and collaborators, on collecting and analyzing data for "Transitional Stages of the Adult Lifespan." Among the principal works produced by this partnership, which lasted from 1969 to 1984, were *Four Stages of Life* (San Francisco: Jossey-Bass, 1975); and *Change and Continuity in Adult Life* (San Francisco: Jossey-Bass, 1990). The contribution that has given Chiriboga the greatest satisfaction has been his attempts to apply lifespan approaches to the study of stress. He has tried to provide more stringent criteria for defining stressors and for understanding mediating factors and stress responses at the micro-, mezzo-, and macro-levels. Stressors, in his view, range from broad-scale social changes and transitions, which are themselves a "chaining of events and experiences," to life events, chronic conditions, and occasional hassles. The exposure to various forms of stress and reaction to stressors both seem to vary with age; some increase, while others decrease in importance. To probe the way differences in response are related to subjects' general condition and specific

circumstances, Chiriboga lately has been assessing the incidence and consequences of stress exposure for younger and older men and women who have
been divorced. See his *Divorce: Crisis, Challenge or Relief?* (New York: New
York University Press, 1992).

In the mid-1980s, Chiriboga collaborated on several studies with Philip G.
Weiler, M.D. Since 1986, Chiriboga has been a senior member of the School
of Allied Health Sciences at the University of Texas Medical Branch, Galveston.
With colleague Kyriakos Markides,* he currently is examining intergenerational
relationships among Mexican-Americans, and examining stress and its consequences in a large (N = 3050) epidemiological study of elderly Mexican-
Americans.

VICTOR G. CICIRELLI. After graduating from Notre Dame (B.S., 1947), Victor Cicirelli earned two doctoral degrees—one in educational psychology at the
University of Michigan (1964) and the second in developmental psychology at
Michigan State University (1971). His interest in aging, however, evolved only
gradually. Until the mid-1970s, Cicirelli worked primarily in the area of child
development psychology. As he became increasingly interested in a lifespan
developmental approach, he began to include some adult and elderly subjects
in his studies. In the 1980s, he began to publish in gerontology-related journals,
though he suspects that "only now [1992] am I reaching the point where I can
make some useful syntheses. I feel that my real contributions to the field lie
ahead of me."

Thus far, Cicirelli's contributions to gerontology fall into two areas. First, he
has studied caregiving of dependent elderly parents by adult children. Cicirelli
has advanced theory-building in this domain by extending the conceptual parameters of "attachment theory" into the adult portion of the lifespan to account
for the sustained helping behavior of adult children who care for dependent
elderly parents. As part of this effort, Cicirelli enlarged the notion of symbolic
attachment as a means of transcending the time and space separations that often
characterize parent-child links in families in the latter stages of their development. He also hypothesized that a complementary system of protective behavior
across generations often arises in an effort to preserve the continued existence
of the attached figure. See Cicirelli's article, "Adult Children's Attachment and
Helping Behavior to Elderly Parents" in the *Journal of Marriage and the Family,* 45 (1983): 815–22; and his essays, "Attachment Theory in Old Age," in
Parent-Child Relations across the Life Span, eds. K. Pillemer and K. McCartney
(Hillsdale, N.J.: Erlbaum, 1991), 25–42; "Feelings of Attachment to Siblings
and Well-Being in Later Life," *Psychology and Aging,* 4 (1989): 211–16; "Attachment and Obligation as Daughters' Motives for Caregiving Behavior and
Subsequent Effect on Subjective Burden," *Psychology and Aging,* 8 (1993):
144–55; and "A Measure of Caregiving Daughters' Attachment to Elderly
Mothers," *Journal of Family Psychology,* in press.

Cicirelli's second major research interest has focused on sibling relationships in adulthood and old age. Once again, he has elaborated ideas from attachment theory to study sibling influence on well-being, sibling gender differences in helping and caregiving behaviors, and filial anxiety related to anticipated caregiving. See his *Sibling Relationships Across the Life Span* (New York: Plenum Publishing, in press); "The Longest Bond: The Sibling Life Cycle," in *Handbook of Developmental Psychology and Psychopathology*, 2nd edn. (New York: Wiley and Sons), 44–59; "Sibling Relationships in Middle and Old Age," in *Sibling Relationships: Their Causes and Consequences* (Norwood, N.J.: Ablex Publishing, in press).

Cicirelli's more recent work has focused on the relationship between ethical beliefs about autonomy and paternalism on the one hand and dyadic family caregiving decision-making on the other. See his *Family Caregiving: Autonomous and Paternalistic Decision Making* (Beverly Hills, Calif.: Sage, 1991); and "Relationship of Personal-Social Variables to Belief in Paternalism in Parent Caregiving Situations," *Psychology and Aging*, 8 (1990): 458–66. Cicirelli has also received a grant from the AARP Andrus Foundation to begin studying the relationship of personality factors to end-of-life decisions in the elderly.

Cicirelli is a member of the Department of Psychological Sciences at Purdue University.

PHILLIP G. CLARK. Phillip G. Clark received a doctor of science degree from Harvard University in 1979. It was there, while an instructor at the School of Public Health, that he was tapped by the head of the university's Division on Aging, Dr. John W. Rowe,* to join a group interested in gerontology and geriatrics.

Since then Clark has been primarily concerned with health care policy and the education of health care workers. He has explored the role that values and ethical principles play in a variety of gerontological contexts, particularly in the area of health care policy. Clark argues that "factual and historical factors are emphasized" without a clear exploration of the principles and values that underlie existing policies and programs. See, for instance, P.G. Clark, "Ethical Dimensions of Quality of Life in Aging: Autonomy vs. Collectivism in the U.S. and Canada," *The Gerontologist*, 31 (1991): 631–39.

Clark has also developed a multidimensional conceptual framework for describing the development of health care teams. This framework is used to describe the way participants evolve as they become "team players" providing service and education. In this area Clark has written with Donald L. Spence and J.L. Sheehan. See, for example P.G. Clark, Donald L. Spence and J.L. Sheehan, "Challenges and Barriers to Interdisciplinary Gerontological Team Training in the Academic Setting," *Gerontology and Geriatrics Education*, 7 (1987): 93–110; and more recently, see P.G. Clark, Donald L. Spence and J.L. Sheehan, "Social, Professional, and Educational Values on the Interdisciplinary Team," *Educational Gerontology*, 20 (1994): 35–51.

In addition, Clark has studied efforts to empower the elderly in the health

82   VIVIAN CLAYTON

care setting. Following his work on values and ethics, he has explored the meaning of empowerment in a gerontological setting. Relevant references include
"The Philosophical Foundation of Empowerment: Implications for Geriatric
Health Care Programs and Practice," *Journal of Aging and Health,* 1 (1989):
267–85; and "Autonomy, Personal Empowerment, and Quality of Life in Long-
term Care," *Journal of Applied Gerontology,* 7 (1988): 279–97.

Clark is currently a professor at the University of Rhode Island, Kingston,
where he directs the Program in Gerontology.

VIVIAN CLAYTON. Vivian Clayton earned her Ph.D. in psychology at the
University of Southern California in 1976. James E. Birren* first attracted her
to the field of gerontology. Birren and K. Warner Schaie* were her primary
teachers and mentors during graduate school. Her primary collaborators to date
have been Birren and Paul B. Baltes.*

Clayton was one of the first researchers on aging to recognize the importance
of "wisdom" as a construct worthy of exploration for gerontology. In 1975,
she presented a paper at the Gerontological Society in which she analyzed commonalities among 165 words she had collected from descriptions of wise people.
She found very few common ties. With Birren, she staked her claim to this area
with "The Development of Wisdom Across the Lifespan: A Re-examination of
an Ancient Topic," in *Life Span Development and Behavior,* eds. Paul B. Baltes
and Orville Brim (New York: Academic Press, 1980), 103–35. On her own,
Clayton elaborated the parameters of a multidimensional model that empirically
defined wisdom in "Wisdom And Intelligence: The Nature and Function of
Knowledge in Later Years," *International Journal of Aging and Human Development,* 15 (1982): 315–20. There, she differentiated "intelligence," which
she defined as the cognitive ability to conceptualize ideas and to think both
logically and abstractly, from wisdom, which she claimed is "the ability that
enables the individual to grasp human nature, which operates on the principles
of contradiction, paradox, and change." Building on ideas from Jean Piaget,
Erik Erikson, and Irene M. Hulicka,* Clayton not only emphasized the differences between expressions of propositional and paradoxical logic, but also stipulated their divergent relationship to time. Social intelligence gathered today is
time-bound; true wisdom, in contrast, is timeless. Wisdom's domain is "human
nature," which included social, interpersonal, and intrapersonal problems.

Currently, Clayton is in private practice in a large geriatric multidisciplinary
medical practice in Walnut Creek, California. She is no longer doing active
research on the subject of wisdom.

RODNEY M. COE. Rodney M. Coe is a central figure among the second generation of researchers on aging, whose names and careers are linked with Washington University and professional gerontology's St. Louis roots. Coe received
his Ph.D. in sociology at Washington University in 1962. He studied primarily
under Albert Wessen and Robert W. Kleemeier,* from whom he gained appre-

ciation for the impact of the environment on the health of the elderly. Harry Rosen, the first executive director of the Gerontological Society, also sparked Coe's interest in this field of inquiry. Two eminent teachers, Erving Goffman and Jules Henry, offered training in ethnomethodology and anthropology, which has served Coe well in his studies and engagement in health care.

Over the course of his career, Coe has produced a series of studies dealing with patterns of utilization of health services by the elderly and the reciprocal practice patterns of health professionals, notably physicians. See, for instance, the books Coe wrote with Henry P. Brehm, *Preventive Health Care for Adults: A Study of Medical Practice* (New Haven: College and University Press, 1973); and *Medical Care for the Aged: From Social Problem to Federal Program* (New York: Praeger, 1980). Coe has written several studies on doctor-elderly patient communications in part to test theories of dyadic and triadic relationships. With Fredric Wolinksy, among others, he also has developed and validated a nutritional risk index for predicting nutrition-related disabilities in older people.

Coe's greatest contribution to gerontology and geriatrics, however, has been to sustain institutions, not generate new theories. As the first wave of giants that made Washington University a prime research center on aging in the 1940s and 1950s (figures such as Edmund V. Cowdry,* Robert Kleemeier, and Albert Lansing) moved on or died, it fell to people like Coe to foster collaborative ties among the remaining strengths in the community and to recruit others to fill in the gaps. During a shake-up in Washington's Sociology Department in 1970, Coe moved across town to St. Louis University School of Medicine. As chairman of the Interdepartmental Committee on Gerontology and Geriatrics and of the Department of Community and Family Medicine, Coe assiduously nurtured a coalition of researchers, practitioners, and educators. In the process, he came to appreciate the contributions that many academic disciplines and professional schools can make to enhancing the well-being of the elderly. See R. D. T. Cape, R. M. Coe, and I. Rossman, eds., *Fundamentals of Geriatric Medicine* (New York: Raven Press, 1983), a volume initially begun as a project under the aegis of the Gerontological Society of America. More recently, Coe and his university colleagues have published a series of books that combine basic science, clinical studies, and behavioral science research on aspects of aging such as nutritional intervention (1984), cancer (1989), endocrine function (1990), quality and cost-effectiveness of care (1991), memory function (1992), musculoskeletal disorders (1993), immune function (1994), and continuous quality improvement in geriatrics (1995).

GENE D. COHEN. Gene D. Cohen received his B.A. from Harvard College in 1966, earning high honors in general studies. He completed his M.D. at the Georgetown University School of Medicine in 1970. He received a certificate in community psychiatry from the Washington School of Psychiatry in 1973. Eight years later, Cohen earned a Ph.D. from the Union Institute, where he designed an independent doctoral program focused on the interface of physical and mental health in geriatrics. Cohen's initial interest in aging dates to 1961, when, as a high school junior, he won first prize in the MIT/Commonwealth of Massachusetts State Fair with a project on aging and oceanography. (Cohen examined the relationship between the age and growth of fish and the health of their ecology.) A decade later, during his psychiatry residency at Georgetown, he found that he enjoyed working in a senior citizens building. A review of the literature on mental health and aging seemed so sparse that Cohen was convinced that he could blaze a new field of inquiry, taking advantage of his multidisciplinary interests.

Since 1971, Cohen has been conducting a community-based descriptive study of older adults who reside in their own homes. In his first major longitudinal study, building on principles of milieu therapy, Cohen studied approximately 300 adults between the ages of sixty and 100 who lived in a Housing and Urban Development senior citizens building. A quarter of this group developed mental disorders. In 1983, he launched a second project, focusing on fifty mentally healthy adults between the ages of sixty-five and 103. Cohen obtained detailed psychological, medical, and social histories of his subjects for a study designed to generate hypotheses as to what contributes to the maintenance and promotion of mental health in later life. From 1975 to 1990, Cohen was primary investigator in a descriptive research study of the manifestation, clinical course, and response to treatment of mental disorders among elderly nursing home residents.

Cohen's investigations have enabled him to advance scientists' understanding of the bio-psycho-social gestalt, especially mental health and physical health interactions at advanced ages. Cohen developed his holistic thesis, including his assertion that biography can be as important as biology in treating older patents with dementia, in *The Brain in Human Aging* (New York: Springer, 1988). Cohen's broad focus also led him to conclude that research on aging offers insights not only into the characteristics of older adults, but provides a new perspective on "development and disorder independent of age." Hence, he believes, well-grounded gerontologic research contributes to an understanding of the human condition in general, across the life cycle. See his "Research on Aging: A Piece of the Puzzle," *The Gerontologist,* 19 (1979): 503–508.

In addition to conducting his own research, Cohen has worked closely with two of his role models, Robert N. Butler* and T. Franklin Williams, in making research on aging a high priority in the National Institutes of Health. From 1975 to 1988, he served as the first chief of the center on aging in the National Institute of Mental Health. In this capacity, Cohen gained national and international visibility for developing a major program in research and training on mental health and aging. He became executive secretary of the Federal Advisory Panel on Alzheimer's Disease in 1986. Cohen served on the initial sub-board on geriatric psychiatry for the American Board of Psychiatry and Neurology. He became deputy director of the National Institute on Aging in 1988 and served as acting director from 1991 to 1993. Cohen left the federal government in 1994.

Cohen took a leadership role in disseminating basic research on mental health and aging. He became founding editor-in-chief of the official journal of the International Psychogeriatric Association in 1989. Four years later, he became founding editor of the *American Journal of Geriatric Psychiatry*. His sense of the "state of the field" can be traced in an early contribution, "Prospects for Mental Health and Aging," in *Handbook of Mental Health and Aging*, eds. J. E. Birren* and R. B. Sloane (Englewood Cliffs, N.J.: Prentice-Hall, 1980); and, more recently, "The Future of Mental Health and Aging," in *Handbook of Mental Health and Aging*, 2nd edn., eds. J. E. Birren, R. B. Sloane, and G. D. Cohen (New York: Academic Press, 1992).

WILBUR J. COHEN. Wilbur Joseph Cohen was born in Milwaukee in 1913. After earning his Ph.B. from the University of Wisconsin in 1934, he went to Washington to work with one of his teachers, Edwin Witte, on the Committee on Economic Security. After Franklin Delano Roosevelt signed the landmark legislation, Cohen joined the staff of the Social Security Administration. He rose through the ranks, serving as director of the system's Division of Research and Statistics from 1953 to 1956. Intending to become an historian rather than a government bureaucrat, Cohen early on showed an academic's penchant for disseminating knowledge. With William Haber, he compiled two books, *Readings in Social Security* (Champlain, Il.: R. D. Irwin, 1948); and *Social Security: Programs, Problems, and Policies* (Champlain, Il.: R. D. Irwin, 1960). He also wrote *Retirement under Social Security* (Berkeley: University of California Press, 1957), which remains one of the most concise historical documents of this fundamental late-life institution.

In 1956, Cohen joined the faculty of the University of Michigan, with which he would maintain some affiliation for nearly the rest of his life. During his tenure as a professor in the School of Social Work, he collaborated with James N. Morgan,* M. H. David, and H. E. Brazer in compiling statistics for *Income and Wealth in the United States* (New York: McGraw-Hill, 1962). The interpretation of poverty in this volume gave weight to the gripping images set forth in Michael Harrington's *The Other America* (New York: Penguin, 1963).

When John F. Kennedy was elected, Cohen returned to Washington to be assistant secretary of the Department of Health, Education, and Welfare (HEW). He assumed greater and greater responsibility during the Johnson administration, and served as secretary of HEW during Lyndon Johnson's last year in office. Cohen was a key, arguably the major, government advocate for the elderly during the Great Society. Historians consider him the architect of the 1965 Medicare legislation. He was also instrumental in securing the Older Americans Act (1965).

In 1969, Cohen went back to Ann Arbor. There, for the next nine years, he served as the dean of the School of Education of the University of Michigan. Cohen continued to write about a variety of social welfare issues. His debate with Milton Friedman was published as *Social Security: Universal or Selective?* in 1972. Five years later, he issued *Demographic Dynamics in America* with

Princeton demographer Charles Westhoff. Cohen also headed the board of over-seers for the university's Institute of Gerontology from 1969 to 1976, recruiting Harold R. Johnson* to be its director. In 1980, he was appointed Sid W. Richardson Professor at the LBJ School of Public Affairs at the University of Texas.

Cohen never really retired. He was active in the American Public Welfare Association in the 1970s, and served on other political and civic boards. In 1977, alarmed by the Carter administration's actions to cut back the rate of growth of entitlements, Cohen joined with his old friend Arthur M. Flemming* in establishing Save Our Security (SOS). The pair of former HEW secretaries used this organization to advocate constructive reforms; both took solace in the fact that the 1983 amendments basically affirmed the fundamental significance of Social Security in American life.

Wilbur J. Cohen died in 1987 while on a speaking tour in Korea.

ALFRED E. COHN. Alfred Einstein Cohn was born in New York City in 1879. Educated at Columbia University (B.A., 1900; M.D., 1904), he did postgraduate studies in Freiburg, Vienna, and London after serving as an intern at Mt. Sinai Hospital (1904–1907). Cohn served as a fellow in pathology at Columbia's College of Physicians and Surgeons (1909–1911) before joining the research faculty of the Rockefeller Institute, where he spent the rest of his career.

Cohn was a cardiologist and internist, best known for his research on the physiology and pharmacology of the heart and circulation. He advised the Veterans Administration and was a member of the board of the Lasker Foundation (1928–1939). His interdisciplinary predilections were evident in his *Medicine, Science, and Art: Studies in Interrelations* (University of Chicago Press, 1931). "The chief reason for writing [these essays] was to make clear to myself the views and opinions and systematic relations of those bits of the world," he wrote.

Cohn merits inclusion in this volume because of his contribution, "Cardiovascular System and Blood," in *Problems of Ageing,* ed. Edmund Vincent Cowdry* (Baltimore: Williams and Wilkins, 1939). There, he addressed the issue of whether aging is a disease, and if not, what constitutes normal or abnormal, usual or atypical, or pathological manifestations. "Normal is not a measurement nor a conception which, like the decalogue, is something given," he said, yet because conceptions of what is "normal" and what is "growth" are essential to any discussion of aging, Cohn found it difficult to separate ailments associated with growth from those occasioned by disease. Nonetheless, on the basis of common sense and his own studies of the heart and of blood, Cohn took the "tentative position" that aging as a normal process of growth does occur in the cardiovascular system.

During World War II, Cohn became very interested in Jewish refugees. After the war he played an active role on the Council of Foreign Affairs. Cohn died in 1957.

THOMAS R. COLE. Thomas R. Cole was born in 1949. He received his B.A. from Yale University in 1975 and his Ph.D. in cultural history from the University of Rochester in 1981, where he studied under Christopher Lasch. The influence of Lasch on Cole's early career cannot be overstated. At a time in which the so-called "new social history" was regnant in leading graduate centers, Cole eschewed quantitative analyses and heavy borrowing from sociological theory. Instead, he followed Lasch's lead and honed his own critical acumen. Like his mentor, Cole considered himself a radical. A member of the New Left, Cole was attracted to the subject of the elderly because he felt that most senior citizens were ignored and their needs were discounted. In studying the origins of ageism and their current needs, he sought to debunk conventional wisdom. Thus, when Cole claims that his entry into the field was greatly influenced by reading W. Andrew Achenbaum's *Old Age in the New Land* (Baltimore: Johns Hopkins University Press, 1978) and *Aging and the Elderly: Humanistic Perspectives in Gerontology,* a collection edited by David Van Tassel, Kathleen Woodward, and Stuart Spicker (Atlantic Highlands, N.J.: Humanities Press, 1978), he does not necessarily mean to be complimentary. Initially, he felt that the contents of both works were quite wrong-headed and ripe for revision.

Upon completing his Ph.D., Cole spent two years on a post doctoral fellowship at Boys Town, Nebraska. He then moved to the newly established Institute for the Humanities at the University of Texas Medical Branch in Galveston. Here, Cole has had the privilege of working with top-flight students of the humanities (including experts in theology, literary studies, and art criticism) as well as having day-to-day interactions with bench scientists and clinicians. Rather than quickly publish his dissertation in order to gain tenure, as historians are wont to do, Cole gambled. During the 1980s, he published a series of incisive essays that probed the cultural history of aging, which appears in the Hastings Center *Report,* in the American Society of Aging's *Generations,* and in an early issue of *Tikkun,* a Jewish intellectual review. He also edited a collection, *What Does It Mean to Grow Old? Reflections from the Humanities* (Durham, N.C.: Duke University Press, 1986) with his colleague Sally Gadow and, with support from the Gerontological Society of America, compiled one of the first annotated bibliographies of recent literature on aging done by experts in the humanities and interpretive sciences. His *Handbook of Aging and the Humanities* (New York: Springer, 1992), co-edited with David Van Tassel and Robert Kastenbaum,* two of his role models, is at once a balanced summary of work in the area and a signal that this subfield has come of age.

In 1992, Cole published *The Journey of Life: A Cultural History of Aging in America* (New York: Cambridge University Press), which was nominated for a Pulitzer Prize. Though less iconoclastic than his mentor's essay on aging in C. Lasch, *The Culture of Narcissism* (New York: Norton, 1979), Cole's monograph had a Lasch-like quality as it excoriated the twentieth-century medicalization and bureaucratization of aging. Weaving together images and themes from

Scripture and classical texts, *The Journey of Life* resonated with a meditative, almost spiritual tone as it reflected on existential issues surrounding the finitude of life and the meaning of death. Along with recent work by Carole Haber* and Brian Gratton,* whose *Old Age and the Search for Security: An American Social History* (Bloomington, Ind.: Indiana University Press, 1994) reflects the latest directions in a social-historical orientation, Cole's work took the history of aging into a more self-consciously self-reflexive mode of inquiry.

In the 1990s, Cole's critique of the culture of aging has been tempered by an awareness of existential and spiritual questions. His anthology, *The Oxford Book of Aging* (New York, 1994), co-edited with Mary Winkler, explores these issues through selections from world literature.

It is not surprising that Cole has become, along with his friends W. Andrew Achenbaum and Harry R. Moody,* a major proponent of "critical" gerontology. Cole urges scientists and practitioners to probe the "meanings" of what they do and how they think about aging. He demands an attentiveness to defining problems and refining methods no less rigorous than that expected in laboratories, yet he is ever mindful of the integrity of humanistic inquiry.

ALEX COMFORT. Alex Comfort is probably best known in the United States as the author of the best-selling *The Joy of Sex* (New York: Simon and Schuster, 1972) and the series of spin-offs that it has inspired. British citizens also recognize him as the author of eighteen works of fiction. He has added lyrics to Pete Seeger's songs, and he served as a staff member of the Center for the Study of Democratic Institutions in Santa Barbara. But Comfort has also done significant research in bio-gerontology to warrant inclusion in this volume.

Born in 1920 north of London, England, Comfort held a scholarship at Highgate School before entering Trinity College, Cambridge, at eighteen with an intent to study the classics. He soon switched to medicine. He won First Class honors in the National Science Tripos in 1940 and a Second Class in the pathology examinations a year later. A conscientious objector during the war, he was temporarily blacklisted for his attacks on Allied policies. During this period he published novels and poetry, but also kept on course with his scientific ambitions. After receiving his bachelor of medicine (1943) and bachelor of surgery (1944) degrees from Cambridge, he earned a diploma in child health from London Hospital. While serving as a resident, he published a textbook, *First Year Physiological Techniques* (London: Staples Press, 1948). In 1949, he earned a Ph.D. in biochemistry for his dissertation on the pigmentation of mollusca.

After serving two years as lecturer in physiology at the London Hospital Medical College, Comfort in 1951 joined the Department of Zoology at London's University College as a Nuffield Research Fellow in gerontology. He held the position for fourteen years, when he became head of the London Medical Research Council Group on Aging. An editor of *Experimental Gerontology* in 1965, he added the title of research director in 1972. In his capacity as a Nuffield Fellow, Comfort began studying the aging process of animals with short lifespans. Guppies, he hypothesized, could grow indefinitely, with appropriate caloric restrictions. In 1961, he summarized the state of theories of aging in an article in the *Scientific American*. Comfort received the prestigious Karger Prize for his work in gerontology in 1969. While still writing plays and novels, Comfort also wrote several books based on his understanding of gerontology. *The Process of Ageing* (New York: New American Library, 1964) and *Biology of Senescence* (New York: Academic, 1972) represented a fuller elaboration of his critique of the field. In 1976, Comfort published *A Good Age* (New York: Simon and Schuster, 1976), which was designed as a gerontologic analog to his paean to healthy attitudes toward sex and sexuality.

Comfort came to the United States in 1972. A year earlier, he wrote for a UNESCO report on aging that American scientists were likely to devise ways to control cancer and heart disease. He also felt that gerontology flourished in this country because most Americans considered old age "an intolerable state, which we are obliged to prevent if possible." Beginning in 1972, Comfort lent his support for the creation of the National Institute on Aging. Ever the reformer, Comfort excoriated the heavy-handed way that U.S. physicians studied diminished mental capacities in late life; see "Non-Threatening Mental Testing of the Elderly," *Journal of the American Geriatrics Society,* 26 (1978): 261–62. In the 1980s, Comfort wrote about the massive loss of neurons that causes progressive dementia in articles such as "Alzheimer's Disease or 'Alzheimerism'?" in *Psychiatric Annals,* 14 (1984): 130–32.

Now retired, Comfort retains an active, though armchair, interest in gerontology.

JOHN M. CORNMAN. Jack M. Cornman, born in suburban Philadelphia, earned his B.A. in English from Dartmouth College in 1955. Beginning his career in the newspaper business, Cornman served as city editor of the (West Chester, Pennsylvania) *Daily Local News.* In 1964, he moved to Washington, D.C., to serve as a congressional fellow under the auspices of the American Political Science Association. From 1965 to 1969, he served as press secretary and then chief legislative assistant to Senator E. L. Hartlett (D-Alaska). For the next six years Cornman served as special assistant and then director of communications for Senator Philip A. Hart (D-Michigan). In addition to overseeing all press relations and policy coordination, he also had staff responsibility for appropriations, arms control, and housing.

After Hart's death, Cornman once again refocused his skills, this time to manage organizations interested in applying theories and ideas to practical policies and programs. In 1975, he became executive director, and then president, of the National Rural Center, a private non-profit corporation engaged in policy research and analysis, information dissemination, and advocacy on rural economic development and service delivery issues. Eight years later, Cornman became executive director of the Gerontological Society of America (GSA). Since 1991, he has served as executive director of the American Anthropological Association, the world's largest organization devoted to scholarly and applied anthropology.

During his tenure at the Gerontological Society, Cornman proved adept at designing and managing multidisciplinary program organizations, fund-raising, and inviting politicians, corporate leaders, and other interested groups to interact with researchers on aging. He insisted that the officers and staff of GSA engage in long-range planning. And he became the first executive director to initiate and participate actively in thinking through issues associated with societal aging.

For instance, with Eric R. Kingson* and Barbara S. Hirshorn, Cornman published *Ties That Bind: The Interdependence of Generations* (Cabin John, Md.: Seven Locks Press, 1986). This volume attempted to rebut claims by organizations such as Americans for Generational Equity that the demands of older members of society undermined the interests of younger men and women. Far from accepting the notion that Social Security's recent financial woes presaged imminent generational warfare, Cornman and his colleagues argued that the nation's largest domestic program was secure in large measure because people of all ages believed in its value and trusted its basic mechanisms. In "Higher Education and Aging Communities: Natural Allies in a Changing World," a major paper in a project that he designed and circulated as *Higher Education and an Aging Society* (Washington, D.C.: Gerontological Society of America, 1989), Cornman stressed the importance of bridging concerns rather than protecting turf.

EDMUND VINCENT COWDRY. Born in MacLeod, Canada, in 1888, Edmund Vincent Cowdry received his B.A. from the University of Toronto in 1909. He earned a Ph.D. from the University of Chicago in 1913, where he remained for another four years in the Department of Anatomy. Cowdry served as an associate professor in anatomy at Johns Hopkins University in 1917, and then became a professor of anatomy at China's Peking Union Medical College. From 1921 to 1927 he was affiliated with the Rockefeller Institute. Cowdry spent most of his career at Washington University, St. Louis, becoming a professor of cytology in 1928, a professor of anatomy in 1941, and professor emeritus in 1961. During his tenure at Washington, he served as a Distinguished Service Professor of the Institution Divi Thomae in Cincinnati, director of St. Louis's Barnard Free Skin and Cancer Hospital (1936–1948) and Washington University's Wernse Research Laboratory (1950–1960).

A grant from the Josiah Macy Foundation enabled Cowdry to assess the state of research on *Arteriosclerosis* (New York: Macmillan, 1933) and led to subsequent Macy funding (in connection with the Union of American Biological Societies, which Cowdry chaired) for a conference at Woods Hole, Massachusetts, in which two dozen bio-medical researchers and social scientists discussed ways to launch gerontology as a field of scientific inquiry. The conference proceedings that Cowdry edited, *Problems of Ageing* (Baltimore: Williams and Wilkins, 1939), remains a classic. Cowdry revised the volume in 1942; A. I.

Lansing issued a third edition of Cowdry's *Problems of Ageing* a decade later. With support from Washington University, the Macy and Forest Park foundations, and the U.S. Public Health Service, Cowdry slowly created organizational networks that would facilitate the exchange of scientific ideas. He was listing himself as chairman of the Research Club on Ageing (American Division) in the mid-1940s. This club evolved into the Gerontological Society (of America), founded in 1945. Cowdry served as president of the Society in 1953, and led the U.S. delegation to the International Association of Gerontology meetings in London in 1954.

Besides promoting research on aging in scientific circles, Cowdry tried to nurture support within the federal community. He was a consultant on gerontology for the U.S. Public Health Service (1938–1946), chaired the VA's advisory committee on aging (1956–1957), and worked with RAND (1961–1964). Cowdry's pioneering work in gerontology was honored with the Bobst Prize (1954) and a medal from the Chinese Ministry of Education (1959). Cowdry the cytologist also worked assiduously in cancer research, integrating his two areas of interest. As he noted in his own contribution to *Problems of Ageing,* "The systematic microscopic investigation of the processes of ageing has barely been commenced. Many techniques are available, yet have not been applied. Cooperation between cytologists and biochemists is essential." For gerontology to live up to its multidisciplinary promise, Cowdry believed, scientists had to master at least two fields of inquiry. Cowdry practiced what he preached.

For more on Cowdry, see Joseph T. Freeman, "Edmund Vincent Cowdry, Creative Gerontologist: Memoir and Autobiographical Notes," *The Gerontologist,* 24 (December 1984): 641–45.

FRANCOISE CRIBIER. Although this volume focuses almost exclusively on North American gerontologists, it does include a few European scholars who have contributed intellectually and otherwise to facilitating research on aging on this side of the Atlantic. French scientists and *literati* have been measuring and pondering the meanings and experiences of aging for centuries, so it can hardly be said, as it can be said of her American counterparts, that Francoise Cribier is a "gerontological pioneer" in her country. Nonetheless, Cribier is one of France's most distinguished social scientists interested in gerontological issues, and she has helped U.S. and Canadian scholars become acquainted with kindred spirits on the continent.

Cribier was educated at the University of Paris, where she studied history, geography, and anthropology; that she could never choose among them attests to her crossdisciplinary predilections. She completed her *these d'Etat,* a more heroic enterprise than the U.S. Ph.D., in 1969; her research focused on places that people tended to go for their month-long vacations between 1950 and 1960, and how they spent their time. Cribier started working in the aging field in 1972, when she began to extend her earlier work by investigating the relatively new phenomenon of retirement communities in France. She was greatly influenced by her colleague, the late philosopher Michel Philibert, who encouraged Cribier's interests and introduced her to the American literature. (Her first field surveys on retirement settlements as a result were done in Florida.) Cribier also admired the French historian Philippe Ariès, whose *Centuries of Childhood: A Social History of Family Life* (New York: Vintage, 1962) revolutionized historical studies of age relations on both sides of the Atlantic. She, too, wanted to reconstruct the lives of ordinary people. Early on, Cribier was also impressed by Bernice L. Neugarten's* work on the Kansas City data sets, and later on, by Neugarten's anthology, *Middle Age and Aging: A Reader in Social Psychology* (Chicago: University of Chicago Press, 1968)—though Cribier was not taken by U.S. "social-class sociology." During the past decade, she has also been influenced by Peter Laslett's work (in her words, "J'adore l'originalite, le serieux, and le non-conformisme") on the Third Age. These scholars fuelled Cribier's own interest in integrating perspectives on middle age and aging into class analysis.

Cribier's research and academic responsibilities fall into two domains. First, she has been reconstructing the lives of Parisian retirees, notably those born in 1907–1908 and 1921–1922. Cribier pays particular attention to residential patterns, family relations, and means of economic support. She does not, however, study retirement communities. Second, she has been studying regional differences in household patterns (especially co-residence) as well as patterns of retirement migration. She makes cross-cultural comparisons between Paris and London. For recent, representative examples of Cribier's work, see "Les vieux parents et leur enfants," *Gerontologie et Societe,* 47 (1989): 35–51; "Les retraites et leur logement," Gerontologie et Societe, 50 (1990): 30–47; "Les mots pour le dire: la vieillesse, les troiseme age, et l'age de nos nations," *Gerontologie,* 76 (1990): 1–8. Cribier also served as special editor of the June 1992 issue *Ageing* devoted to "societies contemporaines."

Cribier created a research unit in 1978 at the University of Paris 7, which has been a major center for doctoral students in gerontology. Historians, anthropologists, sociologists, and geographers have been drawn to it. Cribier herself directs work on social geography. She recently served as editor-in-chief on a series of articles on "Espace Populations Sociétés." Between 1987 and 1991 alone, her group produced roughly 160 publications.

EILEEN M. CRIMMINS. Eileen M. Crimmins received her B.A. in mathematics from Chestnut Hill College in Philadelphia in 1968. She then did her graduate work in demography at the University of Pennsylvania, where she earned her M.A. in 1969 and Ph.D. in 1974. Her disseration focused on "Infant Mortality in New York City: Factors Precipitating the Change, 1950–1960." From 1973 to 1978, Crimmins held appointments at the University of Illinois, Chicago Circle, in the Sociology Department and in the School of Public Health. Since the early 1980s, she has been associated with the Gerontology Research Institute at the University of Southern California (USC). Crimmins has been a professor of sociology and gerontology at USC since 1992.

Many of Crimmins's early papers dealt with a variety of issues associated with mortality trends. See "The Changing Pattern of American Mortality Decline, 1947–1977," *Population and Development Review*, 7 (1981): 229–54. Crimmins has often applied her training in demographic methods to historical data. See, for instance, two essays with G. Condran: "Public Health and Mortality in U.S. Cities in the Late Nineteenth Century" in *Human Ecology*, 6 (1978): 27–53; and "A Description and Evaluation of Mortality Data in the Federal Census, 1850–1900," *Historical Methods*, 12 (1979): 1–23.

Much of Crimmins's research at USC has been done in collaboration with her husband, Richard Easterlin. See, for instance, their book, *The Fertility Revolution: A Supply-Demand Analysis* (Chicago: University of Chicago Press, 1985); and *An Exploratory Study of the 'Synthesis Framework' of Fertility Determination with World Fertility Survey Data* for the National Academy of Sciences, 1983. The conjunction of economic and demographic themes also appears in gerontologically oriented works: Eileen M. Crimmins, "Evidence on the Compression of Morbidity," *Gerontologica Perspecta*, 1 (1987): 45–49; and "Changing Health of the Older Working-Age Population and Retirement Patterns over Time" (with M. Pramaggiore) in *Issues in Contemporary Retirement*, eds. Rita Ricardo-Campbell and E. Lazear (Stanford, Calif.: Hoover Institution Press, 1988).

Lately, Crimmins has been studying the relationship between life expectancy and disability. See, for instance, "Changes in Life Expectancy and Disability-Free Life Expectancy in the United States" (with Yasuhito Saito and D. Ingegneri) in *Population and Development Review*, 15 (1989): 235–67; and "Are Americans Healthier as Well as Longer-Lived," *Journal of Insurance Medicine*, 22 (1990): 89–92; and "Changing Mortality and Morbidity Rates and the Health Status and Life Expectancy of the Older U.S. Population" (with Mark Hayward and Yasuhiko Saito), *Demography*, 31 (1994).

VINCENT J. CRISTOFALO. Vincent J. Cristofalo, who earned his Ph.D. from the University of Delaware in 1962, received rigorous training in biological chemistry and physiology. Those he considers his teachers and mentors (Sidney Weinhouse, John Ward, Raphael Ronkin, David Kritchevsky, and Arnold Clark) made their careers as distinguished bench scientists and administrators; none, to put it as positively as possible, had more than a passing interest in gerontology. Along with his friend (and part-time collaborator, sometime competitor) Richard C. Adelman,* Cristofalo became interested in the then unappealing field of biogerontology because he saw ways of applying basic science to the questions concerning the regulation of senescence. The key, in this instance, was the work of Leonard Hayflick,* who in the early 1960s at the Wistar Institute (where Cristofalo spent much of his career) was demonstrating that cells did not live indefinitely, but tended to divide about fifty times before dying.

Cristofalo has used human cells in culture as a model to study the regulation of senescence at the cellular level. As a result of more than a quarter-century of work, he and his associates and students (including Rosalind Yanishevsky, Arthur Balin, Bryon Rosner, Robert Pignolo, John Ryan, Frank Praeger, Cathy Finlay, Nancy Olashaw, and Bark Keogh) have described in quantitative terms the life history of human cells in culture, focusing on their morphological and physiological changes. They demonstrated that the trajectory of the aging process can be altered by physiologic modulators, such as steroid hormones. More recently, Cristofalo and his colleagues have identified genes that are differentially expressed in different age cells. For an evolution of Cristofalo's own thinking, see V. J. Cristofalo and B. B. Sharf, "Cellular Senescence and DNA Synthesis: Thymidine Incorporation as a Measure of Population Age in Human Diploid Cells," *Experimental Cell Research,* 76 (1973): 419–27; Bryon Rosner and V. J. Cristofalo, "Changes in Specific Dexamethasone Binding During Aging in Wi-38 Cells," *Endocrinology,* 108 (1981): 1965–71; C. R. Carlin, P. D. Phillips, B. B. Knowles, and V. J. Cristofalo, "Diminished *in vitro* Tyrosine Kinase Activity of the Egf Receptor of Senescent Human Fibroblasts," *Nature,* 306 (1983): 617–20; and S. D. Gorman and V. J. Cristofalo, "Reinitiation of Cellular Dna Synthesis in Brdu-Selected Nondividing Senescent Wi-38 Cells by Simian Virus 40 Infection," *Journal of Cell Physiology,* 125 (1985): 122–26. See also his recent review with R. J. Pignola, "Replicative Senescence of Human Fibroblast-like Cells in Culture," *Physiological Reviews,* 73 (1993); 617–37, which brings this subfield and the contribution of his laboratory up to date.

Cristofalo was admired by his peers and non-biologists alike for his no-nonsense approach to science. He had a reputation for building good research teams and for helping others to do the same. The Medical College of Pennsylvania spared no efforts to lure Cristofalo from the Wistar Institute. He became the Audrey Meyer Mars Professor and director of its Center for Gerontological Research in 1990. Although a classically trained bench scientists, he had genuine respect for the value of divergent approaches to gerontologic knowledge.

Cristofalo expected his term as president of the Gerontological Society (1991) to be an opportunity to reinforce the organization's scientific moorings. Emphasizing that GSA is an organization of disciplines, not people, he wanted to strengthen the standing of the Society's bio-gerontologists in the universe of biologists. This meant, he felt, giving prominence to the journals and the annual meeting. Regrettably, Cristofalo early on became the target of those who felt that he and other bio-gerontologists were arrogant in their handling of other people's concerns and unduly territorial in protecting their turf. This exposed rifts within the gerontological community that impeded cross-disciplinary research between fields that did not always share common methods and orientations to problem-solving.

WILLIAM H. CROWN. William H. Crown earned his Ph.D. from MIT in 1982. Among those in his graduating class were several who became prominent figures in the economics of aging (including Joseph Quinn and Richard V. Burkhauser*), social welfare analysts (such as Sheldon Danziger), and high-ranking economists in the Clinton administration (such as Laura Tyson and Alan Blinder). Unlike his peers, Crown has chosen to associate himself primarily with the gerontological community, particularly those affiliated with the Economics and Politics of Aging program in the Florence Heller School at Brandeis University. It is not surprising that Crown considers James H. Schulz* his primary teacher, mentor, and role model. His work, along with Robert H. Binstock's,* drew Crown to research on aging.

Crown's most important work to date has been in the area of the policy implications of demographic change. With Charles F. Longino, Jr.,* he has worked on the implications of national population aging and elderly interstate migration. Having become sensitive to variations that lurk beneath statistical means, Crown has urged scholars to adjust gross measures to take account of factors that affect demographic and economic patterns among the aged. For instance, he has proposed an adjustment of dependency ratios to account for regional variations in economic growth and the elderly's residency patterns. Crown is ultimately working toward a unified, policy-relevant theory of economic status, labor-force participation, and consumption by elderly households. As a first step, he completed a *Handbook on Retirement* (Westport, Conn.: Greenwood, 1994).

NEAL R. CUTLER. Neal R. Cutler majored in English at St. Louis University, and then earned his M.D. from St. Louis in 1975. After completing his residency, he became a staff psychiatrist at the National Institute of Mental Health (NIMH) from 1978 to 1980. In 1979–1980, Cutler worked with Carl Eisdorfer in providing supervision in geriatric psychiatry at Yeshiva University's Albert Einstein School of Medicine in New York; with Frederick Goodwin, scientific director of the NIMH, he supervised work in psychopharmacology during the following two years. (Cutler is board-certified in psychiatry and neurology and board-eligible in clinical pharmacology.) In 1981, Cutler established the section on brain aging and dementia at the National Institute on Aging. For the next four years he served as section chief of the unit and deputy clinical director at the NIA. After a brief stint as director of geriatrics at Cedars-Mt. Sinai Medical Center, Cutler became director of California Clinical Trials in 1987.

Cutler has written over 150 publications. He is a frequent contributor to the *American Journal of Psychiatry,* the *Annals of Neurology,* and the *Annals of Internal Medicine.* In 1986, with P. K. Narang, he co-edited *Drug Studies in the Elderly: Methodological Concerns* (New York: Plenum Press); six years later, the pair co-edited *Pharmacodynamics: Perspectives in Clinical Pharmacology* (New York: Raven Press, 1992).

Cutler's current research falls into three areas: (1) brain imaging techniques in normal aging, Alzheimer's Disease, and Down syndrome; (2) pharmacoki-

netics and pharmacodynamics of drugs in the elderly; and (3) drug therapies in
Alzheimer's Disease and Parkinson's Disease.

STEPHEN J. CUTLER. Stephen J. Cutler, born in 1943, earned his B.A. from
Dartmouth College in 1964, where he studied with Robert Sokol, and received
his Ph.D. in sociology from the University of Michigan five years later. Under
his dissertation adviser, Edward Laumann, he wrote on membership in voluntary
associations and the theory of mass society. Cutler's interest in aging was
sparked by a graduate course in demography taught by Ronald Freedman; his
early work was influenced by that of Ansley Coale, especially Coale's article,
"How a Population Ages or Grows Younger," *Population Development*, 26
(1963).

After teaching for many years at Oberlin College, where J. Milton Yinger
served as a mentor, Cutler now holds the Bishop Robert F. Joyce Professorship
of Gerontology and is director of the Center for the Study of Aging at the
University of Vermont. He served on the Human Development and Aging Study
Section of the National Institutes of Health from 1979 until 1984 and again from
1988 to 1992, chairing the review panel during his last two years. In 1987, he
was chairman of the Gerontological Society of America's Behavioral and Social
Sciences Section, and in 1994–1995 he served as chairman of the American
Sociological Association's section on the sociology of aging. He was also editor
of the *Journal of Gerontology: Social Sciences* from 1989 to 1993.

Cutler has become one of the field's most respected sociologists. He considers
M. Powell Lawton* and George Maddox* to be important role models. Cutler's
most important contributions have come in four areas. He has produced a series
of studies documenting that aging is neither invariably nor inevitably accompanied by attitudinal rigidity. Thus, his work reinforces the findings of political
gerontologists who argue that advancing age does not necessarily presage increasingly conservative sociopolitical attitudes. See, for instance, Nicholas L.
Dangelis and Stephen Cutler, "An Intercohort Comparison of Changes in Attitudes about Race Relations," *Research on Aging*, 13 (1991): 55–73.

A second research interest has been the distribution, correlates, and consequences of voluntary association participation. He summarized his own work
and that of others in this domain in his entry on "group memberships" in the
Encyclopedia on Aging, ed. George L. Maddox (New York: Springer Publishing,
1987), 297–98. Another area of interest to Cutler is the role of transportation in
the lives of older people. See, for instance, Stephen Cutler and Raymond T.
Coward, "Availability of Personal Transportation in Households of Elders: Age,
Gender, and Residence Differences," *The Gerontologist*, 32 (1992): 77–81. Finally, Cutler has published a series of articles that focuses on residence differences in health, household composition, and patterns of assistance. See his
article, again with Coward, "Informal and Formal Health Care Systems for the
Rural Elderly," *Health Services Research*, 23 (1989): 785–806.

Although Cutler's research in these areas has been more concerned with providing solid empirical data than generating theoretical or conceptual contributions, his recent work (with collaborator Lynne Hodgson) has proposed and explored the concept of "anticipatory dementia," that is, how normal age-associated memory change may come to be perceived as a harbinger of dementia. See Lynne Hodgson and Stephen Cutler, "Anticipatory Dementia," *Perspective on Aging*, 23 (1994): 21–22.

Cutler is a member of Sigma Xi, and he is listed in *Who's Who*.

D

DEBRA DAVID. Debra David earned her doctorate from the University of California, Berkeley, in 1981. But it was a human development seminar at University of California at San Francisco team-taught in 1971–1972 by M. Margaret Clark, Donald Spence, and Marjorie Fiske* that drew her to gerontology. The seminar led to her dissertation research on social aspects of reminiscence in old age under the guidance of Arlie Hochschild and Neil Smelser. Her findings were reported in "Reminiscence, Adaptation, and Social Context in Old Age," *International Journal of Aging and Human Development,* 30 (1990): 175–88.

David also completed a two-year National Institute on Aging postdoctoral traineeship in adult development and aging under the auspices of the Midwest Council for Social Research in Aging. She studied at the School of Education at Northwestern University under the guidance of Solomon Cytrynbaum and Bernice L. Neugarten.*

More recently, David evaluated the Personal Autonomy in Long-Term Care initiative of The Retirement Research Foundation. With Martha Pelaez, she translated the theoretical findings of that effort into training materials for professionals working in residential and community-based long-term care. See *Autonomy in Long Term Care: A Training Manual for Nursing Homes* (Washington, D.C.: American Association of Homes for the Aging, 1993). She also drew on George Agich's ideas on autonomy in long-term care, in which an act is defined as autonomous if a person identifies with it. See "Autonomy in Health Care for Elders," in *The Legacy of Longevity: Health and Health Care in Later Life,* ed. S. Stahl (Newbury Park, Calif.: Sage, 1990), 217–31.

This work has led to more current research on multicultural perspectives on ethical issues in health care decision-making.

In addition to research, David has developed a model paraprofessional curriculum in aging and mental health at Elgin Community College, California, a master's degree program at San Jose State University, and a range of academic and continuing education programs for general education students, professionals, and paraprofessionals.

David is currently director of the Gerontology Center and professor of health science at San Jose State University and a member of the core faculty of the Stanford Geriatric Education Center. Her primary collaborators have been Martha Pelaez and Celia Orona. She has also worked with James Ellor, Brian Hofland, and Lela Llorens.

MICHAEL E. DEBAKEY. Michael E. DeBakey, M.D., born in Lake Charles, Louisiana, in 1908, is internationally recognized for his accomplishments as a medical educator, researcher and inventor, surgeon, and medical statesman. While still in medical school at Tulane, DeBakey invented the roller pump, itself an integral component of the heart-lung machine, which launched open-heart surgery. In the early 1950s, DeBakey developed Dacron artificial grafts for replacing diseased arteries. In 1953, he performed the first successful endarterectomy; in 1964, the world's first successful aortocoronary artery bypass operation; and in 1966 the first successful use of the left ventricular assist device. Four years later, he began to perform heart transplants, which he discontinued in 1970, but resumed in 1984, when more effective immunosuppressive drugs and advanced procedures became available. In 1965, in the first use of telemedicine, he operated on a patient in Houston while a group of surgeons in Geneva viewed the event by Early Bird satellite. He is now actively engaged in new telemedicine developments.

DeBakey has been, over the past fifty years, one of the nation's foremost medical spokesmen. An adviser to every president since Franklin Delano Roosevelt, he served on the Medical Task Force of the (President Herbert) Hoover Commission on Organization of the Executive Branch of Government (1949). He was influential in the creation of the National Library of Medicine. President Lyndon Baines Johnson appointed DeBakey to chair the President's Commission on Heart Disease, Cancer and Stroke. He has served as a consultant to numerous heads of state and surgical groups overseas. In 1969, Johnson awarded him the Presidential Medal of Freedom with Distinction, the highest honor an American citizen can receive. In 1987, President Ronald Reagan awarded DeBakey the National Medal of Science. He has received more than thirty-six honorary degrees and innumerable prestigious civic and professional awards, including the Lasker Award for Medical Research.

DeBakey deserves mention in this volume as an eminent cardiovascular surgeon who "early in [his] career" became interested in aging-related work. Influencing him in this direction was his mentor, Dr. Alton Ochsner. In the course of performing more than 50,000 cardiovascular procedures, DeBakey trained more than 1,000 surgeons to distinguish between diseases of an older person's body and "normal" aging. Here, then, is a person who has contributed enormously to gerontology and geriatrics without necessarily being considered (or recognized) as a researcher on aging.

HELEN DENNIS. Helen Dennis earned her B.A. in 1962 from Pennsylvania State University and an M.A. in clinical psychology from California State University, Long Beach, in 1976. Since then she has been affiliated with the Andrus Gerontology Center at the University of Southern California. Reading K. Warner Schaie's* work on aging and cognition, she recalls, sparked her initial interest in aging. Other current and former USC colleagues, such as David A. Peterson, James E. Birren,* and Ira S. Hirschfield, have served as important mentors and role models.

Since 1988 Dennis also has been a consultant to the Conference Board (a private research institute in New York City that serves corporations), directing research and training projects dealing with age issues in management and labor. Her greatest contributions thus far probably lie in this domain. In books and articles, training brochures, management workshops, advocacy, and mentoring, Dennis has focused on employment and retirement issues associated with population aging. Dennis has tried to bridge the interests of business people and experts on aging in promoting industrial gerontology as a viable subfield. She has worked with students, senior citizens, human resource managers, and other executives in developing ways to eradicate ageism in the marketplace, in designing corporate policies that can take advantage of people's added, healthy years, and in making the system more flexible in dealing with people making transitions into and out of retirement. See, for instance, her *Retirement Preparation: What Retirement Specialists Need to Know* (Lexington, Mass.: Lexington Books, 1984).

Dennis has been particularly effective in translating fairly well-known gerontologic principles into boardroom practice. She has refined and promoted the concept that age in itself is irrelevant in the work place. She has also stressed that functional, not chronological, age is what is relevant to job performance. Workers, she documents in vignettes, can learn and adapt at any age. These two principles were central in the Age Issues in Management training program she developed in the mid-1980s, the first of its kind in this country. They also became the basis of her chapter, "Management Training," in *Fourteen Steps in Managing an Aging Work Force,* ed. Helen Dennis (Lexington, Mass.: Lexington Books, 1988).

More than most gerontologists, Dennis has been willing to reach out to help middle-aged and older workers become empowered to manage their own employment and retirement options. For instance, she prepared a video for the American Bar Association, "Downsizing in an Aging Work Force: The Law, Limits, and Lessons Learned."

Dennis served as president of the International Society for Retirement Planners and currently serves as president of Career Encores, a non-profit agency connecting older job seekers with job opportunities. Career Encores takes a "subtle approach" to encouraging employers to hire mature workers.

ROSE DOBROF. Rose Dobrof received her B.A. from the University of Colorado in 1945, and her M.S.W. from the University of Pittsburgh three years later. During the 1950s, while raising a family, she served as a lecturer in the Division of Social Sciences at Indiana University. In 1961, upon moving to New York, Dobrof joined the staff of the Hebrew Home for the Aged. She chose this position largely because the elderly represented the one significant client group with whom she had not worked. For the next decade, she worked closely with Jacob Reingold and Alvin Goldfarb, M.D. From 1963 to 1970, she served as a visiting lecturer in Columbia University's School of Social Work. As she became more of a researcher and mentor as well as a practitioner, Dobrof realized that her next career goal should be to become a professor in the field of social work.

In the early 1970s, Dobrof coordinated various programs in the Hunter College School of Social Work as she pursued her D.S.W. degree at Columbia. Her studies were greatly facilitated by an array of distinguished teachers, including Alfred Kahn and Harold Lewis, her dean. She calls Eugene Litwack her most important teacher and mentor. In writing her dissertation, *The Care of the Aged* (1976), she relied heavily on Litwack's theory of "shared function" as a way of analyzing the task assignments of families and of formal organizations in care of functionally dependent older people. Dobrof also incorporated Litwack's emphasis on the "linkage mechanisms" that are necessary if families and formal organizations are to work together collaboratively. With Litwack, Dobrof wrote a manual, *The Maintenance of the Family Relationships of Older People in Institutions: Theory and Practice* for the Center on Aging, National Institute of Mental Health (1977).

In 1974, Dobrof became founding executive director of the Brookdale Center on Aging at Hunter College, a position that she still holds. Under her leadership, the center has gained a national reputation for its advocacy and training programs on campus and in collaboration with groups such as the American Society on Aging. Dobrof takes special pride in having designed and implemented the Brookdale Social Model of Respite Services and Group Activities Program for people with Alzheimer's Disease and their families. Dobrof's connections with the Brookdale Foundation have grown over time. She became a Brookdale Professor of Gerontology in 1984 and a senior fellow of the Brookdale Foundation a year later. In addition, she serves as co-director of the Hunter-Mt. Sinai Geriatric Education Center with another Brookdale senior fellow, Robert N. Butler.* On the basis of her efforts in geriatrics, she was made a fellow of the New York Academy of Medicine in 1985.

In addition to these responsibilities, Dobrof has served as a consultant to the

New York Community Trust and the Visiting Nurse Service of New York; she co-chaired the committee on Aging of the Federation of Jewish Philanthropies from 1979 to 1981. She also has served on several state and federal advisory councils. Her pattern of commitments resembles that of one of her role models, Jacqueline Wexler, president emerita of Hunter College. Dobrof's board work has enabled her to build bridges between the Brookdale Center and other social service agencies and governmental units. Dobrof resigned this position in 1994.

From 1968 to 1980, Dobrof served on the editorial board of *Omega* and on the advisory board of the Foundation of Thanatology. These experiences convinced her of the need for a specialized journal in her own area of experiences. Accordingly, in 1979, she launched the *Journal of Gerontological Social Work*.

WILMA DONAHUE. Wilma Donahue was born in Mitchellville, Iowa, in 1900. From her parents and childhood experiences, Donahue early on came to appreciate the "serendipitous" yet malleable nature of one's choices. She figured out ways to take advantage of opportunities that presented themselves, but she was equally prepared to cope with disappointments and setbacks. Either way, Donahue claims, she did not "mourn or celebrate the consequences," for she measured growth in how she succeeded in adjusting to changing circumstances. Perhaps this is why she dwelt on the continuing significance of persons and events in Iowa during her adolescence:

> My most important career decision turned out to be one I made when I entered high school. Although I could not dream of attending college, I took college preparatory courses. To be safe I also took Normal Teacher Training. My teachers were extraordinary, college-educated old maids who taught us not only book learning but also the values of a good life.

The paragraph is quite revealing. Even as a teenage girl, Donahue was willing to pursue dreams that required taking risks but nonetheless were within the realm of possibility. She was eager to learn for its own sake, but she also wanted to acquire practical knowledge. So she played it "safe" even though that meant working harder. She had no interest in becoming an old maid; the University of Michigan had to bend the rules for women undergraduates to accommodate her newlywed status! Donahue recognized the gifts her teachers were imparting.

The same patterns continued as Donahue pursued her professional career. That this farm girl managed to earn a Ph.D. at the University of Michigan toward the end of the Great Depression is a remarkable achievement. The feat is even more impressive since Donahue pursued a curriculum that enabled her to become one of the nation's first clinical psychologists. As a specialist in the diagnosis, treatment, and prevention of personality and behavioral disorders, Donahue was well positioned to counsel undergraduates in the Student Health Service and then World War II veterans readjusting to civilian life. That same pioneering spirit was evidenced in her manifold gerontology endeavors.

In 1944, Donahue joined forces with Clark Tibbitts,* who had been hired by the University of Michigan to shape a program for dealing with the "problems" of the elderly through the Institute for Human Adjustment (IHA). With logistical support from the University Extension Service, she and Tibbitts developed a course on "Aging and Living" (1948) for older Detroit residents. A year later the pair taught courses in Detroit, Flint, Traverse City, Bay City, and Windsor, Ontario; they also produced twenty-six radio broadcasts. In addition, they organized three conferences—"Living through the Older Years" (1948), "Planning for the Older Years" (1949) and "Growing in the Older Years" (1950)— in which experts, newcomers, and senior citizens came to Ann Arbor to exchange ideas. These conferences became the prototype for summer institutes that established the University of Michigan as a major center for gerontological training. "Much emphasis has been put by our committees, organizations, and institutions to develop youth into successful adults," Donahue noted in *Living through the Older Years,* ed. Clark Tibbitts (Ann Arbor, Mich.: University of Michigan Press, 1951), "and little thought and less action have been put into programs for the development of adults into successful maturity and old age."

When Tibbitts left Ann Arbor to coordinate aging-related concerns in the Federal Security Agency, Donahue assumed responsibility for IHA's nascent gerontological enterprise. She also stayed on to work on three other projects and attend to her sick husband. "A large part of the Division's work is educational in nature," Donahue observed in "Gerontology at the University of Michigan," *Geriatrics,* 15 (April 1960). With a $200,000 grant from the National Institutes of Health, Donahue in the mid-1950s spearheaded the preparation of three handbooks, James E. Birren's* *Handbook of Aging and the Individual* (Chicago: University of Chicago Press, 1959); Clark Tibbitts's *Handbook of Social Gerontology* (Chicago: University of Chicago Press, 1959); and Ernest W. Burgess's* *Aging in Western Societies* (Chicago: University of Chicago Press, 1960), which became landmarks in the field.

A diminutive woman without tenure faced stiff odds in trying to secure sufficient funds and suitable space for an interdisciplinary venture dismissed as marginal by many senior professors and administrators. Yet, thanks to her persistence, commitment to excellence, repeated successes, and well-placed support, Donahue created an internationally acclaimed center for innovative gerontology in Ann Arbor. In 1965, Governor George Romney created an Institute of Gerontology (jointly housed in Ann Arbor and at Wayne State University in Detroit) "for the purpose of developing new and improved programs for helping older people in this state, for the training of persons skilled in working with the problems of the aged, for research related to the needs of our aging population, and for conducting community service programs in the field of aging."

Donahue emphasized training and service. In 1967, she launched a Specialist in Aging program, which awarded more than 500 certificates over the next thirteen years. A Summer Education Program ran in tandem, registering more than 1,000 students at its peak. Formal curricular arrangements were made with the Schools of Social Work, Architecture, Education, and Public Health. Don-ahue established networks in Michigan that have made the state one of the pacesetters for improving the housing, financial security, and delivery of social services to senior citizens.

In 1970, Donahue formally resigned her posts at the University of Michigan and moved to Washington, D.C. At first she worked closely with Arthur Flem-ming* in planning the 1971 White House Conference on Aging. From 1973 to 1983, she was closely identified with the International Center for Gerontology. After a decade of operations she closed the office in Washington and opened the Center for Social Gerontology in Ann Arbor. She maintained an office in the Institute of Gerontology.

"In my own way, I have not retired," Wilma Donahue wrote in 1991. She continued to attend board meetings of the Center for Social Gerontology, and she met regularly with academics, civic leaders, and public officials here and abroad. "After I read and ponder, I express my opinion by urging the movers and shakers about the way I hope they will proceed," she said.

Speaking on the eve of Donahue's ninetieth birthday, Dr. Robert N. Butler,* the first director of the National Institute on Aging, declared that she "continues to be incisive, even formidable, in intellect and determination. She is one of the great people who have made gerontology grow exponentially in the last 25 years."

Donahue was often honored. She received honorary degrees from St. Thomas' Institute for Advanced Studies in Cincinnati (1965) and Western Michigan University (1970). The Gerontological Society bestowed upon her an Achievement Award (1969) and invited her to deliver the 1976 Kent Lecture. The National Council on the Aging honored her with the Ollie Randall Award (1982), and the Association for Gerontology in Higher Education gave her and Clark Tibbitts leadership awards (1988). The governor of Michigan cited her efforts in pre-senting her with the Michigan Women's Hall of Fame Life Achievement Award in 1983.

Wilma Donahue died in Ann Arbor at the age of 92. Her life and career give witness to the ways men and women can negotiate "social adjustment to old age." Donahue was a paradigm of "successful aging." For her own critique of her significance to the field, see her autobiographical account, "A Survivor's Career," in *Lives of Career Women,* ed. Frances Carp (New York: Plenum Press, 1991), 23–41.

KEN DYCHTWALD. Ken Dychtwald was born in New Jersey in 1950. At age 23, he had completed a B.A. from Lehigh University and was working on his doctorate in psychology and finishing his first book, *Bodymind.* He was living and teaching as a certified yoga instructor at the Esalin Institute in Big Sur, California. Dychtwald was deeply committed to the human potential movement. In 1973, Dr. Jean Houston, president of the Foundation for Mind Research, introduced him to Dr. Gay Luce, who wanted someone to develop a curriculum for her vision of an academy of holistic health and human development. Intrigued by the challenge, Dychtwald moved to Berkeley to develop a human potential program for senior citizens. For the next five years, he co-directed the SAGE project, which was funded in part by the National Institutes of Health.

By the early 1980s, Dychtwald was able to support himself through lectures and royalties from books such as *Millenium: Glimpses into the 21st Century, The Keys to a High Performance Lifestyle,* and *Wellness and Health Promotion for the Elderly.* In 1986, he formed Age Wave Inc., an information and communications firm aimed primarily at members of his baby boom generation, who were growing older. His list of clients included such Fortune 500 firms as American Express, Avon, Bank of America, CBS, Gillette, McGraw-Hill, and Sun Oil. He also served as a consultant for the U.S. Administration on Aging and the American Association of Retired Persons. According to a feature in *New Choices* (December 1988), Age Wave in 1987 turned a profit of $200,000 on sales of $2.7 million.

Age Wave: The Challenges and Opportunities of an Aging America gave the firm and Dychtwald even greater visibility. Published by Jeremy P. Tarcher Inc. in Los Angeles, the book had a first printing of 150,000 copies and a $100,000 promotional budget. Dychtwald's fifteen-city publicity tour was tied in with a CBS news special. Written in plain English, *Age Wave* was intended to communicate reliable information and demolish ageist myths in an effective manner. There were flashes of originality: Dychtwald stressed the importance of living a ''cyclic life'' in which ''(1) second chances are always possible, and (2) with passion and commitment, inner strength and energy can grow with the passing years'' (p. 97). But the book mainly reinforced the message of a ''spellbinding showman,'' who in the late 1980s could command as much ($15,000) for a performance as Henry Kissinger.

E _____

PRISCILLA R. EBERSOLE. After earning a B.S. in nursing at San Francisco State University in 1971, Priscilla R. Ebersole acquired an M.S. in adult psychiatric nursing a year later from the University of California, San Francisco, and a P.M.S. in mental health and aging in 1973. In 1976, she was awarded a Gerontological Nursing Certificate from the University of Southern California, and in 1986, she earned a Ph.D. in health and human services from Columbia Pacific University.

Ebersole, a professor emerita at San Francisco State University, teaches psychiatric nursing, geropsychiatric nursing, and holistic health nursing in the School of Nursing. She also teaches occasional courses in the applied gerontology program and directs graduate students.

Her most recent published work has been nursing texts. Both the third edition of *Toward Healthy Aging: Human Needs and Nursing Response,* co-written with Patricia Hess (St. Louis: C. V. Mosby, 1990), and her own *Care of the Psychogeriatric Client* (New York: Springer Publishing, 1990) were named Book of the Year by the *American Journal of Nursing.* The fourth edition of *Toward Healthy Aging* was published in 1994. Ebersole has also served as editor of the journal *Geriatric Nursing* since 1991.

Ebersole left San Francisco State University in 1988 to occupy the Florence Cellar Endowed Chair in Gerontological Nursing at Cleveland's Case Western Reserve University. She also took leave from 1981 to 1984 to direct field activities of a thirteen-state project to recruit, educate, and support gerontological nurse practitioners in nursing homes. The project was funded by the W. K.

Kellogg Foundation, administered by the Boise, Idaho-based Mountain States Health Corporation, and coordinated with five participating universities.

Ebersole's early work concentrated on collecting the life histories of aged individuals. This interest was sparked, she notes, by the history of her own grandmother's pioneering life of wagon trains and the West. From her interview work Ebersole began to recognize the therapeutic effects of reminiscing for the elderly, which led in turn to gerontological work. She has long been intrigued by the adaptability and life histories of aged individuals.

PHYLLIS EHRLICH. Phyllis Ehrlich has long advocated bridging the gap between gerontological theory and practice. "My professional gerontological career began when only a few practitioners came to GSA meetings," she said. "It was a lonely time for a clinician. It was this paucity of interest by researchers in the application of their work and by practitioners to participate in or utilize research that challenged me."

That statement reflects the obstacles that pioneers in gerontological social work faced even a few decades ago. Ehrlich earned an M.S.S.A. at Case Western Reserve in 1951. She did not return for her Ph.D. until 1978, completing the doctorate in health education from Southern Illinois University, Carbondale, in 1982. In the interim she worked to bridge the gap between research and practice through her own research of, and demonstration projects with, the elderly.

Her first important work brought the plight of the marginal elderly single-room occupant to national attention in the late 1970s. She began with *The Invisible Elderly* (Washington, D.C.: National Council on Aging, 1976). This project was followed by several papers and articles, including the latest, co-written with Ira Ehrlich, "SRO: A Distinct Population," in *Aging and the Human Condition,* ed. Gari Lesnoff-Caravaglia* (New York: Human Sciences Press, 1982).

Ehrlich also developed a community service model for the elderly, the Mutual Help Model, which links academia to service delivery in the community. The model integrates the social work methodology of group work and community organization with the knowledge base of role theory. Her latest article on the subject, "Model Project Reduces Alienation of Aged from Community," can be found in *Aging,* May–June 1982. The model itself is developed in "Service Delivery for the Community Elderly: The Mutual Help Model," *Journal of Gerontological Social Work* 2 (Winter 1979).

Hoping to unify social services, she developed an integrated legal and social work delivery model built on the "concepts, goals and methodologies of both disciplines." See her collaboration with Ira Ehrlich (her primary collaborator) and Robert Dreher, "The Law and the Elderly: Where is the Legal Profession? A Challenge and a Response," *Journal of Legal Education,* 31(3.5), 1982.

Her current effort is to develop a data base for research studies and clinical decision-making through the creation of a clinical/diagnostic recording system. This research is funded through the Older Americans Act.

Together, these projects demonstrate a concern for providing high-quality service to the community based elderly client and an effort to humanize research and practice. Work by Eva Kahana and M. Powell Lawton* on the environmental consequences of institutions has shaped Ehrlich's thinking. Kahana and Rodney M. Coe* have been her role models.

DAVID EKERDT. David Ekerdt credits biochemist Jeremiah Silbert, who directed the Boston VA Normative Aging Study, with teaching him the craft of research. While a sociology graduate student at Boston University (Ph.D., 1979), Ekerdt also worked for Sol Levine as a teaching fellow and gerontologist Jaber Gubrium.* It was at Boston that a senior faculty member told Ekerdt the secret of academic success. "Find a big idea and work it," he was told.

Although he did not originate the notion of retirement as an extended process, refining a developmental view of retirement is Ekerdt's "big idea." Retirement, he argues, has proven to be a process of anticipating, entering, and later adapting to new circumstances. Working with Raymond Bosse and Barbara Vinick, Ekerdt explored workers' changing views on retirement and concluded that readiness for retirement is a dynamic phenomenon marked by more uncertainty than decision models acknowledge. See "Concurrent Change in Planned and Preferred Age for Retirement," *Journal of Gerontology,* 35 (1980): 232–40; and "Orderly Endings: Do Men Know When They Will Retire?" *Journal of Gerontology: Social Science,* 44 (1989): S28–S35.

In other research Ekerdt has examined possible phases of the post-retirement experience, the consistency between expectations and outcomes, and people's efforts to manage the meaning of their experience. See his "An Empirical Test for Phases of Retirement: Findings from the Normative Aging Study," *Journal of Gerontology,* 40 (1985): 95–101.

He has since developed the "busy ethic," which states that moral continuity between work and retirement can be created if retirees hold leisure that is earnest, active, and "occupied" in high esteem. "This is the social and moral management of retirement," Ekerdt says. He developed this concept in his 1986 article, "The Busy Ethic: Moral Continuity Between Work and Retirement." *The Gerontologist,* 26 (1986): 239–44.

In addition to viewing these research efforts as contributions to the academic discipline of gerontology, Ekerdt emphasizes the ways his work benefits his subjects, if indirectly. Retirement is popularly approached with an apprehension that Ekerdt's research dispels.

Ekerdt currently works at the Center on Aging at the University of Kansas Medical Center in Kansas City.

GLEN H. ELDER, JR. Glen H. Elder, Jr. is one of this nation's premier sociologists. He received his Ph.D. at the University of North Carolina, Chapel Hill, in 1961. During his graduate days he was very impressed by the caliber of the faculty and the theories being developed at the University of Chicago's Committee on Human Development. Although he was not a student on the Midway, the committee represented the kind of program that Elder wanted to develop. However, his Chicago connection actually runs deeper. Elder has fashioned his career, especially his style of asking questions and framing issues, after W. I. Thomas, a University of Chicago social scientist renowned for his study of Polish, peasant immigrants. He also has been influenced by two colleagues, John A. Clausen and Urie Bronfenbrenner. The former has been a source of encouragement and support; from the latter Elder has developed some of his ecological perspectives.

After a distinguished career at Cornell University and elsewhere, Elder returned in the late 1980s to his alma mater to become the Howard W. Odum Distinguished Professor of Sociology and Research Professor of Psychology.

Glen Elder came to the field of aging through the kinds of questions that emerged in his program of research. These questions were prompted in part by the aging of cohorts he was studying. Elder began in the early 1960s to do research on the long-term effects of social change. After more than three decades, he is still engaged in his Social Change Project; his subjects are now in their 60s, 70s, and 80s. Thus, while Elder does not view himself primarily as a gerontologist, his theories of the life course have had a profound impact on research on aging.

The Children of the Great Depression: Social Change in Life Experience (Chicago: University of Chicago Press, 1974) remains Elder's signal achievement. It ranks with Philippe Aries's *Centuries of Childhood* (New York: Vintage, 1962) in opening the possibilities for historical sociology. Elder was able to show that it mattered greatly what age people were when certain dramatic events—such as the collapse of the U.S. economy—occurred. Some young people's life opportunities were ruined because they could not go to school, find work, or stay on the job. In contrast, those who were even younger and in school were spared much of the direct impact. *Children of the Great Depression* had a great impact on the thinking of such historians as Tamara Hareven, Daniel Scott Smith, and Maris A. Vinovskis, who in the mid-1970s were beginning to consider the significance of age and aging in past times. They in turn encouraged the current wave of graduate students to digest this seminal work.

Over time Elder has refined his notion of the "life course." He elaborated the perspectives in an essay by that name prepared for *The Encyclopedia of Sociology,* eds. Edgar F. Borgatta and Marie L. Borgatta (Beverly Hills, Calif.: Sage, 1991):

As a concept it refers to age-graded life patterns embedded in social institutions and subject to historical change. The life course consists of interlocking trajectories or pathways across the life span that are marked by sequences of social transitions. As a theoretical orientation, the life course has established a common field of inquiry by providing a framework that guides research in terms of problem identification and interdependent formation, variable selection and rationales, and strategies of design and analysis.

Once again saluting his debt to Thomas, Elder also stresses the significance of social timing and life course variations—referring especially to the pioneering work of Bernice L. Neugarten* and the influential studies of Vern L. Bengtson* and Alice Rossi on interdependent lives across the generations. In his own work, he has stressed the importance of linking mechanisms between changing times and lives, such as the control cycle, situational imperatives, the accentuation principle, the life-stage principle, and the concept of interdependent lives. All of these, Elder contends, have implications for development and aging.

Lately, Elder has broadened his study of social change in life experience by investigating the life course and intergenerational effects of drastic rural change in the American Midwest, using the approach developed in his studies of families in the Great Depression. As in the 1930s, the economic repercussions of the Great Farm Crisis of the 1980s were expressed in family life (mounting economic pressure, emotional distress, marital negativity, and inadequate parenting) and in the lives of parents and children. *Families in Troubled Times,* co-written with R. Conger (New York: Aldine de Gruyter, 1994), reports the initial findings of this ongoing panel study in north central Iowa, a study that brings together what Elder has termed the ''paradigmatic features of life course theory'': human lives in time and place, individual agency in choice making and social constraints, the interdependence of lives across the generations, and distinctions of social timing in lives.

Elder's initial studies of children of the Great Depression who are now in their sixties and seventies raised questions about how so many deprived children could have fared so well in their adult lives. How did they manage to turn their lives around after such unpromising beginnings? To answer this question, Elder turned his attention to World War II, the Korean conflict, and military service in general. For a majority of study men who were born in the 1920s, except possibly those damaged by combat, wartime and military service proved to be a bridge to greater opportunity, developmental growth, and a better life. The service generally came before major social roles and obligations, such as marriage, children, and career. Some American men came to World War II over the age of thirty, however, and they experienced life disruptions that had long-term adverse effects on their health and aging.

These conclusions emerged from his study of elderly men who were members of the Lewis Terman Life Cycle Study of Children with High Ability (1922–1992). Most of the Terman men were born between 1904 and 1917, and thus encountered the 1930s and war years at very different times in life. Writing in ''Talent, History and the Fulfillment of Promise,'' *Psychiatry,* 54 (1991): 251–67, Elder observed that ''perhaps no generation of Americans has embarked on life's journey amidst greater expectations than the young men and women of Professor Terman's study, a sample of the best and brightest after World War

I, who soon faced a massive economic depression and another world war'' (p. 252). The older men entered the job market when there were few good jobs in the 1930s, and over a third were mobilized into the armed forces after the age of thirty. The combined effect of these different times handicapped the early socioeconomic careers of the men, when compared to the careers of younger men. History played an important role in determining whether these men were able to fulfill the promise of their youth. As Elder points out, "Social history is not merely a backdrop for a life study, but rather constitutes an essential dimension of analysis that attends to matters of time, context, and process'' (p. 266).

MERRILL F. ELIAS. Clinical psychologist Merrill F. Elias earned his Ph.D. in experimental psychology from Purdue University in 1963 at the age of twenty-five, three years after graduating from Allegheny College in Meadville, Pennsylvania, with a dual major in psychology and economics. The U.S. Air Force supported Merrill's graduate work at Purdue; he was a second lieutenant from 1960 to 1963, and served three years at Griffiss Air Force Base in Rome, New York, following completion of his doctorate.

Upon his 1966 discharge, Elias returned to Allegheny College as an assistant professor of psychology until taking an NIH postdoctoral position at Duke University in 1969. During the 1970s Elias worked at Morgantown-based West Virginia University and Syracuse University before landing at the University of Maine in 1977, where he remains a professor of psychology. He directed the University of Maine's clinical training program between 1987 and 1990.

Elias's most important work has contributed to the development and integration of health psychology and aging, particularly studies of cardiovascular disease and cognitive functioning across the lifespan. See, for example, M. F. Elias, and M. A. Robbins, "Cardiovascular Disease, Hypertension, and Cognitive Function," in *Perspectives in Behavioral Medicine,* eds. A. P. Shapiro and A. Baum (Hillsdale, N.J.: Lawrence Erlbaum Associates, 1991), 249–86. He also has studied the effects of symptom-reporting anxiety and depression on people who report suffering chest pains.

Elias gave gerontology the journal *Experimental Aging Research,* which he founded in 1975. He served as the executive editor of *Gerontology* in 1984 and as *Growth and Human Development*'s associate editor in 1987.

His more recent work has developed the concept of disease cohorts, as opposed to "disease groups." With W. G. Wood he edited *Alcoholism and Aging* (Boca Raton, Fla.: CRC Press, 1982). This refinement allows the researcher to escape the paradigm of health versus sickness and permits a comparison of subjects according to the severity of disease. Severity is then used as a predictor in aging studies.

In addition to his work with Robbins, Elias has collaborated with Professor of Medicine David H. P. Streeted at the State University of New York, Syracuse.

Elias currently resides in Mt. Desert, Maine.

EARL THERON ENGLE. Earl Theron Engle was born in Waterloo, Iowa, in 1896. He received his B.A. at Nebraska Wesley in 1920 and his M.A. from the University of Colorado (while serving as an instructor in zoology) three years later. Theron earned his Ph.D. in anatomy from Stanford in 1925. After serving as an assistant professor for three years at Palo Alto, he joined the faculty of Columbia University's College of Physicians and Surgeons, where he became a full professor in 1939.

Engle is primarily remembered for his research on the physiology of reproduction. The author of *Diagnosis and Therapy of Gynecological Endocrine Disorders* (Chicago: University of Chicago Press, 1931), he studied the menstrual cycle, ovulation, and pregnancy; he also investigated the physiology and pathology of the testis. On this basis of this latter research, Engle was invited to contribute a chapter, "Male Reproductive System," to *Problems of Ageing*, ed. Edmund V. Cowdry* (Baltimore, Md.: Williams and Wilkins, 1939). Acknowledging that a "decline in sexual activity is taken more or less philosophically as a matter of course," Engle began his review of the literature by noting its relative paucity. He reported that aging was most marked in the prostate and testes. Endocrine deficiencies seemed to account for involution, though unlike women, was not as predictably determined by chronological years. Based on this work, Engle went on to write *Hormones and the Aging Process* (New York: Academic Press, 1956). Engle died in 1957.

CARROLL L. ESTES. Carroll Estes received her A.B. from Stanford University in 1959. Her M.A. thesis from Southern Methodist University was published as *The Decision Makers: The Power Structure of Dallas* (Dallas: Southern Methodist University Press, 1963). From 1961 through 1966, she was mainly associated with the Social Welfare Research Center at Brandeis University.

Estes earned her Ph.D. from the University of California, San Diego, in 1972. Her dissertation, "Community Planning for the Elderly from an Organizational, Political, and Interactionist Perspective," reflects the influence of Arnold Rose. Estes was initially attracted to the field of aging by Rose's work on symbolic interactionism and his notion of aging as a subculture. Among her most significant teachers were Alvin Gouldner, Randall Collins, and Joseph Gusfield.

After working as an assistant professor in the School of Social Work of San Diego State College (1967–1970), where she was named an outstanding teacher, Estes was affiliated with the Department of Psychiatry (1972–1975) and the Department of Social and Behavioral Sciences (1975 to the present) at the University of California, San Francisco (UCSF). Estes became the founding director of UCSF's Aging Health Policy Center in 1979, which six years later was renamed the Institute for Health and Aging. In addition to this position, which she still holds, Estes became a professor in the Department of Social and Behavioral Sciences in the School of Nursing, and the department's chairwoman two years later, in 1981. From 1991 to 1995, she also was associate director of the university's NIA Training Program in Gerontology and Geriatric Medicine.

Although she had written several highly regarded essays in the 1970s—such as her "New Federalism and Aging" for the U.S. Senate Special Committee on Aging's *Developments in Aging: 1974 and January–April 1975* (Washington, D.C.: Government Printing Office) 150–57; "Revenue Sharing: Implications for Policy and Research in Aging," *The Gerontologist,* 16 (1976): 141–47; and "Political Gerontology," *Transaction,* 15 (1978): 43–49—Estes attracted national and international attention with the publication of her *Aging Enterprise* (San Francisco: Jossey-Bass, 1979). Although others had done research on the ways that social policies affect the aged, Estes was a pioneer in introducing a critical perspective into gerontology. She did this by bringing together micro-levels of meaning and experience and macro-level *structural* perspectives. Borrowing from sociology, economics, political science, and history, she offered a political economy paradigm combined with a social constructionist perspective that has become as influential in its own way as had those perspectives on *individual* aging developed by social psychologists.

Throughout the 1980s and 1990s, Estes has extended and amplified her political economy approach to aging. Her research projects were generously funded by multiple federal agencies, including the Administration on Aging, the Health Care Financing Administration, the Agency for Health Care Policy and Research, and private foundations, such as the Pew Charitable Trusts, Commonwealth Fund, Robert Wood Johnson Foundation, and the Andrus Foundation. Sometimes Estes writes alone. Her empirical work has focused on the effects of public policy, particularly in access to home care and long-term care—see, with James Swan and associates, *The Long-Term Care Crisis* (Newbury Park, Calif.: Sage, 1993)—and organizations. See Carroll Estes and James Swan, "Privatization, System Membership, and Access to Home Health Care for the Elderly," *Milbank Quarterly,* 72 (1994): 277–98. Often, she writes books and articles with colleagues in her institute, notably Robert J. Newcomer,* Charlene A. Harrington,* Ted Benjamin, James Swan, Juanita Wood, and Elizabeth Binney. Estes's *Political Economy, Health, and Aging* (Boston: Little, Brown, 1984), co-written with Lenore Gerard, Jane Sprague Zones, and James H. Swan, argues that the economic structure of capitalism and the class structure of Western socioeconomic systems (that is, the United States, Canada, Britain, and France) are responsible for policies and programs that isolate and alienate the aged from society. In contrast to theories of disengagement and other dominant gerontological paradigms, Estes and her colleagues talked in terms of "contradictions" in the system and "crises" (objectively and subjectively produced) in the delivery of health care.

Similarly, in *Fiscal Austerity and Aging: Shifting Governmental Responsibility for the Elderly* (Beverly Hills, Calif.: Sage, 1983), which she wrote with Robert Newcomer and associates at UCSF, Estes boldly conjoined broad policy issues. "Fiscal austerity and old age are inextricably linked," she declared. "The shape and debate of public policy for the aged can best be understood in light of societal perceptions of old age, of the fiscal crisis, and of federal responsibility." It is worth noting how Estes's political economy perspectives on gerontology are infused with her attempts to make explicit the "social construction" of old age and aging and, more recently, its link to critical theory of the Frankfort School. With an obvious debt to Peter Berger and Thomas Luckmann's general work on the social construction of reality, Estes challenges the assumptions that underline dominant gerontological paradigms.

This becomes more evident in two volumes that she edited with Meredith Minkler, *Readings in the Political Economy of Aging* (Amityville, N.Y.: Baywood Publishing, 1984) and *Critical Perspectives on Aging* (Amityville, N.Y.: Baywood Publishing, 1991). Acknowledging that the heretofore underutilized notion of a "moral economy" can enrich the political economy approach to gerontology, Estes's theoretical work has turned to state theory and to feminist theory. Gender issues now are privileged as much as variation by class, race, and age. See C. Estes, K. Linkins, and E. Binney, "The Political Economy of Aging," in *The Handbook on Aging and the Social Sciences*, eds. Robert H. Binstoh and Linda George (New York: Academic Press, 1995).

Biases in the knowledge that is constructed and policies that flow from such constructions are exposed; see C. Estes and E. Binney, "Biomedicalization of Aging: Dangers and Dilemmas," *The Gerontologist,* 29 (1989): 587–96.

Estes has been much honored in a career that has hardly reached its peak. She has served as president of the Association for Gerontology in Higher Education (1981–1982), the American Society on Aging (1982–1984), and has received an honorary degree from Russell Sage College (1986). The Gerontological Society awarded her its Donald Kent Award in 1991 and elected her president for 1995–1996. The AGHE awarded her the Beverly Lectureship (1993), and the American Society on Aging gave her its distinguished Leadership Award (1991). She is one of the few social scientists elected to the Institute of Medicine of the National Academy of Sciences.

LOIS K. EVANS. Lois K. Evans gravitated toward the study of aging during her undergraduate nursing days at Morgantown-based West Virginia University. Following completion of her B.S.N. in 1965, Evans traveled to Washington, D.C., to study at the Catholic University of America, where she earned an M.S.N. in 1970. Evans practiced with the elderly in community and psychiatric nursing before and after earning her master's degree.

It was the teaching of Garland Lewis and David Guttmann in a course on social gerontology that solidified her initial attraction to the field. Forced to develop her own program, she combined doctoral courses in nursing, sociology, and anthropology. She received a doctor of nursing degree in 1979. Her dissertation analyzed social interactions among residents in public housing for the aged. In addition to Lewis and Guttmann, Evans counts Doris Schwartz and Mathy Mezey as important to her continuing development in the field.

Evans has contributed broadly to the evolution of geropsychiatric nursing practice and research. In particular, she did seminal work on the concept of "sundown syndrome" in cognitively impaired elderly. Some 110 institutional elderly were compared by Evans in research supported by the Alzheimer's Disease and Related Disorders Association. See "Sundown Syndrome in Institutionalized Elderly," *Journal of American Geriatrics Society,* 36 (1987): 101–108. Her more recent work on physical restraint of the elderly, done in collaboration with Neville E. Strumpf, has gained wide recognition. See "Tying Down the Elderly: A Review of the Literature on Physical Restraint," *Journal of American Geriatrics Society,* 37 (1989): 65–74; and "Myths About Elderly Restraint," *Image: Journal of Nursing Scholarship,* 22(2) (1990): 124–28. These articles have helped change the practice of routine restraint of the elderly in institutional settings. She recommends that the use of restraints be limited to serious, short-term circumstances. Evans hopes that the design of restraints will be improved and that alternatives will be designed.

Evans is currently an associate professor at the University of Pennsylvania School of Nursing.

F

CHARLES J. FAHEY. Monsignor Charles J. Fahey was born in Baltimore in 1933. As a priest of the Diocese of Syracuse, New York, he was assigned to the field of aging by his superiors. "No choice," he declares, "but love the field just the same." To prepare for this vocation, Fahey earned an M.S.W. from Catholic University (1961) and an M.Div. from St. Bernard's Institute in Rochester, New York (1983). His most important mentors have been Ted Munns, former president of the American Association for Homes for the Aged (AAHA), and Charles Tobin, former executive director of the New York State Catholic Conference. With these men and others associated with Catholic Charities, Fahey developed many long-term care services in New York, including more than thirty-five housing and long-term care units, institutions, and programs. As a consultant to AAHA, Fahey produced the *AAHA White Paper on Ethics,* which focused on corporate ethics in health and long-term care.

Fahey counts among his role models such luminaries as Bernice L. Neugarten,* Robert Ball, Arthur Flemming,* Nelson Cruikshank, and Hobart Jackson, each of whom played a significant role in shaping the direction of federal policies on aging. Like them, Fahey introduced a concept that took hold in both academic and government settings. As a member and then chairman of the Federal Council on Aging, Fahey in 1975–1976 introduced the notion of "the frail elderly" as a way of thinking about that subgroup of older people who are in special need of societal support. Fahey intended the concept to be broader than long-term care because it identifies a group that is at risk as well as in actual need, and because it entails social and economic supports as well as medical interventions. The council, with staff support from Cleonice Tavani, issued a series of interim reports and a final document, that have proved influential in shaping the public discourse and decision-making in this area.

At the same time, Fahey has not ignored issues in long-term care. He co-chaired, with Ellen Winston, a mini-conference on long-term care for the 1981 White House Conference on Aging. He worked with Bartholomew Callopy on a project supported by the Retirement Research Foundation to enhance the autonomy of persons in long-term care.

Fahey also deserves credit for promoting the idea of "the third age" in the United States. The term was first coined in France and then gained currency in Britain to describe educational opportunities offered in university settings for people pursuing higher education opportunities for the first time at a mature age or in retirement. Fahey has broadened the purview of the concept at the research center he established at Fordham University, the Third Age Center. Fahey and his associates, who have included Martha Holstein, seek ways to develop a new construct that takes into account role, status, life events, psychological and intellectual pursuits appropriate to a stage of life few have ever lived long enough to experience. The Third Age, in Fahey's words, "forwards the notion that it is well to attempt to develop a vision to be embodied in culture which is based on the reality of the aging experience, is in accord with the dignity of persons, has social significance, and is congenial to the maintenance of the biosphere for generations yet unborn." Fahey introduced his ideas in "The Church and the Third Age" in *America* (July 1982) and elaborated them in "Toward a Public Dialogue on the Meaning of Age" in *A Good Age,* eds. Paul Homer and Martha Holstein (New York: Simon and Schuster, 1990).

Fahey has also applied his expertise in gerontology in dealing with thorny issues that affect his religious community. With Mary Ann Lewis, the current director of the Third Age Center, he is developing an action plan and training materials for "An Agenda for Religion in the Field of Aging." Fahey has consulted with Catholic Charities in designing the future of the Catholic ministry in health care and long-term care; he helped to develop a blueprint, *A Time to Be Old; A Time to Flourish.* With colleagues at the Third Age Center, Fahey developed a white paper on ways to meet the financial needs of older priests and nuns and contributed to the establishment of fund-raising efforts on their behalf.

Because of his unique gifts and ebullient personality, Fahey has been tapped for several major leadership positions. He has been president of AAHA, the American Society on Aging, and the National Conference of Catholic Charities. He has chaired the organizing session of the Leadership Council of National Aging Organizations. He was a founding officer of the American Association for International Aging, the American Foundation for Aging Research, and the National Stroke Association. Internationally, Fahey was a founding member of Opera Pia International. He has been a consultant to the Helen Hamlyn Foundation (London) and to the United Nations Fund for Population Activities. Fahey was also spokesman for the Holy See at the 1982 World Assembly on Aging.

He served as a member of the work group on ethics on the White House Task Force on Health Care Reform.

Elected to the Institute on Medicine of the National Academy of Science in 1984, Fahey is currently a senior associate at Fordham University's Third Age Center and serves as Marie Ward Doty Professor of Aging Studies.

STEPHANIE FALLCREEK. A *summa cum laude* graduate of the University of Oklahoma, Stephanie FallCreek earned a master's in social work from the University of California at Berkeley in 1974, and a doctorate in social work a decade later. She has had a variety of practical and academic experiences, including work as a parole officer in Norman, Oklahoma, in the early 1970s and as an instructor at the Tacoma, Washington-based Pacific Lutheran University in the 1981–1982 academic year. But her most important work has been at New Mexico State University (NMSU) and for the state of New Mexico.

From 1983 to 1987, she served as director of the Institute for Gerontological Research and Education at NMSU in Las Cruces. From 1987 to 1991, she was the director of the New Mexico State Agency on Aging, working for both the university and the state governor's office. Since 1991 she has worked for the New Mexico Department of Health in Santa Fe, first as director of the Office of Planning and Evaluation, and currently as head of the Division of Long Term Care and Restorative Services.

She has consulted with the Washington, D.C.-based American Association of Retired Persons, the American Medical Association, and the American Hospital Association, among many others. Her current professional activities include sitting on the board of directors for the American Society on Aging, serving as treasurer of New York's Dome Foundation, and on the editorial board of *The Southwestern,* based in Denton, Texas.

It is through this work that she is able to bring the training of a gerontologist to state and national policy questions concerning the elderly. Through the New Mexico State Agency on Aging, she has produced (with Carol Glassman) videos such as *You Can Stop Smoking* (1990) and *Growing Old with Wisdom and Health* (1989). In particular, FallCreek remains sensitive to cultural and ethnic differences among the elderly and encourages service providers and policymakers to be aware of this diversity. She has contributed essays and articles to publications of the National Association of Social Workers.

JOHN A. FAULKNER. John A. Faulkner was born in 1923 in Kingston, Ontario. After serving as a flying officer in the Royal Canadian Air Force (1942–1945), he earned his B.A. in biology from Queen's University in Kingston. After several years of teaching science in local high schools, Faulkner earned an M.Sc. from the University of Michigan's School of Education, before returning to Canada to serve as an assistant professor of physical education at the University of Western Ontario (1956–1960). Named a Burke Aaron Hinsdale Scholar, he subsequently returned to Ann Arbor to earn his Ph.D. in 1962, where he studied with Bruno Balke, Leslie Kirsch, and Robert Kahn.

Faulkner began to move up the professorial ranks in the School of Education at the University of Michigan and to become active in the American College of Sports Medicine. His early publications attest to his increasingly "scientific" orientation. His first publication (with N. Loken), for instance, was "The Objectivity of Judging at the National Collegiate Athletic Association Gymnastic Meet: A Ten-Year Follow-Up Study," in *Research Quarterly,* 33 (1962): 485–86. Five years later, he published (with J. T. Daniels and B. Balke) a paper on the "Effects of Training at Moderate Altitude on Physical Performance Capacity" in the *Journal of Applied Physiology,* 22 (1967): 929–33. As his research orientation changed, Faulkner became an associate professor of physiology in the University of Michigan's Medical School and a full professor five years later. His role model was Horace Davenport, who also straddled two very different domains as a physiologist and historian of medicine.

Faulkner became interested in gerontological research in the late 1970s, when he visited the labs at Indiana University of Bruce Dill, who was investigating age-related changes in former world-class athletes. He subsequently narrowed his focus to the aging of human muscles after conversations with Erling Asmussen and observing the work of Alan McComas and his associates at McMaster University on the remodeling of motor units in muscles of the elderly. The more Faulkner studied and read, the more he realized how much had to be done in this area. Faulkner staked his claim in an article, "Are the Age-Related Changes Observed in Muscle Explained Completely by Muscle Atrophy as Proposed by G. Grimby and B. Saltin," *Clinical Physiology,* 3 (1983): 209–18.

The most important finding Faulkner's laboratory has contributed to the understanding of age-related changes in skeletal muscle is that the decline in maximum force is not just a function of muscle atrophy. Rather, it is due to intrinsic changes in skeletal muscles that result in a 20 percent decrease in the maximum specific force developed per unit of muscle of cross-sectional area. In addition, Faulkner and his associates have demonstrated that skeletal muscles in old animals are more susceptible to injury and regenerate less well than those in young or adult animals. Consequently, Faulkner has hypothesized that contraction-induced injury may contribute to the decrease in the development of maximum specific force by muscles in old animals. See, for instance, John Faulkner, Susan Brooks, and Eileen Zerba, "Skeletal Muscle Weakness in Old Age: Underlying Mechanisms," in *Annual Review of Gerontology and Geriatrics,* eds. Vincent J. Cristofalo* and M. Powell Lawton* (New York: Springer, 1990): 147–66.

Since affiliating with the Institute of Gerontology in 1986, Faulkner's lab has become increasingly gerontologically oriented, and he has encouraged colleagues from the university's medical and engineering schools to engage in cross-disciplinary studies. With anatomist Bruce Carlson, for instance, Faulkner has shown that skeletal muscles regenerate less well in old animals than they do in young ones. In addition, when whole muscles are cross-age transplanted in young-to-old rats inbred for many generations, young and old muscles regenerate equally well in young hosts and equally poorly in old hosts. From this, the authors concluded that muscles have not lost their intrinsic quality to regenerate, but that the old host does not provide a suitable environment for the process of regeneration to occur. Poor regeneration thus is associated with impaired reinnervation. See B. Carlson and J. Faulker, "Muscle Transplantation between Young and Old Rats: Age of Host Determines Recovery," *American Journal of Physiology,* 256 (1989): C1262–C1266.

In 1992, the American College of Sports Medicine awarded Faulkner its highest honors, attesting to the continuing relevance of his research and service to the study of conditioning athletes. Results from Faulkner's laboratories are also being used by a team of University of Michigan geneticists who are trying to solve the mysteries of muscular dystrophy. Faulkner has thus shown that age-related inquiries are not just of interest to bio-gerontologists; they have many practical applications. If more proof is needed, suffice it to say that Faulkner is the best long-distance runner in his age class in Ann Arbor.

KENNETH F. FERRARO. Kenneth F. Ferraro earned his M.A. at Duquesne University in 1978, and his Ph.D. at the University of Akron (1981), where he worked with Charles M. Barresi* and Harvey Sterns. Building on the work of George Maddox,* Ferraro examined the concept of health optimism among older adults. He found, contrary to conventional wisdom, that old-old members, those over seventy-five, of the elderly population may be more optimistic about their health than persons between sixty-five and seventy-four, once controlling for objective health conditions. See his "Self-Ratings of Health among the Old and the Old-Old," *Journal of Health and Social Behavior,* 21 (1980): 377–83.

Ferraro was also one of the first researchers to examine longitudinally the social networks of widows. Taking cues from the pathbreaking studies of Helena Lopata, and using data from before the loss of a spouse and after death, Ferraro (who often collaborated with Charles M. Barresi) found that interactions and social participation do not invariably decline. See his "Widowhood and Social Participation in Later Life: Isolation or Compensation," *Research on Aging,* 6 (1984): 451–68. Ferraro, working with criminologist Randy L. LaGrange, has also questioned the accuracy of the finding that older people are more afraid of crime than are younger people. See, for instance, their "Assessing Age and Gender Differences in Perceived Risk and Fear of Crime," *Criminology,* 27 (1989): 697–719.

Ferraro's penchant for puncturing erroneous ideas about aging, such as questioning the extent of the fear of crime, challenging notions of disengagement, or emphasizing that intergenerational beneficence is more likely than conflict set the stage for his collection of essays in *Gerontology: Perspectives and Issues* (New York: Springer Publishers, 1990). Taking a phrase from C. Wright Mills, Ferraro titled his first chapter "The Gerontological Imagination." There he set out a paradigm for this cross-disciplinary area: (1) aging and causality, (2) aging as a life process; (3) aging as a series of life transitions; (4) aging involves multifaceted change; (5) aging is positively associated with heterogeneity in a population; (6) aging and individual variation in function; and (7) aging and ageism.

In addition to these contributions, Ferraro founded the gerontology program at Northern Illinois University. He currently is professor of sociology at Purdue University, where he is reviving the Center for Aging Research. Ferraro has been a steady contributor to the *Journal of Gerontology: Social Sciences,* and he served on the Human Development and Aging study section at the National Institutes of Health.

CALEB ELLICOTT FINCH. Caleb "Tuck" Finch was born in London on July 4, 1939 to U.S. parents. He majored in biophysics at Yale (B.A., 1961), and earned his Ph.D. in cell biology at Rockefeller University in 1969. His aging-related work began in 1965, when he had to abandon his first Ph.D. project in Edward Tatum's laboratory, a failed attempt to isolate nucleoprotein mutants in *Neurospora.* Finch was generously sponsored by Alfred Mirsky and Eric Davidson to begin his work on the neuroendocrinology of aging in rodents, which proved far more successful. After holding a Public Health Service postdoctoral fellowship, he joined the faculty of the anatomy department at Cornell University Medical College. In 1972, Finch moved to the University of Southern California and in 1985, became the ARCO and William F. Kieschnick Professor in the Neurobiology of Aging and a University Professor four years later.

Finch has been a productive and prolific researcher. By the end of 1991, he wrote more than 225 peer-reviewed scientific articles and edited ten books, including the first two editions of the *Handbook of the Biology of Aging.* His most significant work has focused on the general role of hormonal factors in life history regulation, including the concept that nervous systems contain the pacemakers of aging. See his "The Regulation of Physiological Changes During Mammalian Aging," *Quarterly Review of Biology,* 51 (1976): 49–83 and "Hormones and the Physiological Architecture of Eye History Evolution," *Quarterly Review of Biology* (in press, 1995). Finch has elaborated the concept that cells in an organism generally show age changes in function that reflect regulatory influences through hormones, rather than resulting from autonomous aging. As a major theme of his 1985 Kleemeier Award lecture before the Gerontological Society of America, Finch argued that the neuroendocrinology of aging includes not only responses to hormone deficits, but also result from irreversible effects of hormones on the adult brain. See his "Neural and Endocrine Approaches to the Resolution of Time as a Dependent Variable in the Aging Processes of Mammals," *The Gerontologist,* 28 (1988): 29–42. A precursor of this argument appeared in Finch et al., "Ovarian and Steroidal Influences on Neuroendocrine Aging Processes in Female Rodents," *Endocrine Review,* 5 (1984): 467–97. Finch and his associates have also demonstrated that age-related losses of brain dopamine receptors occur by midlife in humans and rodents, and that they are progressive through the lifespan among healthy individuals. The loss of dopamine receptors became one of the first generally accepted bio-markers of brain aging.

In 1990 Finch published with the University of Chicago Press his first monograph, a 992 page analysis of *Longevity, Senescence, and the Genome*. The book goes far beyond biogerontologists' perennial concern with age-related dysfunctions and mortality risk in humans. Instead, Finch poses grand fundamental questions. Is senescence obligatory in higher organisms? Are there intrinsic limitations in the ways that organisms develop? Are there limits to the influence of the environment on aging? What is the role of the genome in scheduling major events? Boldly extending the comparative approach of those zoologists and botanists who contributed to Cowdry's *Problems of Ageing* a half century earlier, he challenges generalizations about aging based on the study of a few select species, offering a typology of senescence and the first multiphyletic calculations of mortality rate constants. It is the *diversity* of various species' responses to environmental factors that leads Finch to conclude that different genomic influences vary according to the evolutionary history of each organism. If so, then processes of senescence might be modifiable through gene regulation.

Since 1984, Finch has been the principal investigator of the Alzheimer Disease Research Center of Los Angeles and Orange Counties. He has served on agenda-setting committees established by the Social Science Research Council and the MacArthur Foundation Program on Successful Aging. He has served on several national scientific advisory boards, including the Advisory Committee to the Director of the National Institutes of Health (1987–90) and the American Foundation for Aging Research.

MARJORIE FISKE (LOWENTHAL). Marjorie Fiske was born in 1916 in Attleboro, Massachusetts. After graduating from Mount Holyoke College, which honored her with a D.Sc. in 1976, she earned her M.A. from Columbia University. There, she co-wrote two books with Robert Merton, *Mass Persuasion* (New York: Columbia University Press, 1946) and *The Focused Interview* (New York: Columbia University Press, 1948). From 1949 to 1953, Fiske was deputy director of the evaluation staff for the State Department's International Broadcasting Service, which was based in New York. From 1953 to 1954, she was executive director of the Ford Foundation's national planning committee on media research as well as research director of Columbia University's Bureau of Applied Social Research.

In 1955, Fiske moved to the University of California, Berkeley, serving first as lecturer in the Department of Sociology and as director of a book selection and censorship study. In 1958, Fiske became director of the human development research and training program at the University of California, San Francisco. This in turn led her to become founding director of the Department of Psychiatry's Human Aging and Development program, a research and training project that helped shape the development of lifespan studies throughout the United States and Europe.

Fiske's research included pioneering studies in personality development among the elderly and the middle-aged. With P. Berkman, she wrote *Lives in Distress* (1964) and with A. Simon and L. Epstein, *Aging and Mental Disorder in San Francisco: A Social Psychiatric Study* (San Francisco: Jossey-Bass, 1967). For *Middle Age and Aging,* Bernice L. Neugarten's* reader in social psychology (Chicago: University of Chicago, 1968), Marjorie Fiske Lowenthal and Clayton Haven contributed "Interaction and Adaptation: Intimacy as a Critical Variable." There, she stressed not only the importance of gender—a theme that she would elaborate in her 1975 monograph, *Four Stages of Life: A Comparative Study of Women and Men Facing Transitions*—but also the difference between social and psychological instruments for measuring morale. In "The Reality of Social Change," which appeared in *Aging into the 21st Century: Middle-Agers Today,* ed. Lissy Jarvik* (New York: Gardner, 1978), Fiske stressed how perceptions of stress, pending transitions, outlooks on the future, and personal as well as societal resources all helped and hindered efforts of cohorts to cope with changes.

In addition to her membership in a variety of social-scientific professional associations and editorial boards, Fiske served on the boards of the Fromm Institute for Lifelong Learning and the Fielding Institute. Library associations gave her awards for her work in that domain, and the Gerontological Society honored her with the Kleemeier Award in 1973.

Marjorie Fiske died in 1994.

ARTHUR S. FLEMMING. Arthur Sherwood Flemming was born in 1905. He earned his B.A. at Ohio Wesleyan University and his LL.B. from George Washington University. At the age of thirty-four, Flemming was appointed by Franklin Delano Roosevelt to the U.S. Civil Service Commission. Nine years later, in 1948, he became president of his alma mater, Ohio Wesleyan University. For most of his term he commuted to Washington, working in the Office of Defense Mobilization. From 1950 to 1964, he served on the International Civil Service Advisory Board.

In 1958, Dwight David Eisenhower asked Flemming to become his secretary of Health, Education and Welfare (HEW). In that capacity he chaired the first White House Conference on Aging. After the Democrats recaptured the presidency, Flemming mainly engaged in campus politics, serving for seven years as president of the University of Oregon and for a briefer period at Macalester College. However, John F. Kennedy retained his services, appointing him to the National Advisory Committee on the Peace Corps (1961–1965).

Flemming returned to Washington in 1971 to chair the landmark 1971 White House Conference on Aging. Richard Nixon made Flemming a special consultant and then in 1973 his Commissioner on Aging, a position Flemming held until 1978. It was typical of Flemming's sense of public service that he did not mind going down the bureaucratic ladder at HEW in order to serve the needs of senior citizens. Although past the age of mandatory retirement, Flemming's boundless energy and sage advice were well respected by leaders of both parties. Carter's first secretary of Health, Education, and Welfare, Joseph Califano, frequently sought his counsel. In appointing Flemming co-chairman of the 1981 White House Conference on Aging, Jimmy Carter noted that his "accomplishments and his idealism, his commitment and his wisdom are unparalleled, I think, in government."

Ronald Reagan apparently was less impressed with Flemming's liberal Republican tendencies than were his predecessors. The president summarily dismissed Flemming from his post on the U.S. Civil Rights Commission. Undaunted, the septuagenarian formed Save Our Security (SOS) with fellow former HEW secretary Wilbur J. Cohen.*

Flemming also remained an active member of the board of the National Council on the Aging, an organization he had headed from 1967 to 1970 (while serving as president of the National Council of Churches). According to another HEW protege-turned-secretary, Elliott L. Richardson, Flemming's career, still vigorously evident on the eve of his ninetieth birthday, attests to "largeness of mind and spirit. . . . His whole life speaks to the conviction that intractable social, economic, and educational problems will yield to the right combination of energy, ingenuity, and good will."

JAMES R. FLORINI. James R. Florini earned his B.A. in chemistry from Blackburn College in Carlinville, Illinois, and his Ph.D. in biochemistry three years later from the University of Illinois. From 1956 to 1966, he worked for Lederle Laboratories in Pearl River, New York. In 1966, Florini joined the faculty at Syracuse University, becoming a professor of biochemistry in 1970.

Over the course of his career Florini has gained research experience in enzyme kinetics, radioisotope methodology, corticosteroid metabolis, protein and nucleic acid synthesis in muscle, actions of anabolic hormones, biosynthesis of myosin, and muscle cell culture. Early on, this research was relevant to gerontologists. See, for instance, C. B. Breuer and J. R. Florini, "Amino Acid Incorporation into Protein by Cell Free Preparations from Rat Skeletal Muscle. IV. Effects of Animal Age and Androgen-Anabolic Agents on Activity of Muscle Ribosomes," *Biochemistry*, Vol. 4 (1966): 1044–98; V. J. Britton, F. G. Sherman, and J. R. Florini, "Effect of Age on RNA Synthesis and Activities of RNA Polymerases in Liver and Muscle of C57B1/gJ Mice," *Journal of Gerontology*, 27 (1972): 188–92; and two essays by J. R. Florini and R. N. Sorentinio, "Protein Metabolism in Aging," *Special Review of Experimental Aging Research* (1976): 181–97, and "Variations among Individual Mice in Binding of Growth Hormone and Insulin to Membranes from Animals of Different Ages," *Experimental Aging Research*, 2 (1976): 181–97.

In the early 1980s, recognition of the significance of Florini's work in the study of the relationship of protein synthesis and aging afforded him an opportunity to edit the *CRC Handbook of the Biochemistry of Aging* (Boca Raton, Fla.: CRC Press, 1981); to serve as chairman of an NIH panel on "The Influence of Aging on Protein Synthesis," in *Biological Mechanisms of Aging,* ed. R. T. Schmike (NIH Publication No. 2194, 1981), 321–97; and to contribute "Control of Myoblast Proliferation and Differentiation in Purified Proteins Added to Serum-Free Media" to *Altered Endocrine Status during Aging,* eds. Vincent J. Cristofalo,* George T. Baker III,* Richard C. Adelman,* and Jay Roberts (New York: Alan Liss, 1984), 139–61.

Florini's current research interests include the control of muscle cell growth and differentiation, secretion and action of somatomedins, and peptide growth factors—all of which illuminate features of the biology of aging. See, for instance, his "Effect of Aging on Skeletal Muscle Composition and Function," *Review of Biological Research in Aging,* 3, ed. Morris Rothstein (New York: Alan Liss, 1987), 337–58; F. J. Mangiacapra and J. R. Florini, "Alterations in Hormone Synthesis and Secretion with Age," in *Endocrine Functioning and Age,* eds. H. J. Armbrecht, R. M. Cole, and N. Wongsurawat (New York: Springer-Verlag, 1989), 13–25; and with F. J. Mangiacapra, "Problems in Design and Interpretation of Aging Studies: Illustration by Reports on Hormone Secretions and Actions," in *Review of Biological Research in Aging,* 4, ed. Morris Rothstein, (New York: Alan Liss, 1990), 231–42.

Florini has chaired the Biological Sciences Section of the Gerontological Society and served on its finance, fellowship, and publications committees. He served as associate editor of the *Journal of Gerontology* from 1978 to 1992, and held editorial responsibilities for *In Vitro* and the *American Journal of Physiology.* He also has been active in the Endocrine Society and the Tissue Culture Association.

Florini has also been an officer and instructor of the Syracuse Flying Club and Central New York Pilots' Association.

ANNE FONER. Anne Foner, who received her Ph.D. in 1969 from New York University, was brought into the field of aging by her teacher, mentor, and role model Matilda White Riley.* Foner worked with Riley (and with Marilyn Johnson) in evaluating and synthesizing extant research on age and aging, especially from the social sciences. Their analysis appeared in three volumes of *Aging and Society* published by the Russell Sage Foundation (New York, 1968–1972). Foner's work in especially evident in the first and third parts. Volume 1 offered "an inventory of research finding," Volume 3 "a sociology of age stratification."

Foner's contribution to the theoretical understanding of age as a social phenomenon arose from her analysis of the way age is built into the social structure at the societal level and in the domains of family, work, and political institutions. A major concern in her work is the analysis of age as a basis of structured social inequality and of forces promoting or moderating age conflicts. See her "Age Stratification and Age Conflict in Political Life," *American Sociological Review,*

39 (1974): 187–96; "Age Stratification and the Changing Family," in *Turning Points*, eds. John Demos and Sarane Boocock (Chicago: University of Chicago Press, 1978), 340–86; and "Ascribed and Achieved Bases of Stratification," *Annual Review of Sociology*, 5 (1979): 219–42.

In addition, Foner focused on the nature and consequences of certain dynamic age-related processes. She has investigated the ways that age is built into several key transitions over the individual life course and embedded in social institutions, especially those governing work and retirement. See, for instance, Anne Foner and David I. Kertzer, "Transitions over the Life Course: Lessons from 'Age-Set' Societies," *American Journal of Sociology*, 83 (1978): 1081–1104; and Anne Foner and Karen Schwab, *Aging and Retirement* (Monterey, Calif.: Brooks/Cole, 1981). Combining her focus on structure and change, she has explored the interplay between changing lives and changing social structures. See *Age and Structural Lag: Society's Failure to Provide Meaningful Opportunities in Work, Family, and Leisure*, eds. Matilda White Riley, Robert L. Kahn, and Anne Foner (New York: John Wiley, 1994).

Throughout her work Foner has explored the ways broad social theories can help illuminate age-related structures and social processes and how, in turn, a focus on age can contribute to an understanding of social structure and social change in general.

NANCY FONER. Anthropologist Nancy Foner has contributed to two areas in gerontology: the study of cross-cultural aging and nursing home ethnography. It was the work of her mother, Anne Foner,* as well as that of Matilda White Riley* on age stratification that led Nancy Foner toward gerontology. Her dissertation adviser at the University of Chicago (Ph.D., 1971) was Raymond Smith, a Caribbean specialist with interests in stratification and the family. Foner's earliest work is on the Caribbean and Caribbean migration, and she has written extensively on contemporary immigration to the United States. Currently, she is professor of anthropology at the State University of New York at Purchase.

Her most significant work on aging in non-industrial societies is her book *Ages in Conflict* (New York: Columbia University Press, 1984). She applied age stratification to non-industrial societies and examined the implications of age inequalities for relations between young and old in these societies. "By applying the age stratification perspective to the analysis of nonindustrial societies I have been able to show that age inequalities have crucial implications for old people's lives and for their social relations in nonwestern cultures," Foner said.

Her emphasis on the succession of cohorts is particularly useful in highlighting the processes of change in non-industrial cultures. In her book, and an article, "Age and Social Change," in *Age and Anthropological Theory*, eds. David Kertzer and Jennie Keith,* (Ithaca, N.Y.: Cornell University Press, 1984), Foner offers a critical examination of the modernization model as it applies to aging. In *The Changing Contract Across Generations*, eds. Vern L. Bengtson* and W. Andrew Achenbaum (New York: Aldine de Gruyter, 1993), Foner discusses care for the elderly in non-industrial societies when informal contracts fail.

In addition, she has explored the strains and contradictions facing nursing homes aides in an ethnographic study of a New York nursing home. "Nursing home life," Foner writes, "is as much a story of the workers and their worlds as is of the residents, and it is important to be sensitive to the difficulties that workers, as well as residents, face."

In *The Caregiving Dilemma: Work in an American Nursing Home* (Berkeley: University of California Press, 1994), Foner draws on theories of work and bureaucracy to illuminate the dilemmas confronted by nursing home aides. Aides are expected to provide compassionate care and to cope with the many pressures of the workplace and the institution. Foner provides a detailed analysis of the demands that aides experience from a variety of groups in the nursing home, each with its own interests and concerns—patients, administrators, nursing supervisors, patients' families, and co-workers. See also "Nursing Home Aides: Saints or Monsters?" *The Gerontologist,* 44 (1994): 79–86; "Relatives as Trouble: Nursing Home Aides and Patients' Families," in *The Culture of Long Term Care,* eds. J. Neil Henderson and Maria Vesperi (New York: Bergin and Garvey, 1995); and "The Hidden Injuries of Bureaucracy," *Human Organization* (forthcoming).

JAMES L. FOZARD. James L. Fozard was born in 1930. He earned his B.A. in psychology from the University of California, Santa Barbara, and his Ph.D. from Lehigh University in 1961 under Solomon Weinstock. He did a postdoctoral fellowship at Massachusetts Institute of Technology with D. B. Youtema. Fozard was drawn to the field of aging by George A. Talland, who recruited him to work with the Veterans Administration Normative Aging Study. The VA connection was very important. Paul A. Haber,* who headed the VA's Office of Geriatrics and Extended Care, served as an important mentor, especially between 1978 and 1985, when Fozard helped to develop and integrate long-term care programs and geriatric medical practice in the Veterans Administration Department of Medicine and Surgery. Fozard developed the geriatric evaluation unit and guidelines in the VA for caring for patients with dementia.

Much of Fozard's work has focused on the behavioral slowing with age in order to understand age differences in memory and cognitive functioning. The pathbreaking work by James E. Birren* and Alan T. Welford* on the relationship between speed and aging served as a model. Some of this work is summarized in Fozard's "The Time for Remembering," in *Aging in the '80s,* ed. Leonard Poon (Washington, D.C.: American Psychological Association, 1980); "Speed of Mental Performance and Aging: Costs of Aging and Benefits of Wisdom," in *Behavioral Assessment and Psychopharmacology,* eds. F. J. Pirozzolo and G. J. Maletta (New York: Praeger, 1981); and "Normal and Pathological Age Differences in Memory," in *Textbook of Gerontology and*

Geriatric Medicine, 3rd edn., ed. J. E. Brocklehurst (London: Churchill Living-stone, 1984).

Perhaps his signal intellectual contribution has been to redefine M. Powell Lawton's* transactional view of the ways people adapt to their environments. Reflecting his training at Lehigh and MIT, where he came to value the study of basic concepts of human factors engineering, Fozard's work clearly falls into that branch of the applied psychology of aging that depends on basic geronto-logical research. Optimizing conditions is a major theme, which is reflected in Fozard's papers. See his essay (with S. J. Popkin), "Optimizing Adult Devel-opment: Ends and Means of an Applied Psychology of Aging," *American Psy-chologist,* 33 (1978): 975–89; and Fozard et al. "Optimizing the Sensory Perceptual Environment of Older Adults," *International Journal of Industrial Ergonomics,* 7 (1991): 133–62. In "Vision and Hearing in Aging" in the third edition of the *Handbook of the Psychology of Aging* (eds. James E. Birren* and K. Warner Schaie,* New York: Academic Press, 1990), Fozard demonstrated that "older people suffer relatively more than younger ones from stimulus im-poverishment whether achieved by altering the temporal or the spatial aspects of the signal; the level of the end organ is implicated in age differences in seeing and hearing." Because the elderly become expert at inferring the meaning of stimulus events, he recommends greater efforts at training and rehabilitative interventions.

In 1993 and 1994, Fozard spent a year as a visiting professor of gerontech-nology at the Eindhoven University of Technology in The Netherlands, where he probed ideas about manipulating the social and physical environment to en-hance and support the aging and aged.

Following his work on longitudinal studies of aging at the Veterans Admin-istration, Fozard was in 1985 appointed associate scientific director for the Na-tional Institute on Aging's Baltimore Longitudinal Study on Aging (BLSA) conducted at the NIA's Gerontology Research Center in Baltimore. His influence on the study, initiated in 1958, is reflected in an essay (with E. Jeffrey Metter and Larry J. Brant) on "Next Steps in Studying Health and Disease Relation-ships in Longitudinal Studies," *Journals of Gerontology: Psychological Sci-ences,* 45 (1990): P116–P127. Although Nathan Shock* originally designed the BLSA to trace patterns of "normal" aging with characteristics unaffected by pathological manifestations, Fozard believes that the time has come to capture the interplay between disease and processes of aging: "At present, a full de-scription of aging that includes disease does not exist. . . . What is important are the severity of the diseases and their interplay with the aging process."

In other developments, Fozard and colleagues have shown that rates of change in normal physiological and psychological functions are themselves harbingers of later illness. See, for instance, H. B. Carter et al., "Estimation of Prostatic Growth Using Serial Prostate Specific Antigen Measurements in Men With and Without Prostate Disease," *Cancer Research,* 52 (1992): 3323–28.

LAWRENCE K. FRANK. Lawrence K. Frank was born in Cincinnati, Ohio, in 1890. He received his B.A. in economics from Columbia University in 1912. After graduation, he worked for the New York Telephone Company (1913–1920), War Industries Board (1917), and then served as a manager of the New School for Social Research (1920–1922).

Beardsley Ruml recruited him to the Laura Spelman Rockefeller Memorial Fund in 1923. His first task, a survey of the social sciences, concluded that "the growth of science is conditioned by the availability of scientists," particularly those who explored "concrete situations." Over the next thirteen years, Frank invested Rockefeller funds in the training of social scientists interested in the problems of youth and childhood.

Frank established Institutes of Child Welfare, based on the station established during World War I at the University of Iowa, at Columbia (1924), Minnesota and Toronto (1925), Yale (1926), and Berkeley (1927). He supported basic research on adolescent development, including that of Case Western's T. Wingate Todd.* He authorized funds for the National Research Council to support a survey on work in child development in the late 1920s, and in 1933, he provided funds to launch the Society for Research in Child Development. Frank wrote a chapter on "Child and Youth" for the President's Research Committee on Recent Social Trends (1931–1932). In 1931, he became an officer of another Rockefeller philanthropy, the General Education Board. There, Frank helped to found the Society for Research in Child Development in 1933, and sponsored summer programs to bring together scholars to share ideas about what was known of human behavior.

In 1936, Frank became a vice president of the Josiah Macy Foundation, which had been established six years earlier to promote cross-disciplinary, integrative research that promised practical pay-offs. Thanks to input from Edmund Vincent Cowdry,* among others, the Macy Foundation early on became interested in "the processes of aging and degenerative changes." As the foundation put it, "Here was virgin territory with broad implications for many of the biological, medical, and social sciences. Here was an opportunity for a foundation to assist in the development of a new field of science which, by its nature, demanded the integration of data, methods, and concepts from many special branches—a coordinated, multi-professional approach."

Frank was very instrumental in convening the 1937 Woods Hole Conference, and two years later, producing the first U.S. handbook on gerontology, *Problems of Ageing* (Baltimore: Williams and Wilkins), ed. Edmund Vincent Cowdry. "No general theory of aging," Frank's Foreword flatly asserted, "is at present available and the question of human or mammalian senescence must for the present be regarded as a distinct problem, within the larger biological question."

Frank posed three research-relevant questions, which set the tone for all that followed. First, what were the prevailing concepts of senescence in the 1930s? Second, what were the characteristics of the gerontologic "problem?" Third, what obstacles and incentives influenced how experts used scientific knowledge

to deal with social issues? These questions, Frank hoped, would "open up promising leads for investigation . . . and acquaint both the professional and the general reader with the present status of this problem."

Frank was instrumental in convincing the federal government to establish a
gerontology unit in the Public Health Service. (He provided support from the
Macy Foundation in 1939 to pay a director's salary for one year.) In 1945,
Frank helped to found the Gerontological Society. His was the lead article in
the first issue of the *Journal of Gerontology* (1946). "Some of the baffling
problems in the field of aging may also stimulate further critical, reflective thinking," he wrote, "and a greater readiness to consider how we can develop the
new concepts and new methodologies commensurate with these perplexing and
elusive complexities."

Frank directed the Caroline Zachary Institute for Human Development from
1945 to 1950. Thereafter, he taught at Bennington, the Merrill-Palmer School
in Detroit, MIT, Harvard, and Brandeis.

Frank died in 1968.

IRIS C. FREEMAN. Iris C. Freeman attended Barnard College in New York
City and earned a B.A. in English in 1966. In 1977, she earned an M.S.W. in
administration and policy from the University of Minnesota. Freeman has been
working as the executive director of the Minneapolis-based Minnesota Alliance
for Health Care Consumers ever since.

The Minnesota Alliance for Health Care Consumers is a nationally recognized
consumer protection organization for nursing home residents in Minnesota. It is
a membership organization composed predominantly of nursing home residents
and their families. Its services range from individual casework advocacy to resident and family council development, and educational initiatives. In addition,
it is consistently involved in regulatory and legislative policy development. Its
case methods, consumer council publications, and legislative expertise are frequently sought by consumer and professional groups throughout the United
States and Canada. As director, Freeman has accumulated tangible assets and
staff. In her words, "Since most of the stellar ideas are theirs, I will take credit
for intellectual midwifery and synthesis."

But also to Freeman's credit are two state laws unique to Minnesota. One,
which she proposed, is a public-funding mechanism to support the development
and education of resident and family councils in nursing homes. Enacted as state
law MS 144A.33 in 1985, the statute places a surcharge on licensing of nursing
home and boarding care beds to fund consumer education efforts. The second,
which Freeman refined, equalizes public and private pay nursing home rates
(MS 248.B Subd. 1). Equal rates, along with antidiscrimination provisions, have
altered the patterns of admissions.

Freeman also served on the Institute of Medicine's Committee on Nursing
Home Regulation, whose 1986 book, *Improving the Quality of Nursing Homes*

(Washington, D.C.: National Academy Press) has set the agenda for nursing home reform.

JOSEPH T. FREEMAN. Joseph T. Freeman was born in 1908. He earned his A.B. from Harvard in 1930 and his M.D. from Jefferson Medical College in 1934. He worked at Philadelphia General Hospital and Rush Hospital from 1937–1941, was Chief, Department of Geriatrics, Doctor's Hospital from 1942–1947. He was a clinical assistant professor of medicine at the Medical College of Pennsylvania from 1956–1964 and a lecturer in medicine there from 1964–67. He was a professor of medicine in gerontology, University of Nebraska Medical Center from 1971–72. He served as consultant to the Home for the Jewish Aged, 1955–1960, and to the U.S. Senate Special Committee on Aging.

He received the Meyer B. Strouse Award from Moss Rehabilitation Hospital in 1961, the Citation of Merit from the Gerontological Society in 1961, and the AMA Recognition Award in 1971.

Freeman has made important contributions to gerontology through his work as Chairman of the Commission on Geriatrics. This commission was one of the first of its kind in organized medicine in the United States and has been active in practically every area of aging with emphasis on a clinical orientation. His research focuses on medical education in aging, and the history of gerontology. He is a fellow of the Gerontological Society (1960–present), past vice-president of the American Geriatrics Society (1948–1952), Fellow of the International History of Medicine Society. Freeman was president of the Gerontological Society in 1961.

Perhaps Freeman's greatest accomplishment was to advance the status of the arts and the humanities in professional-aging circles. An amateur historian in the best sense of the term, Freeman compiled a series of biographical sketches of major figures in the field. See, for instance, his essays, "Edmund Vincent Cowdry, Creative Gerontologist," in *The Gerontologist,* 24 (1984): 241–45; and "Sona Rosa Bernstein: Gerontologist in Motley," *Journal of the American Geriatrics Society,* 24 (1976): 547–51. He also wrote pieces on the founding of the Gerontological Society and the National Institute on Aging. In addition to encouraging historians such as David D. Van Tassel and W. Andrew Achenbaum to enter the field, Freeman also compiled bibliographies of major works on medical views and popular attitudes toward age and aging. His *Aging: Its History and Literature* (New York: Human Sciences Press, 1979) went into a second addition. He served as an advisor to the Arno Press collection on aging.

Over the course of his long life, Freeman also amassed an impressive collection of books on gerontology. At the time of his death in his early eighties, he owned more than 400 first editions of books, including Cornaro's study of longevity and rare British volumes. Freeman also collected photographs of gerontologic pioneers and some of their holographic letters. His personal bibliography of works on aging, written before 1900, exceeded 5,000 entries. The bulk of his collection was transferred to the College of Physicians of Philadelphia.

132   HIRAM J. FRIEDSAM

HIRAM J. FRIEDSAM. Hiram J. Friedsam cheerfully acknowledges having been
called "the man who brought disaster to gerontology." Born in 1915, he earned
his B.A. from Baylor University in 1939. Upon earning a doctorate in sociology
from the University of Texas in 1950, Friedsam published articles on several
aging-related topics, including inter-regional migration, self- and physician-
health ratings, admissions to nursing homes, and travel as a use of leisure time.
It was his series on older persons as the victims of natural disasters that most
clearly and directly influenced subsequent research by others. His work, "Older
Persons in Disaster," was published in *Man and Society in Disaster,* eds. G.
Baker III* and D. Chapman (New York: Basic Books, 1962).

Friedsam has also played a constructive role in the field. He brought the
theoretical apparatus of sociology to gerontology, using appropriate elements.
For example, he is perhaps the first to have used the notion of "relative dep-
rivation" in aging research. See "Reactions of Older Persons to Disaster-Caused
Losses," *The Gerontologist,* 1 (1961): 34–37.

From 1982 to 1984 Friedsam served as editor-in-chief of *The Gerontologist.*
During that time he broadened the journal's scope to include more international
work and more contributions from the humanities. He also introduced the "Practice Concepts" section, bringing in Barbara Silverstone to edit. The editorial
board was expanded to include persons from "under-represented" disciplines
and professions.

As a faculty member at the University of North Texas since 1948, Friedsam
established the Center for Studies in Aging and developed a master's degree
program in Studies in Aging. The program includes an option in long-term care
administration, which proved significant and popular. A concise statement of
the organization and curriculum of the program can be found in C. A. Martin
and H. J. Friedsam, "A Gerontology-Based Approach to Education for Long-
Term Care Administration," *Gerontology and Geriatrics Education,* 1 (1981):
205–207. He served as president of the Association for Gerontology in Higher
Education in 1977–1978 and received its distinguished educator award, now the
Clark Tibbitts Award, in 1984.

Friedsam is certainly a pioneer of the field. While a graduate student in the
late 1940s at the University of Texas he was intellectually virtually alone. But
the first postdoctoral seminar sponsored by the Inter-University Council on Social Gerontology in Storrs, Connecticut, in 1958 brought him out of the woods.
"Although I had some background in gerontology when I attended, the range
of lecturers and their topics was a revelation," he reports. A different type of
revelation occurred when he served as the "token Texan" on a presidential task
force on the elderly appointed by Lyndon Johnson.

Currently he is professor emeritus at the University of North Texas. In addition to continuing his long-standing participation in AGHE and the Gerontological Society of America, he continues to be active in research and
publications. His most recent publication, written with Mildred M. Seltzer,* is
"An Aging Society: Challenge and Response for Higher Education," in *Ger-*

ontology Program Development and Evaluation, eds. Tom Hickey,* P. K. Still-
well, and Elizabeth B. Douglas (Washington, D.C.: Association for Gerontology
in Higher Education, 1994). A Friedsam chapter in a book edited by Seltzer and
an article, ''Professional Education and the Invention of Social Gerontology,''
are scheduled for publication in 1995.

BRANT E. FRIES. Brant E. Fries was born in Brooklyn, New York, in 1946.
Formerly an Olympic-trained fencer, he majored in mathematics at Columbia
(B.A., 1967). Fries earned his Ph.D. in Operations Research (1972) at Cornell
University, where his thesis involved inventory policy for perishable commod-
ities such as blood. He returned to Columbia for a postdoctoral fellowship,
where he studied operations research problems in health care delivery (1972–
1973), and remained for another five years as a faculty member in the School
of Public Health and Columbia's Center for Community Health Systems. There
he was involved in projects on clinic scheduling and system design for emergency and primary care.

In 1978 Fries joined the faculty of Yale University's School of Organization
and Management and the Yale Health System Management Group. There he
published *The Application of Operations Research to Health Care Delivery Systems: A Complete Review of Periodical Literature* (New York: Springer Publishing, 1981), and worked on his first Veterans Administration grant to develop
a drug information and profiling system to control outpatient drug prescribing.

In 1981 he received a grant from the Health Care Financing Administration
(HCFA) to develop Resource Utilization Groups (RUGs) to differentiate patients
by their functional, social, and behavioral characteristics so that groups would
have similar resource consumption patterns. After moving to Rensselaer Polytechnic Institute in Troy, New York, 1985, he collaborated on the development
of the reimbursement system for New York State nursing homes, using RUG-
II to provide case mix adjustments. This project was funded for $1.8 million by
HCFA over a three-year period. He also worked on case mix classification systems for federal Medicare and New York State home care clients. Beginning in
June 1985, he also collaborated with University of Michigan and VA co-
investigator M. L. F. Ashcraft to develop a patient classification system for
psychiatric and substance-abuse patients.

Since joining the faculty of the University of Michigan in 1985, where he
holds appointments in the Institute of Gerontology and the School of Public
Health, Fries has been developing ever more sophisticated assessment/measure-
ment tools to understand, care for, manage, and finance the elderly in institutional and non-institutional settings. He continues to work on projects for the
VA, HCFA, and New York State. He has done special projects for Michigan,
Pennsylvania, and Texas, primarily involving RUG-III for case mix-based nursing home payment systems. A major product has been the National Resident
Assessment Instrument (RAI), mandated for use in virtually all U.S. nursing

homes, and developed with a team from the Hebrew Rehabilitation Center for the Aged, Brown University, and Research Triangle Institute.

Fries's models and products have attracted international attention. Between 1985 and 1994, he made presentations at more than two dozen conferences on three continents. In 1992, he convened a World Health Organization conference on cross-national comparisons of the elderly in health care institutions, and he now heads an international organization—interRAI—of researchers from fifteen nations interested in uses of the RAI for institutional and home health care.

For recent publications that amplify the scope of Fries's work, see B. E. Fries, D. Schneider, W. J. Foley, M. Gavazzi, R. Burke and E. Cornelius, "Refining a Case-Mix Measure for Nursing Homes: Resource Utilization Groups (RUG-III)," *Medical Care,* 32 (1994): 668–85; S. Clauser and B. E. Fries, "Nursing Home Resident Assessment and Case-Mix Classification: Cross-National Perspectives," *Health Care Financing Review,* 13 (1992): 135–55; and J. N. Morris, B. E. Fries, and D. R. Mehr, "MDS Cognitive Performance Scale," *Journals of Gerontology,* 49 (1994): M174–M182.

G

CHARLES M. GAITZ. Psychiatrist Charles M. Gaitz received his M.D. from the University of Texas Medical Branch at Galveston in 1946, and performed his residency at the Phipps Clinic at Baltimore's Johns Hopkins Hospital from 1949 to 1952. He currently resides in Houston, Texas, where he has been a clinical professor in psychiatry at the Baylor College of Medicine since 1976 and at the University of Texas Medical School since 1983. He also has been the medical director of the Gero-Psychiatry Program at AMI Bellaire Hospital in Houston (1986–1992) and Sam Houston Partial Hospitalization Center (1992–1994), and was a consultant to the city's VA Medical Center from 1957 to 1992. Gaitz is now in private practice.

Gaitz was one of the first American psychiatrists to focus on the elderly. His role models include Alvin Goldfarb, Jack Weinberg,* Alexander Simon,* and Maurice Linden. From 1966 to 1969 he directed an NIMH Demonstration Project, "Comprehensive Care of Suspected Mentally Ill Aged." With subsequent NIMH funding, Gaitz investigated leisure and mental health from 1969 to 1975 to explore cultural and age-related factors. He has long recognized that older people are likely to suffer with physical, social, and psychological problems. Therefore, he encouraged an interdisciplinary approach while heading a program devoted to research and training at the Texas Research Institute of Mental Sciences from 1965 to 1985.

His solo works include: "Multidisciplinary Team Care of the Elderly: The Role of the Psychiatrist," *Gerontologist,* 27 (1987): 553–56; and "Aged Patients, Their Families and Physicians," in *Aging, the Process and the People,* eds. G. Usdin and C. Hofling (New York: Brunner-Mazel, 1978), 206–39.

Much of his recent work has been done in collaboration with Chad Gordon and Nancy Wilson. See, for example, "Comments by a Psychiatrist and a Case Manager," *Gerontologist,* 26 (1986): 606–609; "Organization of Services," Chap. 4 in *Confronting Alzheimer's Disease,* ed. Anne C. Kalicki (Washington, D.C.: American Association of Homes for the Aging, 1987), 51–63; "Dementia: Implications for Patient Care," in *Interdisciplinary Topics in Gerontology,* ed. H. P. VonHahn (Basel: S. Karger, 1984), 185–91.

Gaitz has been active in the Gerontological Society and was president of the organization in 1977. He received the Clinical Medical Section's Joseph T. Freeman award seven years later.

MARGARET GATZ. Margaret Gatz, born in 1944, earned her B.A. in psychology at Rhodes College in Memphis in 1966, where she was elected to Phi Beta Kappa and Sigma Xi. She then spent a year studying psychometrics and social psychology at the University of Illinois. Gatz earned her Ph.D. in clinical psychology at Duke in 1972; as part of her training, she worked as an intern in the Department of Behavioral Medicine and Psychiatry at the West Virginia University Medical Center and the Robert F. Kennedy Youth Center in Morgantown.

Offered a postdoctoral traineeship at the Duke Center for the Study of Aging and Human Development, Gatz became interested in theories of lifespan development, especially those formulated by Klaus Riegel* and Paul Baltes.* While at Duke, Gatz worked with fellow postdoctoral students Ilene Siegler and subsequently with Linda K. George* and Michael A. Smyer,* among others, on several projects. She served as primary investigator on a study of "aging competently" funded by the Administration on Aging.

In the mid-1970s, Gatz was a member of the Psychology Department faculty and an associate in the University of Maryland's Parent Consultation and Child Evaluation Service. In 1979 she became a faculty member in the Psychology Department and a senior research associate at the University of Southern California's Andrus Gerontology Center. Gatz became director of clinical training in 1984 and a full professor of psychology a year later. At USC, Vern L. Bengtson* has been a primary collaborator. She has been a visiting researcher in the Department of Epidemiology of the Karolinska Institute in Sweden, where she is principal investigator on a major study of dementia in Swedish twins, along with Nancy Pederson of the Karolinska Institute.

Gatz has spent much of her career publishing articles that challenge existing wisdom. In an article (with C. Pearson and M. Fuentes) on "Older Women and Mental Health," in *Social and Psychological Problems of Women: Prevention and Crisis Intervention,* eds. A. U. Rickel et al. (New York: McGraw-Hill, 1983), 273–99, for instance, Gatz attacked a series of myths of aging. In a similar vein, she gathered data to suggest that older people should not be considered depressed just because younger people think that their conditions warrant that feeling. See M. Gatz and M-L. Hurwicz, "Are Old People More Depressed?'' *Psychology and Aging,* 5 (1990): 285–90. Again in a revisionist vein, her article (with M. Karel and B. Wolkenstein), ''Survey of Providers of Psychological Services to Older Adults,'' *Professional Psychology,* 22 (1991): 413–15, suggests that there may be more people willing to serve older adults than is generally supposed. In a 1994 ''Forum'' in *The Gerontologist,* 34: 251–55, Gatz and associates argued that understanding Alzheimer's Disease entailed ''Not Just a Search for the Gene.''

Gatz has also been interested in showing the influence of the larger context on some specific problem. In an article on caregiving families for the third edition of the *Handbook of the Psychology of Aging,* eds. James E. Birren* and K. Warner Schaie* (New York: Academic Press, 1990), she, Bengtson and M. Blum went beyond the perspective of the primary caregivers to consider the family network and the recipients' viewpoints. This approach is emblematic of Gatz's concern to point out conceptual parallels between lifespan developmental theory and community psychology tenets that form a common basis about intervention with older adults. For later examples, see F. B. Tyler, M. Gatz and K. Kennan, ''A Constructivist Analysis of the Rotter I-E Scale,'' *Journal of Personality,* 47 (1979): 11–35; and (with Bob Knight and Miriam Kelly), ''Psychotherapy and the Older Adult'' in *History of Psychotherapy,* ed. D. K. Freeheim (Washington, D.C.: American Psychological Association, 1993), 528–51. She also has tried to point out commonalities in mechanisms of change that apply to adults and to psychological intervention with older adults. It is not surprising, then, that Gatz is a charter fellow and founding member of the American Psychological Society, which emphasizes clinical science, and is active in four divisions of the American Psychological Association as well as the Gerontological Society.

Gatz began a six-year term as associate editor of *Psychology and Aging* in 1992.

DONALD E. GELFAND. Donald E. Gelfand was born in New York in 1943. His interest in a research career was sparked by Kurt and Gladys Lang at Queens College, City University of New York, where he earned his B.A. in political science in 1965. He first became interested in aging during his graduate work at Washington University, where he earned his Ph.D. in 1969. Robert J. Havighurst,* visiting on campus, taught the first aging course Gelfand took. Irwin Sanders became ''the model of what a scholar and human being should strive to become.'' After serving as a faculty member in the Department of Sociology at Boston University, where he co-directed the Community Sociology Training Program, Gelfand served as senior research associate (1979–1980) of the Intergenerational Service-Learning Project at the National Council on the Aging. In 1982, he held a Fulbright for research on mental health and aging in Germany, and in 1990, a Visiting Research Fellowship at Australian National University.

Gelfand's major contribution to the advancement of gerontology has been to further the growth of the subfield of ethnicity and aging. His own research has focused primarily on Italians, Russian Jews, Salvadorans, Native Americans, and African Americans. Two collections of readings have been widely used in undergraduate and graduate-level courses: *Ethnicity and Aging,* eds. Donald Gelfand and Alfred Kutzik (New York: Springer, 1979); and *Ethnic Dimensions of Aging,* eds. Donald Gelfand and Charles Barresi* (New York: Springer, 1987). Gelfand's own *Aging: The Ethnic Factor* (Boston: Little, Brown, 1982) offered a judicious overview of the field just as anthropologists were beginning to organize cross-national ethnographic studies. A new book, *Aging and Ethnicity* (New York: Springer, 1994) adds a stronger theoretical base and a focus on the impact of ethnicity on services.

With Barbara W. K. Yee of the University of Texas, Gelfand contributed an article on ''The Influence of Immigration, Migration, and Acculturation on the Fabric of Aging in America,'' *Generations,* 15 (Fall/Winter 1991): 7–11, which argued that future cohorts of minority elders will be less likely to have common immigration histories, socialization patterns, and cultural values than was true earlier in the century.

Perhaps because he spent much of his career at the University of Maryland's School of Social Work, Gelfand has been keenly interested in bridging the gap between basic and applied gerontology. Thus, with the assistance of Jules Berman, he wrote *The Aging Network: Programs and Services,* 4th edn. (New York: Springer, 1993). This work introduces students and service providers to the basic range of income-maintenance, health care, and senior center programs available for older Americans.

While at the University of Maryland, Gelfand also served as associate director of the National Policy Center on Women and Aging. In 1992, he joined the Institute of Gerontology at Detroit's Wayne State University. In 1994, he was appointed chairman of the Sociology Department* at Wayne State University. His research now extends to attitudinal and behavioral differences in cancer screening utilization by older whites and African Americans.

LINDA K. GEORGE. Linda K. George was born in Wadsworth, Ohio, in 1947. She received her B.A. in sociology in 1969 from Miami University in Ohio, where she was elected to Phi Beta Kappa and Sigma Xi. After serving as a case worker in Children's Protective Services in nearby Hamilton, George returned to Miami, where she earned her M.A. in sociology in 1972. Robert C. Atchley* and Mildred M. Selzer* were key figures in this formative stage of her development. Atchley piqued her interest in aging. Issues of role loss and their social-psychological consequences were topics that initially attracted her attention. After spending the 1972–1973 academic year as an instructor in sociology, George moved to Duke University to pursue her doctoral studies. She has remained there ever since.

George earned her Ph.D. in sociology in 1975, and then spent the next two years as a postdoctoral fellow in Duke's Center for the Study of Aging. Her mentor was George Maddox,* who continues to be one of her role models.

(Matilda White Riley* is another.) Beginning her career as a lecturer in the Department of Physical Therapy in the Medical Center, George became associate director for social and behavioral programs in the Center for the Study of Aging and Human Development (1984 to the present), and in 1986, a professor of medical sociology in the Department of Psychiatry and a professor of sociology. (She also has an adjunct appointment in psychology.) In 1988, she became co-director of the Psychiatric Epidemiology and Mental Health Services Research Program in Duke's Department of Psychiatry.

Sociologists who work in first-rate medical centers are expected to raise money for their research and to support their students. George is a master of the art. Her first support came from AARP's Andrus Foundation; she received $15,000 in 1977 to study the meaning and measurement of the well-being of older people. By the early 1980s, she was winning and then renewing awards in six figures from the Administration on Aging to create a data archive and survey laboratory for the study of aging and adult development. The National Institute on Aging and the National Institute of Mental Health have lately been granting her multiyear, multimillion-dollar funding to support her work in psychiatric epidemiology, her demographic surveys of North Carolina's elderly, and her work on geriatric depression. The NIA recently renewed the Duke project on "established populations for epidemiologic studies of the elderly" through 1997 for $4.9 million.

George owes part of her success to her high energy level and the competitive but collegial research environment at Duke. But she has won the admiration of her peers by her ability to produce books and articles that integrate the state of the art in a specific aspect of the field. Her efforts at synthesis—such as "Social Structure, Social Processes, and Social Psychological States," in the *Handbook of Aging and the Social Sciences,* 3rd edn., eds. Robert H. Binstock* and Linda K. George (New York: Academic Press, 1990)—are more frequently cited than most of her empirical studies. George has performed this kind of task in other domains, notably life satisfaction and subjective well-being, self-concept and self-esteem, role transitions, models of change in adulthood, stress and social support, and caregiver well-being. See, for instance, her *Role Transitions in Later Life* (Monterey, Calif.: Brooks/Cole, 1980).

Her most significant conceptual contribution thus far has been to encourage her colleagues to think in terms of "caregiver well-being" rather than "caregiver burden." With L. P. Gwyther, in "Caregiver Well-Being: A Multidimensional Examination of Family Caregivers of Demented Adults," *The Gerontologist,* 26 (1986): 253–59, George empirically documented various relationships of caregiver well-being to caregiving characteristics. She received more than 200 requests for reprints of this article. Although it has had less impact on the field, George considers another of her essays to be her most creative contribution: "Caregiver Burden: Conflict Between Norms of Reciprocity and Solidarity," in *Elder Abuse in the Family,* eds. K. Pillemer and R. Wolf (Dover, Mass.: Auburn House, 1986). This essay is more qualitative in thrust, and it is in a collection of essays whose topic is peripheral to the work of most social scientists working in gerontology.

Increasingly, George has been concentrating on the substantial role played by social factors in the etiology, course, and treatment of physical and mental illnesses in late life. She has been examining illness and its sequelae as biopsychosocial phenomena, making this argument to biomedical investigators who often neglect or disparage the role of social factors in illness. With Dan G. Blazer* and two other colleagues, for instance, she wrote "Social Support and the Outcome of Major Depression," which appeared in the *British Journal of Psychiatry,* 154 (1989): 478–85; and "Social Factors and the Onset and Outcome of Depression," in *Aging, Health Behaviors, and Health Outcomes,* eds. K. Warner Schaie,* James S. House, and Dan G. Blazer (Hillsdale, N.J.: Lawrence Erlbaum Associates, 1992).

It is not surprising that George has held key leadership positions. She was president of the Gerontological Society (1993–1994), and has almost continuously been on the editorial board of the Social Science Section of the *Journal of Gerontology* since the early 1980s. She has also been on the editorial board of the *Journal of Aging and Health* (1988–1992) and a guest editor of *Generations.* She served on study sections for the Administration on Aging, the National Institute on Aging, and the National Institute of Mental Health, as well as the review panel for the Social Sciences and Humanities Research Council of Canada and state-level bodies in Ohio and North Carolina. She also has been an adviser to the Boettner Institute of Financial Gerontology.

ROSE CAMPBELL GIBSON. Rose Campbell Gibson was born in Detroit, Michigan. She majored in mathematics at Wayne State University, receiving her B.A. *magna cum laude,* and completed requirements for medical school admission. After earning her Ph.D. in 1977 at the University of Michigan, she completed a postdoctoral fellowship in statistics at Ann Arbor (1980–1982), specializing in survey research design and methodology. Gibson was attracted to gerontological research by past work on black aging, which she judged "problem-centered and somewhat atheoretical." She nonetheless considered this valuable work that "needed building on." In her efforts to transform minority aging research into a body of integrated knowledge, Gibson has advanced the field of gerontology as a whole.

Gibson has become a major figure in stating the major theoretical issues to be pursued in minority group aging, identifying some of the basic constructs for the subfield, and producing the research paradigms to be revised and clarified through systematic processes of replication. In her state-of-the-art critique of what needs to be done, "Minority Aging Research: Opportunity and Challenge," *Journal of Gerontology,* 44 (1989): S2–S3, for instance, Gibson urged her colleagues to move away from minority-majority group comparisons and single-causation studies. "The challenge before us today is . . . a greater orientation toward theory, more within and between minority group comparisons, and more openness to interpretations of minorities characteristics and strengths,'' she declared. ''Other issues that need attention are distinctions among race, ethnicity and minority-group status; and discussions in manuscripts of limitations of designs, samples, data collection methods, and sources of systematic bias.''

Gibson's concern about methodological issues reflects her own rigorous training and reputation for designing good surveys at Michigan's renowned Institute for Social Research, where she serves as a faculty associate. She also is a faculty associate at Michigan's Institute of Gerontology and a professor in the School of Social Work, where she teaches ''Research Methods'' and ''The Sociology of Aging.'' Her concern over methodological issues is particularly evident in her studies on the health of older African Americans.

Gibson introduced into the gerontological literature evidence that advancing age is more closely associated with death in the older white than older black population. The black-white disparity in health and functioning narrows with age, and this gap is commensurate with the racial gap in mortality. See Rose Gibson, ''The Age-by-Race Gap in Health and Mortality in the Older Population,'' *The Gerontologist*, 34 (1994): 1994.

By taking a life-course approach in her analyses and in her books, *Worlds of Difference: Inequality in the Aging Experience* (with sociologist Eleanor Stoller); *Aging and the Life Course* (Gibson and Stoller); *Health in Black America* (Gibson and Jackson); and in her monograph, *Blacks in an Aging Society*, Gibson has sensitized her colleagues to ways in which unique life experiences shape differently the aging of African Americans. Her contributions to the literature on the life course of black Americans also are evident in her numerous articles and chapters that appear in volumes such as the *Handbook of the Psychology of Aging*, the *Journals of Gerontology*, the *Milbank Quarterly*, the *Annals of Political and Social Research*, and the *Journal of Health and Aging*.

The unique life experiences of older blacks also shape their responses in survey research in a way that is different from the responses of older whites. Gibson found that subjective interpretations of health status are less valid for black than for white elderly, due to a greater infiltration of blacks' non-health concerns. Her model of race differences in the way blacks and whites report their health in national surveys is now used as a foundation for race comparative health research. See Gibson's ''Race and the Self-Reported Health of Elderly Persons,'' *Journal of Gerontology*, 46 (1991). Similarly, the disability reports of older black Americans are more contaminated by economic need for disability pay. See Rose Gibson, ''The Subjective Retirement of Black Americans,'' *The Journal of Gerontology*, 46 (1991): S204–S210. Gibson also introduced the concept of the ''unretired-retired'' into the gerontological literature to refer to those blacks who seem too young to be considered (or to view themselves) as retired, yet who are effectively out of the labor force because of discrimination and disability. This group, effectively screened out of most retirement surveys, is now being included in research.

Although Gibson is adept at powerful quantitative analyses, she is also quite capable of translating her statistical models into ordinary language to explain similarities and differences in the ways that older blacks and whites interpret their lives and experience changes in health status over the life course. A member of the Carnegie Corporation Aging Society Project, where she worked closely with W. Andrew Achenbaum (whom she considers a role model), Gibson made certain that minority issues were not marginalized. At the same time she alerted the group to ways in which population aging was threatening minority family support networks, and in the process, the well-being of the black elderly.

Because of her strengths as a researcher and her ability to grasp the big picture, Gibson was appointed editor-in-chief of *The Gerontologist* in 1993. She is listed in *Who's Who of American Women* and *Who's Who in the Midwest.*

LEO GITMAN. Leo Gitman was born in New York City in 1912. He earned his B.A. from Columbia College in 1933, and his M.D. from the Royal College of Medicine and Surgery in Scotland six years later. In 1942, he was the Stewart Memorial Research Fellow in Endocrinology at the University of Pittsburgh Medical School. During World War II, Gitman served in the Medical Corps. He was an assistant in the research unit of (New York) Metropolitan Hospital after the war.

Gitman then joined the Brookdale Hospital Center in Brooklyn in 1948. He became a senior research associate in 1951, an attending physician in the Department of Medicine in 1960, and chief of the Gerontological Section in 1964. From 1954 to 1960, Gitman also served as medical director and director of the research division of the Hebrew Home and Hospital for the Aged in Brooklyn.

Gitman was very interested in the relationship between aging and endocrinology. In 1967, he compiled and edited *Endocrines and Aging* (Springfield, Ill.: C. C. Thomas, 1968), which communicated findings presented at the seventeenth annual meeting of the Gerontological Society. Gitman's own contribution, which relied heavily on the work of Clive M. McCay,* urged colleagues to move beyond their studies of the physiological effects of urinary secretion. He was particularly interested in the effect of thryroxine and such hormones as insulin and vasopressin, which were thought to transport mechanisms across cell membranes. In 1970, Gitman edited a report on *Research, Training, and Practice in Clinical Medicine of Aging* (New York: S. Karger).

Gitman served as a president of the Gerontological Society in 1963.

BRIAN GRATTON. Brian Gratton received his M.A. (1976) and Ph.D. (1980) from Boston University, where he studied with historians Arnold Offner, Robert Bruce, and Aileen Kraditor. He was first attracted to the field of aging by reading W. Andrew Achenbaum, David Hackett Fischer, and by William Graebner's *A History of Retirement* (New Haven: Yale University Press, 1980). Gratton was particularly impressed by Graebner's interpretation of Social Security as a pivotal event in the history of "modern" old age.

Gratton was a postdoctoral fellow at Case Western Reserve University from 1981 to 1983, where he worked closely with Marie Haug,* a sociologist. His major contributions to the field capitalize on his strengths as a social historian with solid training in quantitative methods. Gratton also has been able to turn his enjoyment of a good intellectual fight into a powerful tool for the revision of prevailing interpretations of old-age history.

In *Urban Elders: Family, Work, and Welfare among Boston's Aged, 1890–1950* (Philadelphia: Temple University Press, 1986), for instance, Gratton provided one of the first case studies of changes in the political, socioeconomic, and demographic status of older men and women living in a highly ethnic, urban-industrial setting during a period of U.S. history that merits far more study. Whereas previous sociologists and historians had suggested that industrialization adversely affected older people, Gratton argued that most older people before 1930 were neither marginal, obsolescent, nor impoverished. Politics (the need to placate Irish working-class voters), not economics, led the Bay State to enact old-age benefits before the enactment of Social Security. In the process, families were protected from covert dependency.

Over the years, Gratton has worked closely with John Myles* and Jill Quadagno.* Like them, he has stressed that attention to *structural* as well as cultural forces is necessary in reconstructing the history of old age. He also shares their interest in the elderly's labor force status and economic well-being. See, for instance, his article with Frances Rotondo, "Industrialization, the Family Economy, and the Economic Status of the Elderly," *Social Science History* (Fall 1991). With Carole Haber,* his collaborator on another case study ("Old Age, Public Welfare and Race," *Journal of Social History,* 20 (1987): 689–910), Gratton tried to make sense of the recent literature on aging and to establish a new research agenda. *Old Age and the Search for Security* (Bloomington, Ind.: Indiana University Press, 1994) divides the social history of the elderly into three eras: preindustrial, industrial, and post-Social Security.

Currently, Gratton is professor of history at Arizona State University.

JILL S. GRIGSBY. Jill Grigsby earned her Sc.B. in applied mathematics from Brown University in 1976, where she was elected to Sigma Xi. There, she worked with Fran Goldscheider. After earning master's degrees in sociology from Brown and Princeton, she earned her Ph.D. from Princeton University in 1983, where she was taught by Ansley Coale. She wrote her dissertation on "the use of contraception for delaying and spacing births in Colombia, Costa Rica, and Korea." The Ansley connection, as well as the interest in population aging expressed by other teachers, attracted Grigsby to the field of aging. Like other demographers, she was greatly influenced by Coale's essay, "How a Population Ages or Grows Younger," and by reading articles by Elaine M. Brody* on parent care and by Alice Rossi on parent-child relations through life.

Postdoctoral opportunities reinforced Grigsby's commitment to research in gerontology. She was a senior research associate at the Policy Center on Aging at Brandeis, where she, Robert H. Binstock,* and T. Leavitt prepared "an analysis of targeting policy options under Title III of the Older Americans Act" for the Administration on Aging. Grigsby also counts as mentors Al Hermalin of the University of Michigan, with whom she worked as a research fellow (1987–1988), and Samuel Preston of the University of Pennsylvania. She was a postdoctoral trainee (1990–1991) at the Gerontology Research Institute of the Andrus Gerontology Center, University of Southern California, where she worked with Eileen Crimmins* and Mark Hayward. Few social science researchers have been so well prepared or well connected to do pathbreaking work in gerontology.

Grigsby is primarily interested in the demographic components of population aging. With S. Jay Olshansky of the University of Chicago, she wrote "The Demographic Components of Population Aging in China," which appeared in the *Journal of Cross-Cultural Gerontology,* 4 (1989): 307–34. She has gained a reputation for her decomposition of population aging by fertility, mortality, and population momentum. See her "Paths for Future Population Aging," *The Gerontologist,* 31 (1991): 195–203, which explains the relationship between demographic transition and population aging. With David Heer, she has also published a textbook for undergraduate use, *Society and Population,* 3rd edn. (Englewood Cliffs, N.J.: Prentice-Hall, 1992), which contains information on aging in several chapters.

Grigsby has been a member of Pomona College's Department of Sociology and Anthropology since 1983. She received an Academic Research Enhancement Award from the National Institute on Aging to study "gender differences in health and longevity" from 1992 to 1994.

JABER F. GUBRIUM. Jaber F. Gubrium earned his M.A. from Michigan State University (1966) and his Ph.D. from Wayne State University (1970). He recalls that Paule Verdet, who was a sociologist at Boston University, was the teacher who first sparked his interest in aging. After spending more than a decade at Marquette University, Gubrium now teaches sociology at the University of Florida.

Cutting across Gubrium's theoretical and empirical work is an enduring aim to make visible the contexts of the aging experience. From an early attempt to resolve some of the conceptual tensions between "activity" and "disengagement" theories (see his *The Myth of the Golden Years: A Socio-Environmental Theory of Aging* (Springfield, Ill.: C. C. Thomas, 1973)) to his heavily descriptive presentation of the multiple worlds of care that affect individual and organizational perspectives in a nursing home (see his *Living and Dying at Murray Manor* (New York: St. Martin's Press, 1975)) and his studies of Alzheimer's Disease (J. F. Gubrium, *Oldertimers and Alzheimer's: The Descriptive Organization of Senility* (Westport, Conn.: JAI Press, 1986)), context has mediated his interpretation of the meaning of life satisfaction, quality of care, strain, person perception, and interpersonal relations. In *Oldertimers and Alzheimer's,* for instance, Gubrium offers fine-grained analyses of conversations and then shows how signs of aging may be assigned "pathological" or "normal" status within alternate frameworks of orientation.

Voice, too, has been a persistent theme in Gubrium's work. In recent ethnographies and narrative accounts, he shows that voice is a concept that cannot, in the final analysis, be relegated to individuals, but must be elaborated to make visible voice's social and organizational contours. See his *Speaking of Life: Horizons of Meaning for Nursing Home Residents* (Hawthorne, N.Y.: Aldine de Gruyter, 1987). His *Mosaic of Care* (New York: Springer, 1991), for instance, uses the concepts of "story," "version," and "local culture" to challenge prevailing "caregiver burden" and "continuum of care" paradigms, thereby showing the social complexity of each individual case.

At the same time, applications and themes have not been limited to the later years. Gubrium has been concerned with the life course as a whole, as a language and framework for constructing human development, stages of experience, maturation, growth, competence, and decline. With his Marquette colleagues James Holstein and David Buckholdt, he outlined a "social constructionist" framework for interpreting change across the life course in *Constructing the Life Course* (Dix Hills, N.Y.: General Hall Press, 1994). Also with James Holstein, Gubrium addressed the ordinary languages and meanings of "family" in relation to family-oriented service organizations; see *What is Family?* (Mountain View, 1990).

Gubrium works with a minimalist understanding of theory; he assiduously limits conceptual elaboration to practice and the ordinary. Empirically, his work, to use Clifford Geertz's apt phrase, is "thickly descriptive." Gubrium makes use of ethnography and narrative to capture the diversity, contradictions, ironies, and fluid categories of aging. He has been advancing such "social constructionism" in a multidisciplinary quarterly he launched in 1987, the *Journal of Aging Studies,* which has quickly become the best qualitative gerontological journal in the United States.

DAVID L. GUTMANN. David L. Gutmann was born on September 17, 1925. He entered the University of Chicago graduate program sponsored through the Committee on Human Development (CHD) at the age of twenty-seven, having performed successfully on the General Education Test and having impressed Bernice L. Neugarten* with his potential. With Neugarten, Gutmann wrote his second article, "Age-Sex Role and Personality in Middle Age: A Thematic Apperception Study," which originally appeared in *Psychological Monographs,* 470 (1958): 1–33, and was reprinted in *Middle Age and Aging,* ed. Bernice L. Neugarten (Chicago: University of Chicago Press, 1968): 58–71.

At the University of Chicago Gutmann placed major emphasis on personality theory and clinical aspects of psychology. On a fellowship from the National Institute of Mental Health, Gutmann began to investigate psychological development in later life. He also completed minor fields in sociology, anthropology, and physiology. Between earning his M.A. in 1956 and his Ph.D. two years later, Gutmann did a pre-doctoral internship in clinical psychology through the Neuro-Psychiatric Institute of the University of Illinois Medical School, Chicago. He also was a research associate in CHD; he investigated psychological developments in late life, with special reference to age-graded patterns of ego defense. Gutmann also served as a postdoctoral fellow in clinical psychology (1958–1959) at the Psychosomatic and Psychiatric Institute at Michael Reese Hospital, Chicago.

After serving as a staff psychologist at Presbyterian-St. Luke's Hospital, Chicago, Gutmann moved to Boston, where he worked from 1960 to 1962 as a staff psychologist at the Massachusetts Mental Health Center in Boston. During this time Gutmann taught sections of courses taught by David Riesman and Erik Erikson, and he conducted a clinical practicum at Harvard. In 1962, Gutmann joined the Department of Psychology at the University of Michigan. He rose through the academic ranks, becoming a full professor in 1970. Gutmann served as a senior staff psychologist in the University's Psychological Clinic for two years; he also maintained a private practice of psychotherapy in Ann Arbor from 1963 to 1976. During the 1974–1975 academic year, Gutmann was a visiting fellow at the Center for Psycho-social Studies in Chicago and held a visiting appointment at the University of Chicago.

In 1964 Gutmann received a Career Development Award from the National Institute of Child Health and Human Development. Over the next decade, this Award supported Gutmann's research on cross-cultural studies of the psychology of aging. This involved collecting interviews and projective data from middle-aged and older Mexican Indian, American Indian, and Israeli Druze subjects of both sexes. Gutmann's analyses attracted attention. See his oft-cited essays, "Aging among the Highland Maya: A Comparative Study," in the *Journal of Personality and Social Psychology,* 7 (1967): 28–35; "The Country of Old Men: Cross-Cultural Studies in the Psychology of Later Life," in *Occasional Papers in Gerontology,* 5 (University of Michigan-Wayne State University: Institute of Gerontology, 1969); "The Premature Gerontocracy: Themes of Aging and Death in the Youth Culture," in *Social Research,* vol. 39 (1972): 416–48; and "Alternatives to Disengagement: Aging among the Highland Druize," in *Culture and Personality,* ed. Robert LeVine (Chicago: Aldine, 1974).

In 1976, Gutmann became professor and chief of the Division of Psychology at Northwestern University's Medical School. He held this position for five years. Concurrently, he was named professor and director of the Older Adult Program, overseeing doctoral and postdoctoral training in clinical geropsychology—responsibilities that he still holds. Since 1980, Gutmann has held a joint appointment as professor in Northwestern's School of Education. He also maintains consultancies at the VA Lakeside Medical Center and the Illinois State Psychiatric Institute, both in Chicago. Since returning to the Windy City, Gutmann has written scientific articles based on his clinical experiences, such as "Psychodynamics of Grandparenthood," which appears in *Grandparenthood:*

Research and Policy Perspectives (Beverly Hills: Sage, 1985). In addition, he explored the psychological dimensions of themes current in public affairs; see, for instance, his "Killers and Consumers: The Terrorist and His Audience," *Social Research,* 45 (1979): 517–26.

Gutmann is probably best known for *Reclaimed Powers: Men and Women in Late Life,* which was published by Basic Books in New York in 1987 and reissued by Northwestern University Press seven years later. In *Reclaimed Powers,* Gutmann summarized his cross-cultural forays in the developmental possibilities of men and women at middle and later paths in their lives. He suggested, based on psychological and anthropological measures, that differences in personality traits and behavioral responses among men and women do begin to narrow with advancing years.

H

CAROLE HABER. Carole Haber received her B.A. *summa cum laude* from Washington University in 1973, where she earned her Phi Beta Kappa key. She earned her Ph.D. in history from the University of Pennsylvania (1979), where she worked with Charles E. Rosenberg, the dean of U.S. medical historians. Her interest in aging arose in the course of her initial forays into medical history. Haber became convinced that the prevailing nineteenth-century model of physical and mental well-being was extremely age-limited. She thus decided to explore what physicians and social scientists thought about the old.

To date, Haber's most significant aging-related concept has been her depiction of the historical development of the medical model of aging in terms of its intellectual roots and its continuing impact upon modern beliefs and practices. In the view of physicians, social scientists, welfare advocates, and businessmen, according to Haber, aging evolved from an accepted stage of life into a disease that requires professional intervention. By the early twentieth century, the old were seemingly trapped by their physiology and psychology. To be elderly was to be deemed both diseased and dependent. Haber developed this argument more fully in a revised version of her dissertation, *Beyond Sixty-Five: The Dilemma of Old Age in America's Past* (New York: Cambridge University Press, 1983). An elegant synopsis of her thesis appears in "From Senescence to Senility: The Transformation of Senile Old Age in the Nineteenth Century," in *International Journal of Aging and Human Development,* 19 (1984): 41–45. Haber tries to situate geriatrics in the culture of medical professions in "Geriatrics: A Speciality in Search of Specialists," in *The Elderly in the Bureaucratic World,* eds.

David D. Van Tassel and Peter N. Stearns (Westport, Conn.: Greenwood Press, 1986), 66–84.

Haber has also tried to challenge gerontologists, especially those who work in the social service arena, to appreciate that old age has a past that predates Social Security and the welfare state apparatus found in most advanced-industrial societies. Her first publication, for instance, highlighted certain age-specific institutional arrangements that existed for widows, spinsters, and old retainers of the urban gentry. See her "Old Folks at Home: The Development of Institutional Care in Nineteenth-Century Philadelphia," *The Pennsylvania Magazine of History and Biography,* 101 (1977): 240–57. She showed the impact of such institutions on public policy in " 'Over the Hill to the Poorhouse': Rhetoric and Reality in the Institutional History of the Elderly," in *Social Structure and Aging: Historical Perspectives,* eds. K. Warner Schaie* and W. Andrew Achenbaum (New York: Springer Publishing, 1993). With Brian Gratton,* her chief collaborator, she offered an invaluable case study of "Old Age, Public Welfare, and Race: The Case of Charleston, South Carolina, 1800–1949," *Journal of Social History,* 20 (1986): 263–79.

Like most historians of aging, Haber relishes the task of revisionism. In her first book, *Beyond Sixty-Five,* she criticized gerontologists, sociologists, and fellow historians David Hackett Fischer and W. Andrew Achenbaum for suggesting that there ever was a period in history in which the elderly were venerated. In her most recent book, *Old Age and the Search for Security* (Bloomington, Ind.: Indiana University Press, 1994), co-written with Brian Gratton, she attacks another fallacy that she thinks is rampant in the literature. Industrialization did not impoverish the elderly, Haber and Gratton argue. Rather, it increased the well-being of the majority and raised expectations about what could be considered "a good old age." Such expectations, in turn, created a broad coalition that supported Social Security and demanded additional old-age entitlements.

DAVID HABER. David Haber's interest in aging was sparked as a graduate student by Maggie Kuhn,* who "made geriatrics come alive." He earned his Ph.D. at the University of Southern California in 1976. Haber worked mainly under Herman Turk in the Department of Sociology, though two members of his dissertation committee, Pauline Ragan (Robinson) and Steven Zarit, were key figures at the time in the Andrus Gerontology Center. Haber cites no mentors or teachers—"much to my disadvantage, I suppose"—but he does consider a fellow USC graduate student, Stephen McConnell, a role model. He has relied on his own instincts and interests, which range from meditation and yoga to exercise, to guide his professional choices. See, for instance, his "Yoga as a Preventive Health Care Program for White and Black Elders: An Explanatory Study" in the *International Journal of Aging and Human Development,* 17 (1983): 169–78; and "Health Promotion to Reduce Blood Pressure Level Among Older Blacks," in *The Gerontologist,* 26 (1986): 118–21.

Part of his dissertation, "Creativity over the Career Course: An Adult So-

150   PAUL A. HABER

cialization Perspective,'' appeared as ''The Broadening of Perspective over the
Career Course: An Exploratory Study of Self-Reported Creative Research
Acts,'' in the *International Journal of Aging and Human Development,* 9 (1978–
79): 305–12. There, Haber analyzed the responses of 157 full professors of
sociology, and reported that most continued to find satisfaction in their careers,
though the sources of satisfaction were shaped by the stages of their career.
While in retrospect he considers this to have been an interesting line of research,
Haber's most significant work has been to emphasize the importance to older
Americans of mutual health groups and other types of empowering for promoting health and for learning about coping with chronic illness. See his *Health
Care for an Aging Society* (New York: Hemisphere Publishing, 1989).

Convinced that older people must take an active, ongoing responsibility for
their own well-being, Haber has shown that the elderly may benefit as much, if
not more, from giving support in mutual-help groups than from receiving assistance. See his ''Promoting Mutual Help Groups among Older Persons,'' *The
Gerontologist,* 23 (1983): 251–53. Haber has encouraged professionals to play
an active role in mutual-help groups and other modalities for empowering clients. See ''A Socio-Behavioral Health Promotion Intervention with Older
Adults,'' *Behavior, Health, and Aging,* 3 (1993): 73–85. To this end, he has
initiated corporate eldercare programs, church-based support groups, and a variety of health promotions efforts in senior centers, congregate housing projects,
religious institutions, and nursing homes. In his recent book, *Health Promotion
and Aging* (New York: Springer Publishing, 1994), Haber provides a conceptually integrated, research-based and pragmatic approach to both individual and
societal health promotion and disease prevention in older adults.

After holding positions at the University of South Florida, the University of
the District of Columbia, and Creighton University Medical School (where he
was director of the Creighton Center for Health Aging), Haber is now in the
School of Allied Health Sciences at the University of Texas Medical Branch,
Galveston.

PAUL A. HABER. Paul A. Haber was born in 1920. He received his B.A. at
the University of Texas in 1941, and M.A. at Columbia University in 1942, and
his M.D. from the University of Texas in 1949. He received an M.S. from
George Washington University in 1968. Paul Haber, then deputy assistant chief
medical director in the VA's Central Office, was chiefly responsible for the
development of the Geriatric Research, Education, and Clinical Centers
(GRECCs) in the Department of Veterans Affairs. These GRECCs, in turn, have
had a substantial impact on the way geriatric medicine has developed and health
care for the elderly is delivered in the United States.

Before Congress enacted Medicare, Medicaid, or the Older Americans Act in
1965, the VA was trying to effect a mix in the continuum of long-term care.
Among other things, the VA in 1964 established a ''satellite laboratory aging
program'' to attract talented medical researchers to its facilities. In the early

1970s, Haber tried to establish a means to offer continuity of care to older veterans. As a result of Public Law 88-450 (1973), Congress mandated that the VA create 2,000 nursing home care beds over the next twelve months. Under Haber's guidance, the VA met this challenge, providing long-term hospital care, nursing home care, and outpatient geriatric services. Since there were not enough beds in the existing system, the VA established a contract community nursing home program as well as a program to help state-level veterans' bureaus construct homes and provide their own care for older veterans. In due course, domiciliaries, hospices, respite, and adult day health care programs were added.

Capping all of this were the GRECCs, which provided the research milieu with a broad educational component necessary to develop and test the actual systems of care. Haber was assisted in this by working with Eugene Towbin, who was chief of the staff of the Little Rock VA Hospital and associate dean of the University of Arkansas Medical School. Towbin insisted that a strong clinical arm also was necessary, and his recommendation quickly bore fruit. Geriatric Evaluation Units (GEUs) were developed at the Little Rock and Sepulveda VA Medical Centers; researchers in these facilities provided specialized diagnoses and ways to manage the elderly's conditions.

The impact of the GRECCs and GEUs can be gauged by the number of board-certified geriatricians who received their training in VA facilities. Roughly a quarter to a third of all articles in the *Journal of the American Geriatrics Society* are submitted by investigators with affiliations to one of the nation's GRECCs.

Haber himself contributed to the scholarly literature. In "Technology and Aging," *The Gerontologist*, 26 (1986): 350–57, he discussed the application of ecological and health care technology to the vision and hearing problems of the elderly, as well as their musculoskeletal disabilities, loss of perception, and dementia. An account of his VA experience appears in "Extended Care: The VA's Program for the Aging," *Generations*, 9 (1985): 16–18. There, Haber discusses the community and nursing home options, hospital-based home care, domiciliary care, and personal care in a rehabilitation-oriented, patient-centered program.

Haber was a member of the National Advisory Council that launched the National Institute on Aging; he was to help bring the VA's perspective to bear. The Gerontological Society awarded him the Donald Kent Award, and the administrator of Veterans Affairs gave Haber the Exceptional Service Award for his work in creating the system's long-term care system.

G. STANLEY HALL. Granville Stanley Hall was born in Ashfield, Massachusetts, in 1846. He earned his B.A. from Williams College in 1867. He then studied at Union Theological Seminary and at universities in Berlin, Bonn, and Heidelberg, before earning his Ph.D. at Harvard University in 1878. He taught at Antioch College (1872–1876), at Harvard, and occasionally at Williams for the next five years, and then at the Johns Hopkins University (1882–1888). In

1888, he became professor of psychology and founding president of Clark University, titles he held until 1920.

Hall is one of the founding figures of U.S. psychology. He established and served as first president of the American Psychological Association (1891). Renowned for his work on educational psychology, psychological testing, and child development, Hall organized the conference that brought Sigmund Freud to the United States for his first and only visit. Hall's two-volume study of *Adolescence* (New York: D. Appelton's Sons, 1904) remains a classic in the field. Hall was the founding editor of the *American Journal of Psychology*. He launched three other scholarly journals: *Pedagogical Seminar; American Journal of Religion, Psychology, and Education;* and the *Journal of Applied Psychology.*

At the age of 78, Hall published *Senescence: The Second Half of Life* (New York: D. Appelton's Sons, 1922). Hall used historical, medical, literary, biological, physiological, and behavioral evidence in an effort to prove that older people had resources that were hitherto underappreciated. "Intelligent and well-conserved senectitude has very important social and anthropological functions in the world, not hitherto utilized or even recognized," he wrote. Although Hall may have exaggerated the novelty of his suggestion, *Senescence* is a benchmark in the history of U.S. gerontology because it was published by a distinguished scientist whose productive years just preceded the first wave of interest of a rising generation of scholars in gauging continuities and changes in personality development over the life course and in measuring declines in cognitive capacities and functioning.

After publishing an autobiographical review, *Life and Confessions of a Psychologist,* in 1923, G. Stanley Hall died a year later in Worcester.

JEFFREY B. HALTER. After two undergraduate years at the University of Minnesota, Jeffrey B. Halter entered the university's medical school. He completed his B.A. in 1966, graduating Phi Beta Kappa and *magna cum laude,* as well as a B.S., and finally his medical degree in 1969. He interned and completed a residency in internal medicine at Harbor General Hospital of Torrance, California, and UCLA Medical School, as well as a residency at the University of Washington School of Medicine in Seattle, which he completed in 1974. Halter became board-certified in internal medicine in 1974, later adding a subspeciality in endocrinology and metabolism (1977). He also served as a physician and surgeon for the U.S. Public Health Service from 1971 until 1973.

From 1975 until 1977, Halter was a fellow at the Division of Metabolism, Endocrinology and Gerontology at the University of Washington and its affiliated Veterans Affairs Medical Center. He remained at Washington until 1984, rising steadily through the ranks. He became an associate professor at the medical school in 1981, and served as the chief of the gerontology section at the VA medical center during 1983 and 1984. He then moved to the University of Michigan, where he became professor of internal medicine and the medical director of the University of Michigan's Institute of Gerontology. In 1987 he was named director of a Geriatrics Center, newly created by the University of Michigan Medical Center. At the Ann Arbor VA Medical Center, he directs a GRECC that was established in 1989.

Halter's most important gerontological research has been his long-term focus on diabetes. The author of more than 200 peer-reviewed articles and book chapters, his most recent work has been in the area of primary research. See, for example, his "Aging and Insulin Resistance: Role of Blood Pressure and Sympathetic Nervous System Activity," *Journal of Gerontology: Medical Sciences*, 48 (1993): M237–M243; and L. A. Morrow, G. S. Morganroth, W. H. Herman, R. N. Bergman, and J. B. Halter, "Effects of Epinephrine on Insulin Secretion and Action in Humans: Interaction with Aging," *Diabetes*, 42 (1993): 307–15.

Halter is one of the editors of the third edition of *Principles of Geriatric Medicine and Gerontology* (New York: McGraw-Hill, 1993). He has received major funding from the National Institute on Aging, the National Institute of Diabetes, Digestive and Kidney Diseases, the John A. Hartford Foundation, Kellogg Foundation, and the Department of Veterans Affairs, among other agencies. He is a member of the board of directors of the American Geriatrics Society and served as chairman of the Clinical Medical Section of the GSA. He has also served as a consultant to the Commonwealth Fund, and Brookdale Foundation, and on several NIH and VA study sections. He is listed in the 1994 edition of *Best Doctors in America*.

CHARLENE A. HARRINGTON. Charlene Harrington earned her B.S. and nursing degrees from the University of Kansas in 1963. She earned an M.A. in community health nursing in 1968 and her Ph.D. in sociology and higher education from the University of California, Berkeley, in 1975. For the next year, she was the director of the California State Licensing and Certification in the Department of Health. Then Harrington served as an assistant to the director of the department. From 1978 to 1980, she was executive director of the Golden Empire Health Systems Agency in Sacramento.

In 1980, Harrington joined the Institute for Health and Aging in the School of Nursing at the University of California, San Francisco. A year later, she became associate director of the institute and a faculty member in the Department of Social and Behavioral Sciences. To these responsibilities were added, in 1989, appointments as a professor and vice chairwoman. In 1993, she became chairwoman of the department.

Harrington's primary mentors and collaborators have been Carroll L. Estes* and Robert J. Newcomer,* her colleagues at the Institute for Health and Aging. In addition to their grant proposals and peer-reviewed articles, the three published *Long Term Care of the Elderly: Public Policy Issues* (Beverly Hills, Calif.: Sage Publications, 1985).

Probably because of her government experience, Harrington has a strong interest in nursing home quality. She has been especially insightful in preparing empirical research that focuses on state policies related to the utilization and expenditures of nursing homes and home care. For the past fourteen years, she has studied long-term care policies and published many articles. See, for instance, C. Harrington, S. Preston, L. Grant, and J. H. Swan, "Trends in Nursing Home Bed Capacity in the States," *Health Affairs,* 11 (1992): 170–80. Harrington was co-principal investigator with Robert Newcomer on the National Evaluation of the Social Health Maintenance Organization Demonstration Projects, financed by the Health Care Financing Administration, from 1985 to 1991. She has reported some of her findings in an article with Robert J. Newcomer, "Social Health Maintenance Organizations' Service Use and Costs," *Health Care Financing Review,* 12 (1991); and C. Harrington, C. M. Lynch, and R. J. Newcomer, "Medical Services in Social Health Maintenance Organization," *The Gerontologist,* 33 (1993): 790–800. In 1994, she and Robert Newcomer began providing technical assistance in the development of the second generation S/HMOs sponsored by the Health Care Financing Administration along with Robert L. Kane* and colleagues at the University of Minnesota.

Harrington served as a member of the Institute of Medicine's Committee on Nursing Home Regulation, whose 1986 report led to congressional enactment of the Nursing Home Reform Act of 1987. Since that time, she has been studying nursing home quality and regulatory issues, and is conducting a small study of nursing home quality regulation across states. She is also working on a study of AIDS caregivers with Leonard Pearlin.

Harrington uses a political economy approach to her research on aging. She likes to focus on public policies and their effects on cost, access, and quality of care. In this area, Harrington has looked at the market for long-term care services and for health maintenance organizations.

RAYMOND HARRIS. Raymond Harris was born in Albany, New York, in 1919. He earned his B.A. from Cornell University in 1940 and his M.D. from Albany Medical College three years later. Harris was an intern at the Metropolitan Hospital in New York (1943–1944) and did his residency as well as a fellowship in cardiovascular disease at Michael Reese Hospital in Chicago (1944–1949).

From 1950 until his death, Harris was an attending cardiologist and chief of cardiovascular medicine at St. Peter's Hospital in Albany. In 1950, he also became an assistant medical director of the Ann Lee Home and Hospital, which primarily cared for senior citizens. In 1969, he accepted appointments as a clinical associate professor of medicine at Albany Medical College and as an attending cardiologist at the Albany Medical Center Hospital.

Harris's interest in aging arose from his training and professional experiences. He focused on cardiovascular diseases and senescence as well as non-invasive graphic recordings in cardiovascular diseases. In an op-ed piece, "Geriatric Cardiac Intervention," *The Gerontologist,* 7 (1967): 82, 141, Harris challenged conventional wisdom and emphasized that older persons suffering from heart disease should and could be restored to their best functional capacity. To accomplish this objective, he recognized on the basis of programs conducted by the Cardiac Rehabilitation Committee of the New York State Heart Assembly, would require indoctrinating professional and non-professionals alike and in acquainting them with the community resources at their disposal as well as a better understanding of the aging process.

Harris also wrote more general pieces. In "Maintaining the Geriatric Patient's Identity," *New York Journal of Medicine,* 75 (1975): 1252–55, Harris discussed the interpersonal and professional relations between patient and physician in the context of family dynamics and the health care setting. He also stressed the importance of workers in fostering friendships in institutionalized settings, so as to prevent mental deterioration.

Harris served as vice president of the Gerontological Society in 1968. A year later he founded the Center for the Study of Aging in Albany.

A. BAIRD HASTINGS. A. Baird Hastings was born in Bellevue, Kentucky, in 1895. He earned his B.S. from the University of Michigan in 1917; the school bestowed an honorary Sc.D. upon him in 1941. Hastings earned his Ph.D. from Columbia in 1921, while serving as a chemist with the U.S. Public Health Service.

After working at the Rockefeller Institute (1921–1926), the University of Chicago (1926–1928), and as a professor of biochemistry at the Lasker Foundation for Medical Research (1928–1935), Hastings joined the faculty of Harvard University. There, until 1959, he served as Hamilton Kuhn Professor of Biological Chemistry. As one of the pre-eminent researchers of his day, Hastings is best known for his research on the physiology of fatigue (the eighth edition of a book by that title was issued in 1949), the use of isotopes as biochemical tracers, and biological oxidations. Hastings served as editor of the *Journal of Biological Chemistry* from 1941 to 1959 and was closely affiliated with the Brookhaven National Laboratory.

Hastings's interest in research on aging did much to give the fledgling field credibility. He supported Nathan W. Shock's* appointment to the Gerontology Research Center in 1941. With Oliver Lowry, he published "Histochemical Changes in Aging" in the second edition of *Problems of Ageing,* ed. Edmund V. Cowdry* (Baltimore: Williams and Wilkins, 1942), 728–55. Elaborations of this research, as it affected skeletal functioning, appeared in the *Journal of Biological Chemistry.* With Lowry and Clive M. McCay,* Hastings discussed "Histochemical Changes Associated with Aging: Liver, Brain, and Kidney in the Rat" in the first volume of the *Journal of Gerontology* (1946): 345–57. As a member of the National Advisory Cancer Council (1943–1946) and of the scientific advisory committee of the Nutrition Foundation (1947–1961) as well as various advisory committees of the Public Health Service, he supported work in gerontology. He served on the national advisory committee for the 1971 White House Conference on Aging.

After retiring from Harvard, Hastings headed a laboratory for metabolic research at the Scripps Clinical and Research Foundation in La Jolla (1959–1966), and then served as an emeritus member until his death in 1987.

MARIE HAUG. A 1935 Vassar *cum laude* graduate, Marie Haug received her Ph.D. in sociology in 1968, at the age of fifty-four, from Case Western Reserve University. Her major teacher was Marvin B. Sussman.* Haug's interest in aging arose from her prior research on physician authority in relationships with patients, authority that seemed to have begun eroding in the 1960s in the United States and abroad. Haug noted that older patients were more willing than younger ones to accept the physicians' power. Realizing that the area was understudied, she decided to investigate why elderly patients may have special problems in dealing with doctors. With Amasa Ford, a geriatrician at Case Western, as a colleague, Haug organized a symposium in 1979, the proceedings of which were published as *Elderly Patients and Their Doctors* (New York: Springer, 1981). Her insights were reported in "Doctor-Patient Relationships and the Older Patient," *Journal of Gerontology,* 34 (1979): 852–60.

Later, with Marcia G. Ory,* she explored the ways that demographic and psychological characteristics of doctors and patients affect power relationships between them. See Haug and Ory, "Issues in Elderly Patient-Provider Interactions," *Research on Aging,* 9 (1987): 3–44. In exploring why people avoid using a doctor and engage in self-care, she has done research on this phenomenon in the United States and Japan (Haug et al., *Social Science and Medicine,* 33 (1991): 1011–22. Currently, she is studying, in her NIA MERIT award project, how elderly people who note a bodily change may decide that it represents an illness ("Stresses, Strains and Elderly Physical Health"). She will be publishing a paper (in 1995) on the "Effects of Physician/Elder Patient Characteristics on Health Communication."

Haug's future research plans, from now to the year 2000, focus on what she calls "the hidden patient." This concerns the role of the physician of an elderly patient in attending to the needs of that patient's caregiver(s), an unstudied feature of the stress-support-health paradigm.

BETTY J. HAVENS. Betty J. Havens, born in Omaha in 1936, earned her B.A. in psychology and sociology from Milwaukee Downer College in 1958. Her interest in aging preceded her formal schooling. A close relationship with her grandfather nurtured her "fascination with the wisdom and knowledge of my elders." Havens, in fact, had only one course with "gerontology" in the title, which she took with Vivian Wood. She has spent most of her career introducing her interest in aging-related research and program development related to aging and health care into "traditional" educational and policy niches, which made every course she took a gerontology course and every policy sensitive to aging.

Havens spent four years as a social worker in Winnipeg's Norquay Neighbourhood House. Returning to Milwaukee from 1962 to 1971, Havens worked as a program coordinator in the Convent Hill Housing Project for senior citizens,

as a psychometric technician, and an instructor in Milwaukee Junior College
and Adult High School, among other things, as she pursued graduate work. She
earned her M.A. in sociology from the University of Wisconsin-Milwaukee in
1965. From 1968 to 1971, Havens was the instructional resources coordinator
at the Milwaukee Area Technical College. Moving back to Winnipeg, she was
initially self-employed, working as a consultant on research methodology.

In 1972, Havens became director of research for the Department of Health
and Social Development in the Province of Manitoba, a position she held for
the next decade. In this capacity, she developed and began to maintain what
have come to be known as the "Aging in Manitoba" data sets, which now
include almost twenty-five years of data on more than 9,000 older Manitobans.
This longitudinal data base is widely recognized as one of the most scientifically
rigorous and comprehensive sources of demographic, socioeconomic, and psychosocial data on the needs and health of aging persons. The information has
been analyzed by many researchers, policymakers, and program developers.

Havens was instrumental in creating "the Manitoba Model of Continuing
Care." See, for instance, E. Thompson and B. Havens, *Aging in Manitoba: A
Study of the Needs of the Elderly and Resources Available to Meet Needs,* 9
vols. (Manitoba Health and Social Development, 1977); Ellen Winston and
Betty Havens, *Aging in North America* (Washington, D.C.: National Council on
the Aging, 1982); and Eloise Rathbone-McCuan* and Betty Havens, *North
American Elders* (Westport, Conn.: Greenwood Press, 1988). In analyzing the
data she had begun to gather in 1971, Havens became struck by the notion of
"mirror images," in the ways that the needs of older persons were defined and
the ability of resources to fulfill those needs.

Over time, Havens has been using her Manitoba data base to clarify other
concepts in the gerontological literature. For instance, she reminds demographers
and sociologists that "living alone" should not be interpreted as "loneliness"
in the sense that psychologists might use the term. She also emphasizes that
"disposable income" is not the same thing as "discretionary income," especially for retirees. Thus, Havens plays an important role in bridging basic and
applied research. See N. P. Roos, E. Shapiro, and B. Havens, "Aging with
Limited Resources: What Should We Really Be Worried about?" in *Aging with
Limited Health Resources* (Ottawa: Economic Council of Canada, 1987). In
addition to helping to train rising Canadian stars such as Neena Lane Chappell*
and John Myles,* Havens has also found an intellectual home interacting with
members of the (U.S.) Midwest Council for Social Research on Aging. See Betty
Havens, "Individual Needs and Community Resources" in *Research Instruments in Social Gerontology,* 3, eds. David J. Mangen and Warren A. Peterson
(Minneapolis: University of Minnesota Press, 1984).

In 1982, Haven was appointed provincial gerontologist of Manitoba, which
made her a major liaison between government, voluntary agencies, senior citizens' organizations, and individuals in meeting the needs and concerns of Manitoba's aging population. A founding member of the Canadian Association on

Gerontology, Havens served as president from 1979 to 1983; she is also a fellow of the Gerontological Society of America. Havens has also held prominent offices in the International Association on Gerontology and both the International and the American Sociological Association. In 1991, she became assistant deputy minister of the provincial Continuing Care Programs Division.

In 1994, she received a D.Litt. from the University of Waterloo and returned to academia on a full-time basis as professor in community health sciences, University of Manitoba with a Visiting Research Fellowship from Statistics Canada. In this capacity she continued to elaborate issues relevant to sample mortality and the use of large data bases especially related to longitudinal research questions and secondary analyses. She is evaluating techniques to enable national surveys and provincial survey and administrative data to better inform researchers and policymakers through mutual interaction across jurisdiction and data sources.

Havens has also served as a consultant for the United Nations, the World Health Organization, and the International Institute on Aging in Malta.

ROBERT J. HAVIGHURST. Robert James Havighurst was born in DePere, Wisconsin, in 1900. The grandson of a distinguished German Methodist minister and the son of a history professor at Lawrence College, Havighurst attended public schools in Wisconsin and Illinois before taking his B.A. at Ohio Wesleyan University in 1921. Three years later, he earned his Ph.D. in chemistry from Ohio State University and then was a postdoctoral fellow in physics, on a National Research Council fellowship, at Harvard University from 1924 to 1926.

After a promising start as an assistant professor of chemistry at Miami University (1927–1928) and as an assistant professor of physics at the University of Wisconsin (1928–1932) Havighurst made the first of several career shifts. After four years of serving as an adviser in the University of Wisconsin's Experimental College (established by Alexander Meikeljohn), Havighurst's interest in education grew. He accepted an appointment as an associate professor of science education at Ohio State (1932–1934). He then spent the rest of the decade working for the Rockefeller Foundation, supporting innovative general education programs at the secondary and college levels. There he worked directly with Lawrence K. Frank,* who directed the foundation's program in child and adolescent development. When Frank joined the Josiah Macy Foundation, Havighurst assumed his responsibilities as program director, and thus began his lifelong interest in processes of human growth and development.

In 1940, Havighurst was invited by Ralph W. Tyler to join the faculty of the University of Chicago as a professor of education and executive secretary of its prestigious Committee on Human Development (which three years earlier had changed its name from the Committee on Child Development, to reflect the faculty's broad interests.) Apart from Fulbright professorships at the University of Canterbury and the University of Buenos Aires, and visiting appointments at

Fordham and Princeton Theological Seminary, Havighurst remained at the University of Chicago for the rest of his career.

Havighurst was engaged in many types of investigations with colleagues in anthropology, sociology, and education (including Allison Davis, W. Lloyd Warner, Helen Koch, Carl Rogers, and Bruno Bettelheim) and with graduate students in the Committee on Human Development. Some involved studies of social class and child-rearing practices. With the U.S. Office of Indian Affairs, Havighurst engaged in cross-cultural studies, paying particular attention to the personality development of children in various Native American tribes. With Bernice L. Neugarten,* one of his prized students and future colleague, he published *American Indian and White Children: A Sociopsychological Investigation* (Chicago: University of Chicago Press, 1955). He also engaged in longitudinal studies of adolescent personality and character development. Between 1944 and 1954, Havighurst wrote six major books, of which *Human Development and Education* (New York: David McKay Co., 1953; rev. edn., 1972) is the best known.

Havighurst's interest in research on aging began as a result of a conversation in 1944 with his colleague Ernest W. Burgess,* a professor of sociology who had been invited by the Social Science Research Council to survey the state-of-the-art of research on aging in the social sciences. Together, Burgess and Havighurst organized a Committee on Human Adjustment. (For their blueprint, see Otto Pollak, *Social Adjustment in Old Age* (New York: Social Science Research Council, 1948).) "A study of social adjustment in old age" was listed in the committee's research program in the University of Chicago's 1946–1947 *Announcements.* In the spring of 1948, Havighurst and Burgess offered a graduate course on the topic, and a year later sponsored a two-day "institute on problems of old age."

By the end of the decade, Havighurst and Burgess were undertaking studies to determine how ministers, YMCA officials, teachers, and recipients of old-age assistance were adjusting to retirement. Results were quickly disseminated. In 1949, Ruth Shonle Cavan published *Personal Adjustment in Old Age* (Chicago: Science Research Associates, 1949), which analyzed patterns of adjustment and social problems faced by 3,000 white, English-speaking, mentally competent, middle-class people over the age of sixty. Cavan relied on a survey instrument, the Activities and Attitudes Inventories, which had been designed by Havighurst and Burgess.

With Ruth Albrecht, Havighurst issued *Older People* (New York: Longmans, Green, 1953). A year later, with E. A. Friedmann, he published a collection of essays, *The Meaning of Work and Retirement* (Chicago: University of Chicago Press, 1954), which explored attitudes among such diverse occupational groups as steel workers and coal miners, department store clerks, skilled craftsmen, and elderly physicians. Both volumes stressed that there was a definite relationship between an older person's activity and his or her ability to adjust to old age. "The personal problem of retirement for the average person will be made easier if our society provides more facilities and greater assistance for older people to learn to enjoy the leisure arts,'' Havighurst concluded in *The Meaning of Work and Retirement.*

By the end of the first postwar decade, thanks in large measure to Havighurst's initiatives, the Committee on Human Development (CHD) had emerged as one of the nation's best centers to study social and psychological aspects of the aging process. In the early 1950s, as chairman of CHD, Havighurst invited his colleagues W. Lloyd Warner, Everett Hughes, David Reisman, and Ethel Shanas* "to secure the kind of knowledge which may assist aging persons on such questions as employment, health, civic participation, and the use of leisure of time." With initial support from the Carnegie Corporation, CHD faculty and graduate students embarked upon a decade-long investigation of middle age and aging that came to be known as the Kansas City Studies. From this project emerged Elaine Cumming and William Henry's *Growing Old* (New York: Basic Books, 1961). Developing "an inductive theory of aging to fit [their] data," Cumming and Henry stipulated that "aging is an inevitable, mutual withdrawal or disengagement, resulting in decreased interaction between the aging person and others in the social system he belongs to."

At first privately and then publicly, other members of the CHD research team, such as Bernice L. Neugarten, Martin Loeb, Sheldon S. Tobin,* and Havighurst himself, expressed reservations about the "disengagement theory," especially the ways that Cumming and Henry manipulated and interpreted their data. In a 1963 paper delivered at the Congress of the International Association of Gerontology, Havighurst, Neugarten, and Tobin concluded that "the aging individual may or may not disengage from the pattern of role activities that characterize him in middle age. It is highly doubtful, however, that he ever disengages from the values of the society which he has so long internalized. It is even more doubtful that the aging individual ever disengages from the personality pattern that has so long been the self" (paper reprinted in *Middle Age and Aging,* ed. Bernice L. Neugarten (Chicago: University of Chicago Press, 1963)).

Four years later, Havighurst presented the Gerontological Society's Kleemeier lecture, the same year in which he served as the Society's president. In his Kleemeier lecture, he suggested that adjustment to old age should not be dichotomized in terms of activity or disengagement. Rather, the process of growing older involves a process of adaptation to biological and social changes that occurs with the passage of time. The paper, according to Bernice Neugarten, "stands as a milestone in the field" (paper published in *The Gerontologist,* 5 1965). Extending his work on the Kansas City data and earlier occupational studies, Havighurst published *Adjustment to Retirement: A Cross-National Study* (Chicago: University of Chicago Press, 1969), which incorporated case studies of teachers and steel workers from Britain, France, Austria, and Poland.

While pursuing research on aging, Havighurst did not abandon his other intellectual interests. For instance, he carried out a ten-year study of youth development. His cross-cultural studies of childhood and youth extended to

Argentina, Brazil, Italy, Germany, Japan, Mexico, New Zealand, and Yugoslavia. He also has served as an adviser to UNESCO and to the Ford Foundation. Havighurst's fascination with Latin American educational systems resulted in several books in the field of comparative education.

In the 1960s, Havighurst began to receive a series of honors for his many accomplishments. He received honorary degrees from Hofstra University and from his alma mater, Ohio Wesleyan. The American Psychological Association's Division of Educational Psychology awarded him its Thorndike Memorial Award in 1969. The University of Michigan named him one of the nation's "10 Pioneers in Gerontology." Havighurst served as a director of the National Council on the Aging, was an adviser at both the 1961 and 1971 White House Conferences on Aging, and served on several civic committees in Chicago.

Well into his eighth decade, Havighurst maintained an active professional career. He began to study philanthropic organizations and renewed his inquiries into the impact of English culture on Native American societies. He became a visiting professor of sociology and anthropology at the University of Notre Dame.

Robert J. Havighurst died in 1993.

For more, see Bernice L. Neugarten, "Robert J. Havighurst, a Pioneer in Social Gerontology," *Sonderdruck aus "Zeitschrift fur Gerontologie,"* 8 (March/April 1975): 81–86.

LEONARD HAYFLICK. Leonard Hayflick was born in Philadelphia in 1928. After serving in the U.S. Army, he earned all of his degrees at the University of Pennsylvania: his B.A. in microbiology and chemistry (1951), an M.S. in medical microbiology (1953), and his Ph.D. in medical microbiology and chemistry (1956). After serving as a McLaughlin Research Fellow in Infection and Immunity in the Department of Microbiology at the University of Texas Medical Branch, Galveston, from 1956 to 1958, Hayflick returned to his home town, where he became a member of the Wistar Institute of Anatomy and Biology.

There, working with Paul S. Moorhead, he made what some biogerontologists consider one of the field's most important discoveries. Since the early 1900s, cell culturists had accepted Alexis Carrel's claim that there was an inverse relationship between the "growth rate" of embryonic chicken fibroblasts cultivated in plasma clots and the age of the chicken supplying the plasma. This idea was overturned in later years. Studies by Alfred E. Cohn* and others, moreover, suggested that with increasing age, there was a longer latent period preceding the appearance of migrating cells. From about 1920 onward, Alexis Carrel thought it would be possible to keep cultured fibroblasts from chicken embryo heart tissue proliferating indefinitely. It was for this reason that biogerontologists believed that aging was not due to any intrinsic failure within cells but was caused by extracellular events.

Contrary to Carrel's hypothesis that normal cultured cells might live indefinitely, however, Hayflick and Moorhead found, using cultured, normal human fibroblasts, that normal cells underwent a finite number of population doublings and then died. They initially published their finding as "The Serial Cultivation of Human Diploid Cell Strains," in *Experimental Cell Research*, 25 (1961): 585–621, because experts who first reviewed the paper for the *Journal of Experimental Medicine* refused to believe that the sixty-year-old dogma that cultured normal cells were immortal was wrong. This publication, and his simultaneous discovery that a mycoplasma was the cause of human primary atypical pneumonia (walking pneumonia), put him in line for a Career Development Award from the National Cancer Institute (1962–1970). Now, his cell culture paper is considered a gerontological classic.

Hayflick was not influenced by the research conducted by investigators who were identified with Cowdry's *Problems of Ageing* or with Shock's group at the Gerontology Research Center. Rather, as he noted in "Origins of Longevity" in *Modern Biological Theories of Aging* (ed. H. L. Warner (New York: Raven Press, 1987), 21–34), he was inspired by cytologists such as August Weissman and Charles Sedgwick Minot as well as by such biogerontologists as George Sacher* and Bernard L. Strehler.*

After spending two years as an assistant professor of research medicine at the University of Pennsylvania (1966–1968) simultaneously with his Wistar Institute appointment, Hayflick became a professor of medical microbiology at Stanford University's School of Medicine. In addition, he served as a senator-at-large for Basic Medical Sciences (1970–1973) and chaired the general research support grant committee (1972–1974). Hayflick also played a major role in California's planning for the 1971 White House Conference on Aging, and served on various blue ribbon panels for the National Cancer Institute, World Health Organization, and the National Institute of Child Health and Human Development.

Because of his achievements as a bench scientist and his visibility in national networks, Hayflick was offered the first directorship of the National Institute on Aging, which he turned down for family reasons. Around the same time, an intellectual property-rights dispute arose over the WI-38 cells that Hayflick had used in his research. The controversy took years to resolve, but Hayflick won in an out-of-court settlement. This victory is often mentioned by biologists who subsequently established what is now a flourishing biotechnology industry.

Hayflick was appointed in 1975 as a founding member of the National Advisory Council of the NIA. He resigned his position at Stanford in protest against that university's unwillingness to support him in his argument with the U.S. government. Later, Stanford embraced the position that Hayflick had taken and became an advocate for the intellectual property rights of its faculty. (For more on this, see Bernard L. Strehler, "Hayflick-NIH Settlement," *Science*, 215 (1982): 214–15.)

From 1976 to 1981, Hayflick served as a senior research cell biologist at Children's Hospital in Oakland, California. For the next six years, he was a professor of zoology, microbiology, and immunology at the University of Florida; he also directed its Center for Gerontological Studies. Since 1988, Hayflick has been a professor in the Anatomy Department of the University of California, San Francisco School of Medicine.

Hayflick co-edited with Caleb E. Finch the first edition of the *Handbook of the Biology of Aging* (New York: Van Nostrand Reinhold, 1977), contributing a chapter on the cellular basis for biological aging. He is editor-in-chief of *Experimental Gerontology,* and has been an editor of the *Journal of Gerontology,* the *Journal of Bacteriology,* the *Journal of Virology, Mechanisms of Aging and Development,* and *Gerontology and Geriatrics Education.*

Hayflick won the Kleemeier Award in 1972 and served as president of the Gerontological Society in 1983. He has been on the board of directors of the American Federation of Research on Aging since 1981. Hayflick has received many other awards, including the Samuel Roberts Noble Foundation Research Recognition award (1984), the Brookdale Award (1990), and the Sandoz Prize from the International Association of Gerontology (1991). He has recently written *How and Why We Age* (New York: Ballantine Books, 1994) which received widespread notice in professional and popular periodicals.

JON HENDRICKS. Jon "Joe" Hendricks was born in 1943. He was first attracted to the field of aging by Donald P. Kent,* one of his teachers and one of social gerontology's deans of blending basic and applied research. Hendricks also took notice of training initiatives developed during the early years of the U.S. Administration on Aging. Thus, after receiving his M.A. from the University of Nevada (1968) and Ph.D. from Pennsylvania State University (1971), he was very well prepared to pursue a career that has made him one of the important idea-generators and master teachers in gerontology.

Early on, while teaching at the University of Kentucky, Hendricks saw the need for another introductory gerontology textbook. Whereas Robert C. Atchley* tried to reflect the state of the art in *Social Forces in Late Life* (Belmont, Calif.: Wadsworth Publishing), emphasizing the latest work across domains without imposing his own imprimatur on the field, Hendricks (with C. Davis Hendricks) sought in *Aging in Mass Society* (Cambridge, Mass.: Winthrop Publishers, 1981) to offer a multidisciplinary perspective on aging informed by his interest in theory building: "It may turn out that, for the time being, the questions raised are even more salient than any of the tentative answers. Accordingly, the primary goal of this work is to offer a contextual overview of aging in modern mass societies, knowing full well no definitive conclusions can be forthcoming."

Hendricks devoted the first chapters of his text to "thick" descriptions of demography and history. He also used his text to develop a "personal resource model," which was his approach to the economics of retirement and the social and health care networks available to older people. This same penchant for putting a slightly different spin on ideas was evident in his specification of the concept of "moral economy" (in language that paralleled but also deviated from the meanings of the phrase as used by the anthropologist James Scott), which appeared in his *Critical Perspectives on Aging* (Baywood, 1991).

In the years since the series appeared, the authors, including W. Andrew Achenbaum, Carroll L. Estes,* John Myles,* Jennie Keith,* Ted Koff, Linda Breytspraak, Paul Costa, and Robert McCrae, have assumed positions of intellectual leadership within the field. Hendricks's contributions have continued to stimulate conceptual development in social gerontology, and his 1992 "Generations and the Generation of Theory in Social Gerontology" in the *International Journal of Aging and Human Development,* 38 (1993) spurred inquiry into the linkages between theorizing and career tracks for gerontologists. In these and in other contributions, Hendricks seems to have emulated the style of the gerontological figure who served as his mentor and role model, Klaus F. Riegel.*

Hendricks was elected the 1995 president of the Association of Gerontology in Higher Education. The Gerontological Society has also honored him for his achievements.

BETH B. HESS. Beth B. Hess was born in 1928 and graduated *magna cum laude* from Radcliffe in 1950. As a graduate student in sociology, she was working as a teaching assistant when her mentor, Matilda White Riley,* was invited by the Russell Sage Foundation/Ford Foundation to inventory the state of gerontological research in the social sciences. While earning her Ph.D. at Rutgers University (1972), Hess worked closely for five years with Riley and her research team. Hess spent the first several years gathering articles published by researchers on aging. She analyzed their contents for conceptual clarity, methodological adequacy, and substantive results. The findings of the Rutgers team appeared in a codification of the field, published as the first volume of *Aging and Society: An Inventory of Research Findings* (New York: Russell Sage Foundation, 1968). As a member of Riley's work group, Hess had a hand in refining what came to be called the "age stratification model."

Applying ideas that she learned in this discussion, Hess contributed an analysis of "friendship and aging" to Volume 3 of *A Sociology of Age Stratification* (New York: Russell Sage Foundation, 1972), which is considered a pioneering work. Friendships, she noted, were based in part on shared cohort experiences and mutual current concerns. Patterns of friendship, moreover, vary by sex. Men through middle age tend to have broader networks of friends that are rather superficial. Women, in contrast, are more likely than men to describe relationships in terms of intimacy, self-disclosure, and emotional closeness. These differences seem to reflect variations in the ways that men and women adapt their social bonds over the life course.

Hess continued to collaborate with members of the Rutgers group after she assumed a teaching position at the nearby County College of Morris. With Joan Waring, for instance, she published an article on "Changing Patterns of Aging and Family Bonds in Later Life," which appeared in the *Family Coordinator* (October 1978): 304–14. Hess also has published several editions of leading articles in the field, *Growing Old in America,* co-edited with Elizabeth W. Markson.* Over time, Hess became increasingly interested in applying the concept of gender stratification as it related to various aspects of aging. See, for instance, her "Aging Policies and Old Women," in *Gender and the Life Course,* ed. Alice S. Rossi (Chicago: Aldine, 1985).

Hess's major contribution to the professional mores of the field has probably been her advocacy, early on, for a feminist consciousness in gerontology. She organized an informal women's caucus in the Gerontological Society in the 1970s. Hess played a major role in getting the society's annual meeting in 1978 moved from New Orleans, which was in a state that had declined to vote for the ratification of the Equal Rights Amendment, to Dallas, where civic leaders had demonstrated greater sensitivity to the concerns of many groups for gender-based issues. A secretary and chairwoman of the Gerontological Society's Behavioral and Social Science Section, Hess has also demanded, "futilely, for the most part," for enhanced influence and representation for the section, which represents roughly 40 percent of the organization's membership.

TOM HICKEY. Tom Hickey was born in California in 1939. After attending the University of Santa Clara, he received his B.A. with honors in philosophy and psychology from Gonzaga University (1963). After earning an M.A. in psychology from California State University, Los Angeles, Hickey transferred to UCLA, where he earned an M.P.H. (specializing in behavioral sciences/gerontology) in 1968 and his Dr.P.H. in 1970. Hickey's graduate studies were underwritten from 1967 to 1970 by a U.S. Public Health Service Research fellowship. During his last two years at UCLA he taught psychology at California State, Los Angeles, and (with Richard A. Kalish) published his first two papers. See, for instance, Hickey and Kalish, "Young People's Perceptions of Adults," *Journal of Gerontology,* 23 (1968): 215–19. In 1970, Hickey was initiated into the Delta Omega National Honorary Society in Public Health.

Hickey became an assistant professor of human development at Pennsylvania State University after completing his doctoral studies. He chose to begin his career at this institution because of the presence there of Donald P. Kent,* who was the first gerontologist Hickey had met. Hickey was strongly influenced by Kent's multiple talents as a scholar whose work was firmly anchored in the reality of public policy and practice. Kent's encouragement, Hickey recalls, influenced his graduate work. It is also evident in his subsequent intellectual and professional contributions. The Pennsylvania Department of Public Welfare, for instance, awarded him two grants in excess of $600,000 to train researchers and practitioners in the field. In 1973, he won the first of six research and training grants from the U.S. Administration on Aging during the decade.

In addition to writing "Catholic Religious Orders and the Aging Process," *The Gerontologist,* 12 (1972): 17–21, Hickey contributed many articles on ways to develop comprehensive programs in gerontology. See, in addition to works in *The Gerontologist,* his "Continuing Education for Allied Health," *Journal of Allied Health,* 4 (1975): 5–12. More important than these refereed reports, however, were the five widely used practitioner training manuals that Hickey developed. He traveled extensively in the early 1970s, consulting with states and foundations regarding the implementation of Title III of the Older Americans Act. In 1976, Hickey received the National University Extension Association's award for his ability to translate research into practice.

After six years in University Park, Hickey became an associate professor in the community health programs of the University of Michigan's School of Public Health, rising to a full professorship five years later. During the 1980s, Hickey directed the school's Health Gerontology Program. He has been associated with Michigan's Institute of Gerontology since 1981. Particularly in the 1980s, Hickey provided substantive leadership in defining self-care and aging. He convened an international conference on the subject at Oxford University in 1983. See his contribution, "Health Behavior and Self-Care in Late Life" in *Self-Care and Health in Old Age,* eds. K. Dean, T. Hickey, and B. Holstein (London: Croom Helm, 1986), 1–11. Much of this work was done in collaboration with his former colleague, William Rakowski.

Although Hickey did not introduce the concept of self-care, his application of the notion to an older population, especially his description of the process the aged go through in making treatment decisions about their health, has proved quite influential. This line of investigation also led him to study mistreatment of the elderly in the community. Two essays that he published with Richard L. Douglass—"Neglect and Abuse of Older Family Members" in *The Gerontologist,* 21 (1981): 171–76; and "Mistreatment of the Elderly in the Domestic Setting," *American Journal of Public Health,* 71 (1981): 500–507—became the basis for articles in the popular media and congressional hearings, and inspired others to study the topic.

Hickey's current work focuses on the health effects of low-intensity exercise. The relevance of this inquiry is especially evident for a largely ignored group— chronically impaired individuals. He finds that even modest amounts of physical activity, when extended over time, have significant effects on blood pressure, mobility, and the reduction of muscle and joint pain, which help chronically impaired older persons maintain their independence in community settings and delay or avoid institutionalization.

Hickey's efforts in advancing aging issues through national professional organizations have made him a major spokesman in the field. He was president of the Association for Gerontology in Higher Education in 1976–1977, a body that he helped to found and continues to serve. Hickey also was elected president of the Gerontological Society of America (1991–1992). He has served on the major gerontological publications' editorial boards, and remains on the *Journal of Aging and Health.*

Hickey continues to receive major training grants. He serves as co-investigator on "Social Research Training on Applied Issues of Aging," supported by the National Institute on Aging.

NANCY R. HOOYMAN. Nancy R. Hooyman received her M.S.W. from the University of Michigan in 1970 and her Ph.D. in sociology and social work from Michigan's joint-degree program four years later. She is currently professor and dean at the University of Washington School of Social Work.

Her initial catalyst for involvement in gerontology occurred after her graduate training, when she confronted ageism in the health care system as her mother was dying. Hooyman has not taken formal course work in the field per se. Rather, she obtained her training through workshops at annual meetings of the Gerontological Society, the American Society on Aging, and the Association for Gerontology in Higher Education and through workshops sponsored by various university centers on aging. She has been greatly influenced by the writings and example of Eugene Litwak; she has tried to apply his "balance theory" to the study of family and community relationships. She considers Gerontological Society leaders Carroll L. Estes* and Amy Horowitz* to be among her role models, as well as the late Tish Sommers, whom she met through her work with the Older Women's League.

Hooyman considers the writing of widely used textbooks to be her major contribution to the field. With Asuman Kiyak, she published *Social Gerontology: A Multidisciplinary Perspective* (Boston: Allyn and Bacon, 1988, 1991, 1993). This book has been adapted for the Annenberg telecommunications course on aging, "Growing Old in a New Age." With Wendy Lustbader, she wrote *Taking Care of Aging Family Members* (New York: Free Press, 1986, 1988, 1994), which delves sensitively into some of the most complex issues facing family caregivers, eschewing a superficial "cookbook" approach. With Judith Gonyea, she is currently completing a book for Sage Publications, *Family Care, Policy and Gender Justice: Feminist Perspectives on Caring for Adults with Developmental Disabilities, Mental Illness, and the Frail Elderly.* In these works, Hooyman emphasizes gender inequities in the care of dependents, showing how discrimination on the basis of sex results in economic inequities across the life course.

Hooyman's most important aging-related contribution to date has been her insistence that caregiver burdens be differentiated according to objective and subjective indexes of stress. See, in particular, two articles she co-wrote with Rhonda Montgomery and Judith Gonyea: "The Impact of In-Home Services Termination on Family Caregivers," *The Gerontologist,* 25 (1985): 141–45; and "Caregiving and the Experience of Subjective and Objective Burden," *Journal of Family Relations,* 34 (1986): 19–26.

AMY HOROWITZ. Amy Horowitz earned her B.A. in sociology from Boston University in 1971 and her M.S.W., with emphasis on research and social work practice, from Fordham University's Graduate School of Social Services in 1974. During the next four years she served as a senior research assistant for New York's Community Service Society. There she assisted in the design and training of interviewers for a city-wide survey of elderly welfare recipients. She became acquainted with Janet Sainer and Mary Zander, who awakened her interest in aging in general.

Awarded a Brookdale Doctoral Fellowship (1978–1979), Horowitz then pursued her D.S.W. at the Columbia University School of Social Work, receiving her degree in 1982. She served as principal investigator at the Brookdale Center on Aging at Hunter College in two projects on family caregiving. The first, "The Role of Families in Providing Long-Term Care to the Frail and Chronically Ill Elderly Living in the Community," was funded by the Health Care Financing Administration. The Administration on Aging underwrote her research on "Commitment to Caregiving: The Consequences for Aged Family Members and Governmental Services of Women Working." Abraham Monk and Eugene Litwak served as her major advisers.

During the next two years, Horowitz directed the research component, New York City Home Care Project, through the city's Department for the Aging. Horowitz directed all phases of this research/demonstration project, utilizing an experimental-comparison group and longitudinal research design. In 1984, she joined The Lighthouse Inc., a private organization committed to research, education, and services for the visually impaired and is currently vice president for research and evaluation, directing demonstration projects for the blind. There, she works closely with a former Gerontological Society president, Barbara Silverstone, president of The Lighthouse Inc. During this time she has also held adjunct positions at the New School for Social Research and at Yeshiva University and has been an associate professor at Fordham University.

Horowitz's early research focused on family caregiving, especially the consequences for adult children. She focused on gender differences and other factors that influenced family behavior, as well as analyzing the structure and dynamics of stress. See, for instance, her essays, with L. W. Shindelman, "Reciprocity and Affection: Past Influences on Current Caregiving," *Journal of Gerontological Social Work,* 5 (1983): 5–20; and "Social and Economic Incentives for Family Caregivers," *Health Care Financing Review,* 5 (1983): 25–33.

"Caregiving consequences" is a pivotal concept in Horowitz's work. She is interested in the positive and negative emotional, financial, and social aspects of caregiving for family members. A good example of her work on gender differentiation is "Methodological Issues in the Study of Gender Within Family Caregiving Relationships," in *Gender and Family Care of the Elderly,* eds. J. W. Dwyer and R. T. Coward (Beverly Hills, Calif.: Sage, 1992). For articles Horowitz wrote on aging and vision, see "Development of a Vision Screening Questionnaire for Older People," *Journal of Gerontological Social Work,* 17 (1991): 37–56; and with J. E. Terisi and L. A. Cassels, "Vision Impairment and Functional Disability among Nursing Home Residents," *The Gerontologist,* 34 (1994): 316–23. Her current work focuses on adaptation to chronic disability and on the role of social support in geriatric rehabilitation.

Horowitz has been active in the Gerontological Society. She chaired the Research, Education and Practice Committee (1987–1988) as well as the Social

Research, Policy and Practice Section (1991–1992). She has been on the editorial board of *The Gerontologist* since 1989.

ROY G. HOSKINS. Roy Graham Hoskins was born in Nevinville, Iowa, in 1880. He earned his B.A. and M.A. from the University of Kansas in 1905; five years later, he earned his Ph.D. from Harvard University. From 1910 to 1913, he was an associate professor of physiology at Starling-Ohio Medical School in Columbus. He spent the next seven years at Northwestern University Medical School.

Hoskins then went to medical school at the Johns Hopkins University, earning his M.D. in 1920. He spent seven years as head of the Department of Physiology at Ohio State's medical school. In 1927, he returned to Harvard, where he was director of the Memorial Foundation for Neuro-Endocrine Research for the next twenty years; he also served as a research associate in physiology in the Harvard Medical School. From 1950 until his death, Hoskins served as a research professor at Tufts University.

Hoskins is best known for his research on endocrinology and insanity. With Llewylyn F. Barker and H. O. Mosenthal, he edited *Endocrinology and Metabolism* (2 vols., 1922). Hoskins was editor-in-chief of the *Journal of Endocrinology* from 1917 to 1940. His *Endocrinology: The Glands and Their Functions* was first issued in 1941 and expanded and reissued by W. W. Norton in 1950. He viewed the book as a complement to his *Tides of Life* (1933), with an eye to the needs of biologists, psychologists, premedical students, and physicians who did not require an overly technical introduction to the science of hormones. Recognizing that the practical applications of endocrinology lagged far behind anatomical and physiological knowledge, he urged researchers to study the impact of hormones in older humans.

Because of his interest in multidisciplinary studies, it is not surprising that Hoskins would have been attracted to emerging ideas in gerontology. He served as the Gerontological Society's second president (1946). A member of Phi Beta Kappa, Sigma Xi, and the American Academy of Arts and Sciences, he also was president of the Society for Research in Psychometric Problems in 1944.

IRENE M. HULICKA. Canadian-born Irene M. Hulicka earned a master's degree from the University of Saskatchewan in 1949. Following completion of a Ph.D. in experimental psychology at the University of Nebraska (Lincoln) in 1954, she pursued research and published prolifically on learning. Postdoctoral work as an intern at Buffalo's VA Hospital led to a position there as first a clinical psychologist (1960–1963), and then a research psychologist (1963–1965). Her important early work examined factors contributing to the cognitive efficiency of older adults (I. M. Hulicka and R. Weiss, "Age Differences in Retention as a Function of Learning," *Journal of Consulting Psychology*, 29 (1965): 125–29). What conventional wisdom took to be bad memory in older people, Hulicka attributed to poor learning as a result of, among various factors, inadequate opportunities for learning.

Two important studies co-written by Hulicka suggested that there might be differences among age groups for preferred or spontaneously selected strategies for learning and recall. See I. M. Hulicka and J. Grossman, "Age Group Comparisons for the Use of Mediators in Paired Associate Learning," *Journal of Gerontology*, 22 (1967): 46–61; and I. M. Hulicka, H. Sterns, and J. Grossman, "Age Group Comparisons of Paired Associate Learning as a Function of Paced and Self-Paced Association and Response Times," *Journal of Gerontology*, 22 (1967): 274–80. These studies also indicated that the learning and recall efficiency of the elderly might be enhanced through instruction and training. In addition to laying out a course of study for further research, they provided background for cognitive intervention research and training. Hulicka has followed up with recent study into the fears of older adults.

Concluding from a long course of research that there is a prevailing tendency among caregivers to underestimate the elderly, Hulicka has sought out variables that interfere with cognitive efficiency and, in her clinical work, identified the assets and strengths of individuals and structured opportunities for success. True to this conviction, when asked to identify her mentors, Hulicka responds, "My 'teachers' have been the elderly people with whom I have interacted professionally."

Similarly, Hulicka's teachings to nurses, physicians, and other health care providers have stressed the importance of treating each elderly person as a unique individual, rather than relying on unfounded and negative stereotypes. Her call is to attend to potentials and aspirations rather than simply the deficits of the elderly.

In addition to research, publishing, and teaching—as a longtime member of the psychology faculty at New York's State University College at Buffalo (1965 to the present)—Hulicka has lectured avidly. Her primary collaborators to date include former student Harvey Sterns and colleague Susan K. Whitbourne. Finally, she has worked at the national level on gerontological education, developing workshops to train psychologists who work with the elderly.

MARGARET HELLIE HUYCK. Margaret Hellie Huyck received her B.A. from Vassar College in 1961, and did her graduate work under Bernice L. Neugarten* and Morton Lieberman in the Committee of Human Development at the University of Chicago, where she also earned her Ph.D. in 1970. Huyck dates her attraction to the field of aging to the intellectual ferment generated in the famous "adult development" program on the Midway. Robert J. Havighurst* and William Henry were senior members of the committee, and Sheldon S. Tobin* was a rising star. Huyck learned much from fellow graduate student David Gutmann, but it was Neugarten who served as her primary mentor and role model.

Although she considers herself a "relatively late starter," Huyck (with William Hoyer) made an early splash with an integrative textbook that offered a coherent view of the field: *Adult Development and Aging* (Belmont, Calif.: Wadsworth, 1982). Since then, Huyck has worked on the sort of detailed community case studies made famous by the Chicago schools of sociology and interdisciplinary studies. Based on her analysis of "Parkville," a Midwest city, she has engaged in a systematic, qualitative field study comparing midlife and young adult members of "normal," "hard-core" families. Of particular note is her decision to investigate generational relations by focusing on subjects who have passed through adolescence yet have not become frail elders. See her "Midlife Parental Imperatives," in *Midlife Loss,* ed. Richard A. Kalish (Newbury Park, Calif.: Sage Publications, 1989).

Huyck's intellectual contributions to date lie in clarifying the nature of gender-linked attributions and experiences in shaping the life course. For instance, she has refined the notion of "accommodative mastery," as opposed to "passive mystery," in clarifying characteristics of "feminine" style in Gutmann's* model of life course change. In so doing, she has questioned whether androgyny is the ideal manifestation of late-life human development. Huyck questions whether there is a "cross-over" in attitudes and behavior with aging. She debunks unisex models, which suggest that there are repressed aspects of the self that are added to an existing substrata of a person's gender-congruent identity. Thus, in analyzing how people face death, Huyck is beginning to suggest a very different gestalt than that presented by Kübler-Ross. See her "Final Parental Imperative," in *Midlife Loss.*

J

HOBART C. JACKSON. Hobart C. Jackson was born in 1917. He is best known for his work on the black elderly, particularly in the area of housing. "There is a lack of awareness of how [the black elderly] are treated in this country," he told *Ebony* magazine in 1973. "They don't understand how racism really works. There's a tendency among black people in general, and especially among older blacks, to accept what we have as being enough." At the National Conference on Senior Centers, Jackson reported that most black aged in senior centers are treated very poorly, partly due to the racial attitudes and poor training of the staff. See, for instance, "Overcoming Racial Barrier in Senior Centers," National Conference on Senior Centers, 2:20–28.

As head of the National Caucus on the Black Aged, Jackson cooperated with the U.S. Senate Special Committee on Aging in the early 1970s to establish a usable database of information on the black elderly, including life styles, geographical distribution, income, illness, life expectancies, employment, housing, and the effectiveness of federal programs in providing assistance.

Ultimately, Jackson has sought radical solutions to the problems of the black aged. He argued that a redistribution of income and wealth would be critical to freeing the black elderly from the oppressive poverty that so many endure. In short, he called for "power for the powerless" to help the black aged. See, "Housing and Geriatric Centers for Aging and Aged Blacks," Proceeding of Black Aged in the Future, ed. Jacquelyne J. Jackson (Durham, N.C.: Center for the Study of Aging and Human Development, Duke University, 1973): 23–33.

JACQUELYNE JOHNSON JACKSON. Jacquelyne Johnson Jackson is considered by many to be the leading authority on elderly African Americans. She was born in 1932 in Winston-Salem, North Carolina, and earned her B.S. in 1953 and a masters in 1955 from the University of Wisconsin. She completed her Ph.D. at Ohio State University in 1960 and went on to pursue postdoctoral work at the University of Colorado, Boulder; Duke University; and the University of North Carolina, Chapel Hill. Her academic career has included work at Southern University of Baton Rouge, Jackson State College. She joined the faculty of Howard University as an assistant professor in 1964 and served there as a full professor from 1978 until 1985. She then returned to Duke, where she remains. Much of her most important work has originated from Duke's Center for the Study of Aging and Human Development.

Jackson's first important work was her doctoral dissertation, published in 1962 as *These Rights They Seek* (Washington: Public Affairs Press). Her emphasis has been on the unique needs of the black aged and on the importance of government involvement in meeting those needs. Her subsequent work, *Minorities and Aging* (Belmont, Calif.: Wadsworth Co., 1980), echoed this theme, though it expanded to include other minority groups. It was called at the time the most complete work on minority aging. Her first priority in the late 1960s was to point to the lack of empirical data on the black aged that could be used to direct research and policy. See, "Social Gerontology and the Negro: A Review," *Gerontology*, 7 (1967): 168–78. To help fill this gap, Jackson began research on older black women, finding that, in the aggregate, black women faced an exacerbation of problems seen earlier in life as a result of racism, economics and isolation. See, for example, "Comparative Life Styles and Family and Friend Relationships Among Old Black Women," *Family Coordinator*, 21 (1972): 477–85; and, "The Plight of Older Black Women in the United States," *Black Scholar*, 7 (1976): 47–55.

In addition to voluminous research and publications, Jackson has served a number of organizations. She was on the board of directors of the Carver Research Foundation of Tuskegee from 1970 until 1987, she has been the director of the National Council on the Black Aging since 1975, and she has served on the board of the National Council on Aging. Along with accolades from the American Psychiatric Association, she has twice been an NIH Fellow, a National Science Foundation fellow, and a John Hay Whitney fellow.

JAMES S. JACKSON. James S. Jackson earned his B.A. at Michigan State, his M.A. at the University of Toledo, and his Ph.D. (1972) at Wayne State University. His primary focus has been to develop theoretical orientations and methodological approaches in establishing a National Survey of Black Americans (NSBA). His related work on the National Study of Three Generation African-American Families has resulted in important contributions to aging, human development, and social gerontology. These studies broke new ground in the study of the life course of African American individuals and families. His current work, a thirteen-year longitudinal four-wave panel study of the original NSBA, shows similar promise. He has edited two volumes on the subject: *Life in Black*

America (Newbury Park, Calif.: Sage Publications, 1991), and *Aging in Black America,* co-edited with Linda C. Chatters and Joseph R. Taylor (Newbury Park, Calif.: Sage Publications, 1992).

Not only has Jackson contributed to the refinement of a life course development framework of aging among African Americans, but he has also been able to carry this construct over to work on other racial and ethnic groups. With Kyriakos S. Markides* and Jersey Liang, Jackson prepared ''Race, Ethnicity, and Aging: Conceptual and Methodological Issues,'' for the third edition of the *Handbook of Aging and the Social Sciences,* ed. Robert H. Binstock* and Linda K. George* (New York: Academic Press, 1990). See also his related handbook chapter with Toni C. Antonucci* and Rose C. Gibson,* ''Cultural, Racial and Ethnic Minority Influences on Aging,'' for the third edition of the *Handbook of the Psychology of Aging,* eds. James E. Birren* and K. Warner Schaie* (San Diego: Academic Press, 1990). See also his ''Race: What Implications for Adult Development?'' in *The Encyclopedia of Adult Development,* ed. Robert Kastenbaum* (Phoenix: Oryx Press, 1993).

Jackson has trained a number of researchers conducting work on racial and ethnic aspects of aging and human development in his labs at the University of Michigan's Program for Research on Black Americans Institute for Social Research. He has served on the Gerontological Society of America's Task Force on Minority Issues in Gerontology. In his editorial, ''Race, Ethnicity, and Psychological Theory and Research,'' *Journal of Gerontology,* 44 (January, 1989): P1–P2, Jackson stressed that ''current psychological theories and research paradigms neither encompass nor address the behaviors observed in racial ethnic populations. . . . The importance of having cross-disciplinary involvement cannot be overstated.'' He also produced a series on empirical studies of African Americans for broader dissemination.

Jackson won the Gerontological Society's 1994 Kleemeier Award.

LISSY JARVIK. Lissy F. Jarvik was born in The Hague, The Netherlands. She graduated *cum laude* from Hunter College in 1946. Jarvik earned her M.A. (1947) and Ph.D. (1950) from Columbia University and received her M.D. at Case Western Reserve University in 1954.

From 1946 to 1972, Jarvik was affiliated with the New York State Psychiatric Institute in New York City, rising in rank from research assistant to Psychiatrist II. A diplomate of the American Board of Pediatrics, she also served in varying capacities at the Vanderbilt Clinic (1957–1958, 1962–1972). Concurrently, from 1956 to 1972, Jarvik was on the faculty of Columbia University's College of Physicians and Surgeons.

In the early 1970s, Jarvik relocated to the West Coast. From 1970 to 1982, she served as chief of the psychogenetics unit of the Brentwood Veterans Administration Medical Center in Los Angeles; in 1982, she became chief of the psychogeriatric unit. In addition, Jarvik has been a professor of psychiatry at UCLA's medical school since 1972. She also has been chief of the section on neuropsychogeriatrics at UCLA's Neuropsychiatric Institute and Hospital. Since 1987, Jarvik has been a Distinguished Physician in the Department of Veterans Affairs.

Jarvik has published more than 300 scholarly articles and books. Her work has been interdisciplinary in scope, generally concerned with changes in intellectual functioning. See, for instance, her collection (with Carl Eisdorfer and June E. Blum*), *Intellectual Functioning in Adults: Psychological and Biological Influences* (New York: Springer Publishing, 1973). She also contributed a chapter on "The Impact of Immediate Life Situations on Depression: Illnesses and Losses," in *Depression and Aging: Causes, Care, and Consequences* (New York: Springer, 1983). Often, her work takes a biological turn, as in her study of changes in the central nervous system among twins, "Organic Brain Syndrome and Aging" (with R. Vineta and S. S. Matsuyama), *Archives of General Psychiatry,* 37 (1980): 280–86.

With Robert Neshkes, Jarvik discussed two extremes of affective disturbance in the elderly—mania and depression—in "Affective Disorders in the Elderly," *Annual Review of Medicine,* 38 (1987): 445–56. Suggesting that specific studies of the elderly were lacking in the literature, Jarvik put forward general principles for the use of antidepressants among older patients, noting likely side effects.

Jarvik was founding co-editor of *Alzheimer Disease and Associated Disorders—An International Journal.* She also was a founder of the American Geriatrics Society and a president of the American Association for Geriatric Psychiatry. She has received many honors for her accomplishments, including the Jack Weinberg Memorial Award from the American Psychiatric Association in 1986 and, the same year, the Gerontological Society's Kleemeier Award. In 1988, Jarvik won the American Federation for Research on Aging's Irving S. Wright Award.

COLLEEN LEAHY JOHNSON. Medical anthropologist Colleen Leahy Johnson has focused on the American family system and its members' adaptation to change since completing her graduate work at Syracuse University (Ph.D., 1972). In particular, she initially focused on correlations between ethnic and social class variations as they related to family solidarity.

Her interest in aging and the late life family came when she explored the family's ability to support elderly parents. Subsequent research centered on the role of grandparents and how their position was redefined during the post-divorce reorganization of their child's family. This longitudinal study with white, middle-class, suburban families also followed kinship systems as they adjusted to frequent marital change. Her interest in comparative study led Johnson into research on health care of the inner-city, minority elderly. "The major research questions have examined the extent to which the health care system is serving latent social needs of this at-risk and socially disadvantaged population," Johnson explains.

Since 1988, Johnson has had a NIA MERIT Award that examines the adaptation and competencies necessary for the advanced aged to continue community living. See Colleen L. Johnson and Lillian E. Troll,* "Family Functioning in Late Life," *Journal of Gerontology,* 47 (March 1992): 566–72; and the special issue, "Social and Cultural Diversity of the Oldest Old," *International Journal of Aging and Human Development,* 39 (1994): 1–12.

Her insights are reported in the books *Growing Up and Growing Old in Italian American Families* (New Brunswick, N.J.: Rutgers University Press, 1985), and *Ex Familia: Grandparents, Parents and Children Adjust to Divorce* (New Brunswick, N.J.: Rutgers University Press, 1988).

Johnson is currently working with the Medical Anthropology Program at the University of California, San Francisco (UCSF). Her primary collaborator and mentor has been Lillian Troll* at UCSF. Johnson has also worked with Leonard Pearlin and Robert J. Newcomer.*

HAROLD R. JOHNSON. Harold R. Johnson was born in 1926 in Windsor, Ontario. After serving as a sergeant in the Royal Canadian Armoured Corps in the European Theater during World War II, he graduated with a B.A. from the University of Western Ontario (Assumption College) in 1950. There, he was named the Senior Class Award-winner in psychology. He worked for seven years as executive director of the Windsor Labour Committee for Human Rights and International Representative of the International Union of United Brewery, Soft Drink and Distillery Workers of America, AFL-CIO.

After receiving his M.S.W. in social work from Wayne State University in 1957, Johnson held increasingly more visible roles in community action programs at a time in which the federal and state governments became more attentive to urban affairs and the plight of minorities in urban America.

From 1957 to 1961, Johnson was a planning consultant to the United Community Services of Metropolitan Detroit. For the next eight years he was associate director of Detroit's Neighborhood Service Organization. In this capacity Johnson developed a network of programs (health evaluation, clinics, food services, counseling services, consumer education projects, and recreation services, among other things) for the aged as well as services for emotionally disturbed and delinquent children. In 1970, Michigan Governor William G. Milliken asked Johnson to organize the Office of Youth Services, to plan a program for this new state agency, and to recruit its first permanent director.

Meanwhile, Johnson began to focus his attention on higher education. From 1959 to 1966, he was a lecturer in the School of Social Work at Wayne State. He became a lecturer in the School of Social Work at the University of Michigan in 1966, and then three years later joined the faculty on a full-time basis as professor of social work and head of its Community Practice Program (1969–1974). During the 1974–1975 academic year, Johnson was a divisional coordinator in the school.

In 1975, Johnson became director of the Institute of Gerontology at the University of Michigan; he was charged by the provost to "develop as broad a base as possible for [his] programs." Expanding on the institute's original mandate to be a pioneer in education, research, and service, Johnson developed academic ties to seventeen schools and colleges. He and his staff built on the institute's expertise on older workers, milieu therapy, and housing and community programs in applying for research grants; they initiated efforts in the arts and humanities. By 1980, more than fifty University of Michigan professors were listed as faculty associates, and summer training programs drew students and professional from across the nation. The institute responded to requests for assistance from federal and state agencies, area agencies on aging, health planning councils, retired senior volunteer programs, and Native American tribes.

"The totality of gerontological activity here is difficult to quantify," Johnson declared in a summary of his first five years in office. "Although the Institute initiates and coordinates University programs in aging, it also encourages instructional and research units to develop such activities independently. Many of its resources are expended in quiet diplomacy intended to assist other units to develop gerontological projects in keeping with their own scholarly priorities." During his tenure, Johnson helped U.S. and Canadian universities develop and assess gerontology programs and assisted North American and European government officials in evaluating their policies. He also chaired a blue-ribbon panel on "Foundations of Gerontological Education: Collaborative Project of the Gerontological Society and the Association for Gerontology in Higher Education," which was published in *The Gerontologist,* 20, Part II (June 1980).

From 1981 to 1993, Johnson served as dean of the University of Michigan's School of Social Work. Since then he has been special counsel to the university president in addition to serving as a professor of social work and professor of health behavior and health education in the School of Public Health. On July 1, 1994, he was appointed secretary of the University of Michigan.

In 1984, Johnson was awarded an honorary doctorate from Yeungnam University, Korea, for his extensive work with the government of the Republic of Korea and his role as adviser to several Korean universities. He also received the Wilbur Cohen award from the University of Michigan in 1984. A former president of the Association for Gerontology in Higher Education (1978–1979), he received that organization's Clark Tibbitts Award in 1991, and has been part of a team developing ways to coordinate efforts between the Gerontological Society and the Association for Gerontology in Higher Education.

K _____

ROBERT L. KANE and ROSALIE A. KANE. Rosalie and Robert Kane are not the only husband-and-wife team in gerontology. Neither is theirs the longest-standing intellectual partnership: That tribute belongs to Jack and Matilda White Riley.* But in our opinion, only Steve and Elaine Brody* have been so closely identified as a couple working with the same sets of research problems. In filling out a questionnaire for this dictionary, both of "the Kanes" (as they are known in the field) referred to the other as his or her respective teacher and primary collaborator.

The Kanes met at the University of Toronto. Robert, born in the United States, earned his M.D. from Harvard Medical School in 1965; Rosalie, a Canadian, earned her D.S.W. from the University of Utah in 1975. Rosalie did her thesis on interdisciplinary teamwork. Robert claims that he "got into aging literally on a dare" in 1972. After recommending that family practitioners take care of nursing home patients, colleagues urged him to set up a model. Rosalie's interest in long-term care issues were fuelled while serving on the faculty of the University of Utah's School of Social Work. In the late 1970s, the Kanes became affiliated with the Rand Corporation. (In addition, Robert served as a professor of geriatric medicine and public health at UCLA; Rosalie became a lecturer in the university's School of Social Welfare.) With support from the National Center for Health Services Research and the Henry J. Kaiser Family Foundation, the two worked with other members of Rand's Geriatric Manpower Policy Task Force, including David Solomon, John Beck, and Emmett Keeler on a series of research projects and publications. Some explored ways to measure functional status in long-term care, while others focused on personnel needs in geriatrics.

In 1981 Rosalie and Robert Kane published *Assessing the Elderly* (Lexington, Mass.: Lexington Books). As its subtitle indicated, theirs was "a practical guide to measurement" for physicians, nurses, gerontologists and other researchers, policy analysts, and evaluators, as well as case managers and therapists of all kinds. "A major attribute of long-term care is the way providers define the reality of old people—a reality that they help to shape," the Kanes stated. "Any strategy for altering the health status of the elderly requires a technology for first assessing the health status and then detecting increments of progress."

The Kanes, in a cautionary tale, discussed issues of assessment and outcomes in various North American long-term-care systems. They described abuses of various measurements in long-term care, and worried about indiscriminate uses. They stressed the benefits of greater utilization of such instruments for measuring physical functioning as Sidney Katz's Activities of Daily Living (ADL) and Instrumental Activities of Daily Living (IADL). The Kanes also evaluated various measures of mental and social functioning as well as instruments designed to assess patients according to several dimensions. Throughout their analysis, which is illustrated with concrete examples, the Kanes emphasized the value of precise descriptions rather than inconsistent, facile labels. However, the pair fear that their book "has been used more as a catalogue of such measures."

"Assessments" and "outcomes" are key words that the Kanes have tried to refine in their research and writing. Empirical researchers rather than armchair theorists, they have tried to merge quantitative components with fundamental principles of geriatric care in encouraging the use of stringent designs to test the effects of geriatric interventions and the appropriate interpretation of their effects. The Kanes are also concerned with measuring social values in domains such as residents' satisfaction and affect. See Robert L. Kane, Robert M. Bell, and Sandra Z. Riegler, "Value Preferences for Nursing Home Outcomes," *The Gerontologist,* 26 (1986): 303–308. To them, the value of outcomes depends on the reliability and validity of the measurement instrument.

The Kanes have also offered comprehensive assessments of the ways health care for the elderly is organized, financed, and evaluated in the United States. Their "Health Care for Older People: Organizational and Policy Issues," in the third edition of the *Handbook of Aging and the Social Sciences,* eds. Robert H. Binstock* and Linda K. George* (New York: Academic Press, 1990), for instance, offers a succinct overview of functional status, funding and form, the use of services, the supply of services, and deals with such issues as continuum of care, insurance options, and dementia. The Kanes also have made explicit comparisons with the Canadian system and programs elsewhere. See, for instance, their *Improving Health in Older People: A World View* (New York: Oxford University Press, 1989).

Currently, the Kanes are in the School of Public Health at the University of Minnesota. They have championed new forms of long-term care that would "uncouple" the housing and services represented by the dominant nursing home model. In addition to their collections of essays on principles of geriatrics and long-term care, Robert remains preoccupied with outcomes of care, while Rosalie focuses on ethical issues. Rosalie has served as editor of *Health and Social Work* and *The Gerontologist;* Robert has been editor of the *Journal of Community Health.*

OSCAR J. KAPLAN. Oscar J. Kaplan's professional interest in aging began in 1937, when he was completing a B.A. in psychology and writing an M.A. thesis on "Some Aspects of the Psychophysiology of Aging" (1938) at the University of California, Los Angeles. His initial curiosity actually dates earlier. As a lad of fourteen-years, contemplating a career in medicine, Kaplan was impressed by the fact that cancer seemed mainly to be a disease of later life. He decided that he wanted to learn all he could about the biomedical aspects of aging.

Kaplan earned his Ph.D. in psychology at the University of California, Berkeley. There, he studied with Harold E. Jones, whose longitudinal studies of children and adolescence were attracting international attention. He spent the 1940–1941 academic year working as a research associate in Jones's Institute of Child Welfare. After spending five years at the University of Idaho, Kaplan in 1946 became a professor of psychology and director of the Center for Survey Research at San Diego State University, where he remained for the rest of his professional career. He introduced a course on "Psychology of Later Maturity" in 1950, one of the first in the nation.

Kaplan has been called the "father of geriatric psychology" because of his interest in the relationships among behavioral, physiological, and pathological processes of the brain. In 1945, he published the first edition of *Mental Disorders in Later Life* (Stanford, Calif.: Stanford University Press; 2nd edn., 1956), which was the first book on geriatric psychiatry in any language. In the late 1940s and 1950s, with grants from the U.S. Public Health Service, Kaplan did pioneering research on the health knowledge, attitudes, and behavior of older persons. In 1960, with support from the National Institute of Mental Health, he conducted one of the first major studies of the psychology of the senile dementias. From this work emerged Kaplan's "cumulative insult theory" of senile dementia. This holds that, in some cases, late-life dementia is the result of brain damage experienced even as early as the prenatal period. While each case is individual, cumulative insults (due to disease, trauma, vascular, and nutritional problems) are imposed upon a nervous system in which neuronal changes associated with "normal" aging are going on. See his edited collection, *Psychopathology of Aging* (New York: Academic Press, 1979).

Institution-building characterizes Kaplan's career even more than his research accomplishments. Kaplan was the first behavioral scientist in the field of aging appointed to a National Institutes of Health study section. From 1946 to 1950, he served on the NIH's Gerontology Study Section, which launched an extramural grants program for research on aging. In 1949, influenced by the success of the White House Conferences on Children and Youth, Kaplan proposed to Harry S Truman, in a letter transmitted by San Diego Congressman Clinton

McKinnon, that the president convene a White House Conference on Aging. Kaplan helped Edmund V. Cowdry,* Clark Tibbitts,* Oscar Ewing, and others plan the First National Conference on Aging in 1950.

Kaplan also played a critical role in building old-age professional organizations. In 1953, concerned that some Gerontological Society members from the behavioral and social sciences found little of interest in the *Journal of Gerontology*, the leadership established the *Newsletter of the Gerontological Society*, which was to include an annotated bibliography and invited articles. From 1954 to 1960, Kaplan produced the *Newsletter* without compensation or help. He wrote most of the copy and took each issue to the Post Office to mail. In 1960, when the GSA decided to establish a second journal, *The Gerontologist*, Kaplan was named editor-in-chief. He served in this capacity through 1966.

In addition, Kaplan has served for fifteen years on the editorial advisory board of the *Journal of Gerontology*, most recently in 1986–1987. In the 1970s, he was on the board of *Geriatrics*.

Finally, Kaplan was instrumental in establishing the Western Gerontological Society. Looking upon the Western Psychological Association as a model in the early 1950s, Kaplan felt that it would relieve the burden of time and money for scholars located west of the Rockies. In 1955, while serving as president of Division 20 (now called the Division of Adult Development and Aging) of the American Psychological Association, which was meeting that year in San Francisco, Kaplan convened a meeting of what he called the Western Gerontological Society as the first regional society on aging in the United States. He served as president of the group in 1956–1957. From the start, Western's survival was very much in doubt; membership hovered around 150. Under the leadership of Gloria Cavanaugh, the organization became dynamic, attracting many professionals to its annual meetings and subscribers to its lively publications. To reflect its growing prominence, the group changed its name to the American Society on Aging in the 1980s.

Thus, Kaplan, who filled an important niche in gerontology's formative years, was instrumental in shaping many of the field's most important institutions for disseminating knowledge. What makes this accomplishment all the more impressive is that Kaplan had another career that he was pursuing with equal vigor. In some circles, he is best known as a survey researcher, not a gerontologist. Kaplan, for instance, edited the monthly *Bulletin* of the Economic Research Bureau of San Diego from 1957 to 1969. In addition, he produced a series of reports on housing, voluntary health organizations, and economic prospects for the local community. When to this is added his considerable service to his university and his extensive work in the media, it becomes very hard to keep track of all that Kaplan has done over a long and productive career.

Kaplan died in 1994.

MARSHALL B. KAPP. Marshall B. Kapp was born in 1949. He received his B.A. in 1971 from Johns Hopkins University and graduated from the George

Washington University Law School in 1974. He became interested in dependent populations for rather personal reasons: He has a brother who is mentally retarded. After completing his master's degree in public health (MPH) at Harvard in 1978, Kapp took a job with Janice Caldwell, who was then in charge of the Health Care Financing Administration's Division of Long-Term Care regulating intermediate-care facilities and nursing homes. It was there that his interest in long-term care and, specifically, aging developed.

Combining his doctor of law and MPH expertise, Kapp has analyzed and explained legal and ethical aspects of delivering health care services to older persons. He has devoted particular attention to issues of informed consent, confidentiality, guardianship, and protective services. He has also looked at long-term care financing, resource rationing, abuse and neglect, treatment decisions for critically ill patients, and liability issues in geriatrics and gerontology. A second edition of his *Geriatrics and the Law* was issued in 1992 (New York: Springer Publishing). This and his *Preventing Malpractice in Long-Term Care* (New York: Springer, 1987) provide legal background for health care providers.

Rather than overwhelm health care workers with the law and potential liability risks, Kapp tries to provide a realistic perspective and, in his words, "to explain to health-care professionals that successful risk management is fully consistent with respect for older patient autonomy, sound ethical judgment, and good clinical practice." Hence his *Legal and Ethical Aspects of Health Care for the Elderly*, edited with Harvey Pies and A. Edward Doudera (Ann Arbor, Mich.: Health Administration Press, in cooperation with the American Society of Law and Medicine, 1985), included chapters by physicians, and public health experts as well as lawyers. See also, for example, his "Our Hands Are Tied: Legally Induced Moral Tensions in Health Care Delivery," *Journal of General Internal Medicine,* 6 (July/August, 1991): 345.

Kapp is currently with the Departments of Community Health and Psychiatry, Wright State University School of Medicine in Dayton, Ohio, where he also serves as director of the Office of Geriatric Medicine and Gerontology. Additionally, he teaches a course of law and aging at the University of Dayton School of Law.

ROBERT KASTENBAUM. Robert Kastenbaum entered the University of Southern California on a graduate scholarship in philosophy but emerged with a Ph.D. in clinical psychology in 1959. His interest gradually centered on time, aging, death, and creativity. Inspiration came from Lawrence K. Frank's* pioneering article on time perspective, Lawrence LeShan's study of time orientation and social class, and Herman Feifel's explorations of attitudes toward death. As a graduate student Kastenbaum contributed a chapter on the concepts of time, aging, and mortality in adolescence to Feifel's *The Meaning of Death* (New York: Harper, 1959), a book often credited with opening the death awareness movement.

Kastenbaum's commitment to gerontology was established during an NIMH postdoctoral research experience at Clark University's Institute of Human Development. One day he visited a geriatric hospital in the vicinity and was immediately engrossed both by the anguish and resourcefulness of the residents. Soon he was director of Cashing Hospital's Department of Psychology and co-principal investigator in a series of funded studies. J. Sanborn Bockoven and Constantine Gherondache, respectively, superintendent and medical director of the Framingham, Massachusetts, facility, opened Kastenbaum's eyes to the challenges of doing "real world" service and research. Applying new time-perspective techniques, Kastenbaum provided a richer and livelier view than previously existed concerning how people reorient themselves through a time lens that recalibrates their sense of the past, present, and future.

Sociologist Philip Slater served as a consultant on some of his studies of drug effects and on his early dying-death projects, bringing "worldly sophistication" and helping Kastenbaum make the "transition from textbookish research designs to complex real-life studies." Existential psychiatrist Avery D. Weisman later joined the research team as a consultant, offering his expertise in the interaction among medical, personality, and socio-environmental influences. One of their major publications from this period was the Weisman-Kastenbaum monograph, *The Psychological Autopsy: A Study of the Terminal Phase of Life.* Kastenbaum also undertook a series of studies that involved the use of alcoholic beverages to create a therapeutic milieu within a geriatric facility. Although some people regarded this approach with alarm, the results were positive and confirmed by research and demonstration projects carried out at various sites by subsequent investigators. At Cashing Hospital, the "Captain's Chair"—a "geriatric socialization chamber" that much resembled a neighborhood pub—became the center of the facility's social life.

Kastenbaum quickly fell into the habit of starting new endeavors. In 1970 he founded two journals that are still going strong: *International Journal of Aging & Human Development,* and *Omega, Journal of Death and Dying,* the latter with the collaboration of Richard A. Kalish, who served as its first editor. Kastenbaum continues to serve as editor of both journals. He was co-founder of the National Caucus for Black Aging and consultant for the U.S. Senate Special Subcommittee on Aging for minority and ethnic issues. At Wayne State University he established the Center for Psychological Studies of Dying, Death and Lethal Behavior, the first university-based interdisciplinary program on that topic. Kastenbaum returned to Cashing Hospital as its director (1976–1980) with the hope of introducing further upgrades in its therapeutic and rehabilitation programs.

In the 1980s he participated in writing the proposal that launched the National Hospice Demonstration Study, an HCFA-financed project that helped to establish hospice care as a viable enterprise in the United States. He also helped to train interviewers and to analyze and report the results. He was elected president of the American Association of Suicidology.

It is not easy to synthesize the recurring themes in Kastenbaum's prolific writings, but several are perhaps salient. First, Kastenbaum has been interested in formulating a contextual theory of the development of "old behaviors" (or "behaving oldly") in which the markers of "old" behaviors, attitudes, cognitions, and relationships are generated through symbolic interactions. See his earlier essay, "Getting There Ahead of Time" in *Psychology Today,* December 1971. Lately, he has focused on creativity, which Kastenbaum acknowledges can be viewed as an ability, but which he thinks more appropriately is understood in terms of contextualized functions and meanings. Creativity, he contends, is an attitude and philosophy of life as much as it is a set of cognitive and aesthetic skills. Far from being an end in itself, in acts of creation, we re-create ourselves. For more, see "The Creative Process: A Life-Span Approach," in *Handbook of the Humanities and Aging,* eds. Thomas R. Cole,* David D. Van Tassel,* and Robert Kastenbaum (New York: Springer, 1992).

Second, Kastenbaum has emphasized "habituation" as a partial model of lifespan development and aging. He locates the origin of both cognitive development and proto-aging in the process and phenomenon of habituation observed in the first few weeks of postnatal life. Habituation is itself a significant, positive element in normal development. What will be recognized as "oldness" in the negative sense after many years actually begins in youth for many people as excessive filtering-out of new opportunities and a commitment to stasis-maintenance operations. Parallel but distinguishable developmental difficulties in the realm of primary relationships can augment the "progeria" effects of hyperhabituation. See his "Habituation as a Partial Model of Human Aging," *International Journal of Aging and Human Development* 12 (1980): 159–70; and "When Aging Begins: A Lifespan Developmental Approach," *Research on Aging,* 6 (1984): 105–18.

Third, in exploring the structure of hyperhabituation, Kastenbaum has been studying the creation of a "fortress-self" in later adulthood. To cope with stress, loss, mixed signals from others, as well as one's own reduced capacities to process information, he hypothesizes that people rely increasingly on stereotypes, routinized cognitive operations, and self-narratives to establish "the view from the fortress." Very often, this contributes to the bigotry evidenced in old age. See, for instance, his "Racism and the Older Voter," *International Journal of Aging and Human Development,* 32 (1991): 199–210; and "Encrusted Elders: Arizona and the Political Spirit of Postmodern Aging," in *Voices and Contexts,* eds. Thomas R. Cole, W. Andrew Achenbaum, Patricia L. Jacobi, and Robert Kastenbaum (New York: Springer, 1993).

Fourth, he has focused repeatedly on the human encounter with mortality, believing this to be a crucial test of both the individual and society. See, for instance, *The Psychology of Death,* rev. edn. (New York: Springer, 1992), and *Death, Society, and Human Experience,* 5th edn. (Boston: Allyn & Bacon, 1995).

In recent years Kastenbaum has supplemented his research approach with an attempt to examine issues of time, aging, death, and creativity within a dramatic framework. Eight of his short plays and an essay on theory and methodology are presented in *Defining Acts: Aging as Drama* (New York: Baywood, 1994). *Dorian Graying: Is Youth the Only Thing Worth Having?* includes his libretto for the opera, *Dorian* (scheduled for its premiere in February 1995, Hofstra University), and discussion of the quest for prolonged youth from ancient times to our own.

SHARON R. KAUFMAN. Sharon R. Kaufman's first book, *The Ageless Self: Sources of Meaning in Late Life* (Madison, Wis.: University of Wisconsin Press, 1986), began as a doctoral dissertation at the Medical Anthropology Program of the University of California, San Francisco. Her Ph.D. was awarded by UCSF in 1980. The project was inspired by earlier work on the relationship between aging and culture conducted by her teacher, Margaret Clark. Kaufman collected detailed life histories from middle-class Californians between the ages of seventy and 100 to explore notions of identity, culture, values, and community in late life.

The Ageless Self argues that old Americans do not perceive meaning in aging itself; neither is identity frozen in the past. Kaufman found that old people do not relate to aging or chronological age as a category of experience or meaning. Rather, the ageless self maintains continuity through a symbolic, creative process in which the past is interpreted and recreated as a resource for being in the present. The book uses the voices of old people to develop theory about adult development and aging. Identity in late life is shown to be ongoing, continuous, and creative.

Kaufman has conducted research in collaboration with UCSF's Gay Becker. Funded by the National Institute on Aging, Kaufman focused on stroke rehabilitation, decline, and dependence in late life, and the relationships among medical practice, ideology, and the chronic illness experience. In these studies she has been particularly interested in the different ways health practitioners and patients perceive rehabilitation and recovery, and in cultural constructions of frailty and risk. Based on participant-observation in acute-care hospitals, rehabilitation centers, and geriatric assessment services, and in-depth interviews with physicians, rehabilitation specialists, Kaufman explores how people confront disability in late life, and are affected by the cultural sources of expectations about recovery from illness and autonomy in late life. See her "Toward a Phenomenology of Boundaries in Medicine: Chronic Illness Experience in the Case of Stroke," *Medical Anthropology Quarterly*, 2 (1988): 338–54; "Illness, Biography, and the Interpretation of Self Following a Stroke," *Journal of Aging Studies*, 2 (1988): 217–27; "Old Age, Disease, and the Discourse on Risk: Geriatric Assessment in U.S. Health Care," *Medical Anthropology Quarterly*, 8 (1994): 76–93; and, with Gay Becker, "Content and Boundaries of Medicine in Long-Term Care: Physicians Talk about Stroke," *The Gerontologist*, 31 (1991): 238–45.

Kaufman's second book, *The Healer's Tale: Transforming Medicine and Cul-*

ture (Madison, Wis.: University of Wisconsin Press, 1993), is an inquiry into the crisis of values and goals in late twentieth-century American medicine. Through life histories of seven eminent physicians over the age of 80, whose careers spanned most of this century, the book explores medicine's changing definition and the fact that its emerging technologies have produced widespread social and moral dilemmas. The doctors' narratives are used as cultural and historical documents to make explicit medicine's transformation from an occupation of help and care to a profession of cure and finally, to a pursuit of extending and re-creating human life.

JEANIE KAYSER-JONES. Jeanie Kayser-Jones earned her Ph.D. from the University of California, Berkeley, in 1978. As with many anthropologists who were attracted to studies of the aged in the 1970s, she credits the 1967 work of Margaret Clark and Barbara Gallatin Armstrong, *Culture and Aging: An Anthropological Study of Older Americans* (Springfield, Ill.: C. C. Thomas), for sparking her interest.

Kayser-Jones did an early cross-cultural comparative study of institutional care of the elderly in the United States and Scotland. Hers was one of the first full-scale anthropological studies of nursing homes in the United States. She was also one of the first anthropologists to conduct an ethnographic study of nursing homes. This study presents a new understanding of the interrelationships between the structural characteristics of the institutions and the historical and social-cultural milieu within which they are situated. Using interactional analysis, Kayser-Jones analyzed not only how structural characteristics influenced the quality of care, but also the symbolic and functional value of gift and service exchanges between residents and staff. She extended social exchange theory by describing how the exchange of small gifts for service affects the quality of care in nursing homes. See her *Old Alone and Neglected: Care of the Aged in the United States and Scotland* (Berkeley: University of California Press, 1981, 1990).

Her subsequent research, funded by the National Institute of Aging, investigated the treatment of acute illness in nursing homes. This study analyzed the clinical and social-structural factors that contributed to the hospitalization of nursing home residents. Kayser-Jones argues that the 216,000 nursing home residents who are hospitalized annually could be treated in nursing homes if adequate staff and services were provided. In this research, conducted with Carolyn Wiener and Joseph Barbaccia, Kayser-Jones argued that some $1 billion could be saved. See "Factors Contributing to the Hospitalization of Nursing Home Residents," *The Gerontologist* 29 (4): 502–10.

Environmental influences on the aged have been another focus of her research. In particular, she has examined how the environment influences the quality of care in nursing homes. See her "The Environment and Quality of Care in Long-Term Care Institutions," in *Indices of Quality in Long-Term Care: Research and Practice* (New York: National League for Nursing Homes, 1989); and

"Open Ward Accommodations in a Long-Term Care Facility: The Elderly's Point of View," *The Gerontologist,* 26 (1986): 63–68.

Her current research, "The Behavioral Context of Eating and Nutritional Support," funded by the National Institute on Aging and the National Institute of Dental Research (1993–1997), investigates the social, cultural, environmental, and clinical factors that influence eating and the nutritional status of nursing home residents. In this research, she is also investigating the use of feeding tubes and the consequences of feeding tubes for the elderly and their families.

Kayser-Jones has also pressed for the creation of a Institute of Gerontology to promote advanced study, research, and education in elderly care. An associated center, modeled on the British Geriatric Service, could provide a complete range of professional services to the elderly. See her "Institute of Gerontology: A Comprehensive Approach to the Care of the Elderly," *Educational Gerontology: An International Journal,* 12 (1986): 43–55.

JENNIE KEITH. Jennie Keith was drawn to gerontology as an anthropology graduate student at Northwestern University. Curious about retirement communities that were springing up in California in the mid-1960s, Keith came across the work of cultural anthropologist Margaret Clark, who has been influential in the anthropology of aging with her 1967 book, written with Barbara Gallatin Armstrong, *Culture and Aging* (Springfield, Ill.: C. C. Thomas). Keith also recalls Irving Rosow's* *Social Interaction of the Aged* and Frances Carp's *Victoria Plaza: New World for the Elderly* as critical to the early stages of her work on old age.

Keith's doctoral studies were completed in 1968 under the direction of Paul J. Bohannan, a major figure in cultural anthropology. Keith credits Bohannan with encouraging her to pursue the then unconventional topic of aging. Her dissertation documented and interpreted the emergence of old age as a distinct social category in the United States. This primarily archival research included interviews with residents in California retirement homes, and Keith viewed the study as preparation for her first major fieldwork in France in 1969–1970. Her choice of France as a site was influenced by Ethel Shanas* at the University of Illinois, Chicago Circle, who put Keith in contact with French colleagues such as Paillat and Huet. Her participant observation in a French retirement residence led to a book about age as a basis of community formation, *Old People, New Lives: Community Creation in a Retirement Residence* (Chicago: University of Chicago Press, 1973, 1982).

Keith has consistently argued for the importance of qualitative data for understanding experiences of aging, as in *New Methods for Old Age Research,* which she edited in collaboration with Christine L. Fry of Chicago's Loyola University (South Hadley, Mass.: Bergin and Garvey, 1986). She also collaborated with David Kertzer of Brown University to organize an NIA workshop on "Age and Anthropological Theory," which led to their book of the same title, published in 1984 (Ithaca, N.Y.: Cornell University Press). Keith also highlights

188   DONALD P. KENT

the intellectual—and practical—dangers of viewing old persons in isolation from people of other ages or from their social and cultural context. See Keith's chapter, "Age in Social and Cultural Context," in *Handbook of Aging and the Social Sciences,* eds. Robert H. Binstock* and Linda K. George* (New York: Academic Press, 1990).

In *Old People as People* (Boston: Little, Brown, 1982), Keith's effort was to understand the experiences, attitudes, and behaviors of old people by first coming to grips with the cultural and social mechanisms affecting all members of society. "We should not begin by assuming that the behavior or attitudes of older persons are a result of their age," Keith warns. "Community formation by older people in some industrial societies, for example, can be described and explained by the same theoretical principles as community formation by urban squatters, nation states or utopian experimenters."

Believing that fuller understanding of the conditions promoting different meanings of age required systematic and comparative research, Keith and Christine Fry organized Project AGE, which was supported by the NIA and carried out by a team of seven anthropologists in Africa, Ireland, Hong Kong and the United States. This research is reported in *The Aging Experience* (Thousand Oaks, Calif.: Sage Publishers, 1994) by Keith, Fry, and the other members of Project AGE, Charlotte Ikels, Anthony Glascock, Jeanette Dickerson-Putman, Henry Harpending, and Patricia Draper.

To fulfill a research agenda oriented toward viewing old people in their full social and cultural context, Keith has brought cross-cultural and qualitative perspectives into the mainstream of gerontological research. She has exerted influence as a study section reviewer for the National Institute on Aging and through her roles in the Gerontological Society. She is equally proud, however, of her efforts to encourage students and younger scholars to take up the study of aging and the elderly.

Keith, long a professor of anthropology at Swarthmore in Pennsylvania, now serves as the college's provost.

DONALD P. KENT. Donald Peterson Kent was born in Philadelphia in 1916. He earned his B.A. from Pennsylvania State University in 1940 and an M.A. from Temple University in 1945. While working toward his Ph.D. (1950) at the University of Pennsylvania, Kent served as an instructor in sociology.

From 1950 to 1957, Kent served as an associate professor of sociology at the University of Connecticut; his first academic monograph, *The Refugee Intellectual,* was published in 1953. Increasingly, however, his interests focused on the ways families coped with social change, which in turn sparked his interest in the aged. From 1957 to 1961, he headed the university's gerontology center; he also chaired the Connecticut Commission on Services for Elderly Persons. During the Kennedy administration, Kent served as a special assistant to the U.S. Secretary of Health, Education and Welfare and as vice chairman of the President's Council on Aging. From 1963 to 1965, he directed the U.S. Office of

Aging, prior to the enactment of the Older Americans Act. He worked closely with state executives in aging, and conducted workshops for such officials after leaving government. (See his *Institute in Social Gerontology for State Executives in Aging* (Idyllwild, California: State of California, 1966).)

In 1965, Kent was appointed head of the Department of Sociology and Anthropology at Pennsylvania State University. He held that position until his death in 1972. His *Research, Planning and Action for the Elderly: The Power and Potential of Social Science* (New York: Behavioral Publications, 1972) attests to the practical and intellectual insights he gained by combining careers in academia and government.

Kent was very active in the Gerontological Society. He served as editor of *The Gerontologist* from 1967 to 1970. His valedictory publication, "Planning-Facilities, Programs, and Services: Government and Non-Government," *The Gerontologist,* 12 (1972): 36–48, reported on forty-one recommendations from the 1971 White House Conference on Aging, which dealt with advocacy, delivery of services, and the need to involve older persons in developing an adequate concept of aging. As always, Kent stressed the importance of using appropriate methodological tools to conduct research.

The Gerontological Society now awards the Donald Kent Award each year to those who exemplify "the highest standards of professional leadership in gerontology through teaching, service, and interpretation of gerontology to the larger society."

GARY M. KENYON. Gary M. Kenyon was born in 1949 in Montreal, Canada. He earned a B.A. in business administration and an M.A. in philosophy at Concordia. He received his Ph.D. in interdisciplinary studies in gerontology from the University of British Columbia in 1985, where he studied with Michael Chandler and Kjell Rubensson. After completing his Ph.D., Kenyon spent a year as a postdoctoral fellow with James E. Birren* at the University of Southern California and another six months at the University of Linkoping, Sweden. Attracted to the fields of activity theory and adult intelligence by what he saw as implicit assumptions in the literature, Kenyon has brought the insights of philosophers such as Hans Gadamer and the existentialists to the theories of aging and strategies of intervention.

Most existing theories of aging, in Kenyon's view, assume that there is only one real mechanism of aging, either biological or social. These lead to the view of human aging as decrement, and to negative stereotyping of the elderly as well as "paternalistic" intervention strategies. In place of such assumptions, Kenyon begins with existential thinking that emphasizes both the finitude and interpersonal nature of human beings. The result is an emphasis on the role that meaning plays throughout life. More concretely, his line of argument calls for a more "contextual or situational orientation" when considering intervention, whether through policy, treatment, or research. Training of gerontologists, therefore, ought to highlight critical thinking, specific research, and particular practice.

Kenyon's more recent work has focused on the role that metaphors and life-stories play in the field of aging through collaborative interdisciplinary efforts. His goal is to bring the humanities to bear on the study of aging through a dialogue with scientific disciplines.

Along with his research and teaching activities, Kenyon works to bring meaningful activity and independence to the local community of seniors, with outreach efforts that bring the community of seniors, professionals, and students together. His own network of collaborators reflects this commitment to transgenerational intellectual journeys. His partners include James E. Birren,* Torbjorn Svensson, Jan-Erik Ruth, Wilhelm Mader, and Phillip G. Clark.* Kenyon maintains active scholarly collaborations in Holland, Sweden, Finland, Germany, and the United States.

Kenyon's recent writings include, "Basic Assumptions in Theories of Human Aging," in *Emergent Theories of Aging,* eds. James E. Birren* and Vern L. Bengtson* (New York: Springer, 1988); *Metaphors of Aging in Science and the Humanities* (New York: Springer, 1991); "The Humanities in Gerontology," in a special issue of the *Canadian Journal on Aging,* 8 (1993); and an edited volume, *Aging and Biography: Explanations in Adult Development* (New York: Springer, 1995). He has created a certificate and degree program at St. Thomas University in New Brunswick.

PAUL A. KERSCHNER. Paul A. Kerschner was born in 1942 in California. From 1965 to 1967, he was a Peace Corps Volunteer in Nigeria, West Africa; he later served as a senior consultant to the Peace Corps. Kerschner earned his M.A. and his Ph.D. at the University of Southern California's School of Public Administration. His dissertation focused on "Organizational Placement: A Case Study of the Administration on Aging."

In 1973, James E. Birren* hired Kerschner to direct the Community Programs Division at the University of Southern California's Andrus Center. As he assumed more leadership responsibilities, Kerschner became instrumental in launching the Leonard Davis School and in teaching courses on administration and public policy. In 1978, he moved to Washington, D.C., to become associate director of the American Association of Retired Persons. In addition to these administrative tasks, he became executive director of a commission on nursing homes in Maryland. As a result of his efforts, the state's aging and long-term care services were substantially reorganized.

From 1985 to 1989, Kerschner served as director of the National Foundation for Long Term Health Care. For the next three years, he was the senior vice president at the National Council on the Aging. In 1992, Kerschner became executive director of the Gerontological Society. Among other things, he helped Bob Blancato and his staff develop an agenda for the 1995 White House Conference on Aging. He also chaired the Coalition for Consumer Protection/Quality in Health Care Reform.

Tragically, Kerschner died after a short illness in 1994.

ERIC R. KINGSON. Eric R. Kingson received his B.A. from Boston University in 1968. During the next four years, he was associated with the Elizabeth Peabody House in Somerville, Massachusetts. His interest in aging began in 1972, when he was serving as an in-help coordinator for the Eastern Middlesex County Retired Senior Volunteer Program. That experience raised his interest in issues of work, leisure, retirement, and meaningful roles for elders. An Administration on Aging fellowship (1975–1977) made graduate school possible.

While working during the summers for the Commonwealth's Department of Human Resources, Kingson earned an M.P.A. from Northeastern University in 1976. Three years later, aided by a Department of Labor dissertation grant, he completed his Ph.D. dissertation, ''Men Who Leave Work Before Age 62: A Study of Advantaged and Disadvantaged Very Early Retirement,'' at Brandeis University's Florence Heller Graduate School for Advanced Studies in Social Welfare. There, he worked primarily under James H. Schulz,* though he also formed professional bonds with Robert H. Binstock* and Robert Hudson, among others.

From 1979 to 1986, Kingson was an assistant professor in the School of Social Work and Community Planning at the University of Maryland at Baltimore. He took his teaching and community involvement in policy-relevant organizations very seriously. But it was his two leaves of absence that put into motion connections that established Kingson's presence in the field. Kingson served on the staff of the National Commission on Social Security Reform, which proved to be the vehicle for the enactment of the landmark 1983 Social Security amendments. There, he worked very closely with former Social Security Commissioner Robert Ball. Toward the end of the decade, Kingson worked with Ball and others in establishing the National Academy of Social Insurance, which is designed to advance research on Social Security and other social welfare and health care issues.

Kingson has written several books designed to help Americans understand their rights and the workings of the Social Security system: *Social Security and You* (World Almanac Publications, 1984); *What You Must Know about Social Security and Medicare* (New York: Pharos Books, 1987); with Edward Berkowitz and F. Pratt, *Social Security in the U.S.A.: A Discussion Guide to Social Insurance with Lesson Plans* (Washington, D.C.: Save Our Security Education Fund, 1989); and with Edward Berkowitz, *Social Security and Medicare: A Policy Primer* (Westport, Conn.: Auburn House, 1993).

Kingson took a second leave for eighteen months to serve as director of the Emerging Issues Program at the Gerontological Society. In this capacity, he worked closely with John M. Cornman,* GSA's executive director, and Linda Krogh Harootyan, the society's media director, to think through the demographic, economic, political, social, and ethical dimensions of an aging society. This project was supported with funds from the Allied Corporation, AARP Andrus Foundation, John A. Hartford Foundation, and the National Institute on Aging.

With John Cornman and Barbara Hirshorn, Kingson published *Ties That Bind: The Interdependence of Generations* (Cabin John, Md.: Seven Locks Press, 1986), which received considerable media attention because of its reasoned assault on the specter of generational inequities. This work led, in turn, to his involvement in a series of projects with the Andrus Foundation and AARP, notably its New Roles in Society project.

Since 1986, Kingson has been affiliated with the Graduate School of Social Work at Boston College. He has directed a Minority Management Training Grant for the Administration on Aging since 1990.

VIRA R. KIVETT. Vira R. Kivett was first attracted the early developmental stage of gerontology in 1970. In 1976 she completed her Ph.D. in family studies at the University of North Carolina at Greensboro, where she continues to teach and conduct research. She is affiliated with the Department of Human Development and Family Studies within the School of Human Environmental Sciences.

Kivett's most important research has been on the various blood and marriage ties in the families of older rural adults. This work has ranged from older parent-adult child solidarity and exchanges to those of grandparent and grandchildren. Her current research has been in the areas of very old rural survivors, studying cultural differences and similarities in the importance and function of the grandparent role, and the family supports and relationships of older adults migrating to the Southeast. See her "The Importance of Emotional and Social Isolation to Loneliness among Very Old Rural Adults," *The Gerontologist,* 34 (1994): 340–46; and "Racial Comparisons of the Grandmother Role: Implications for Strengthening the Family Support System of Older Black Women," *Family Relations,* 42 (1993): 165–72.

Kivett has also tested, and found wanting, some important models through her work in rural gerontology. In an 1986 article with M. Atkinson and Ruth Campbell,* Kivett challenged the intergenerational theory of family solidarity first advanced by Vern L. Bengston* and colleagues. Examination of the untested theory showed little support. While the model was found to be useful in explaining objective solidarity, it was not useful in explaining subjective solidarity (consensus and affection). See "Intergenerational Solidarity: An Examination of a Theoretical Model," *Journal of Gerontology,* 41 (1986): 408–16.

In 1992, Kivett, writing with Edward A. Powers, modified the kin selection principle, posited by Van der Berge and Barash. Kivett argued that the rank order of help provided does not follow blood lines alone, but follows both consanguineous and affinal ties. See "Kin Expectations and Kin Support among Rural Older Adults," *Rural Sociology,* 57 (1992): 194–215.

Kivett's interests continue to reflect those she shared with her mentor, Ellen Winston, who was commissioner of welfare under John F. Kennedy. Kivett counts her own students as her primary collaborators. Among them are B. Jan McCulloch of the University of Kentucky, Texas Technical University's Jean Pearson Scott, and Beth Dugan, currently at the University of North Carolina at Greensboro.

MORTON H. KLEBAN. Morton H. Kleban was born in 1931. He graduated from City College of New York in 1953, earned an M.A. from the State University of Iowa in 1955, and completed his doctoral work in psychology at the University of North Dakota five years later. He is currently director of psychometrics for the Philadelphia Geriatric Center, a post he has held since 1966. He has also worked as a research scientist for the Norristown State Hospital, in Norristown, Pennsylvania, since 1966, and advanced to the position of senior statistician there in 1990. His research career has been supported completely by federal grants.

It was in 1966 that Kleban first turned to aging-related work. He was recruited in the Behavioral Research Laboratory of behaviorist M. Powell Lawton* at the Philadelphia Geriatric Center. Working with biochemists Henry Altschuler and Martin Gold, Kleban conducted studies of the biochemical relationships among RNA, DNA, brain proteins and escape and avoidance learning. "There had been much controversy about these experiments at the time, and funding sources began to disappear," Kleban recalls.

He has published widely with a number of colleagues. In general, his studies have focused on psychobiology in animals, mental impairment, excess disability, caregiving, and healthy human aging. He has also advanced gerontological methodology with work on statistical power programs and the application of covariance analysis to gerontological problems.

Kleban's most important theoretical construct is the refinement of Q-type factor analysis suited to the study of a small group of subjects across a large number of variables. He outlined a method for converting subject factors into information about the contribution of variables to the subject factors. Although not widely used since, this methodology remains available as a tool, clearly outlined in "Q-Technique Methodology in the Study of Healthy Aged Men (Part I)," *Experimental Aging Research*, 5 (1979): 109–35; and "Q-Technique Methodology in the Study of Healthy Aged Men (Part II)," *Experimental Aging Research*, 6 (1980): 69–109.

Kleban served as a consulting editor of the *Journal of Gerontology* from 1979 to 1984 and then on the *Journal of Gerontology* editorial board for a three-year term. From 1980 to 1986, he also served on the editorial board of *Experimental Aging Research*. Kleban has also been active in the American Psychological Association and in the Pennsylvania Psychological Association.

ROBERT W. KLEEMEIER. Robert W. Kleemeier was born in Cincinnati in 1915. He received his B.A. from Ohio Wesleyan University in 1938, and then studied psychology at the University of Michigan, where he earned his M.A. in 1939 and his Ph.D. in 1941. While pursuing graduate work, Kleemeier taught at Ohio State and Michigan; he also served as a clinical assistant in the University of Michigan's psychology clinic.

After serving for a year as a clinical counselor and instructor of psychology at the University of Illinois, Kleemeier joined the faculty of Northwestern University (1942–1949). In 1949, Kleemeier was named the first director at the Moosehaven Research Laboratory for Gerontology in Orange Park, Florida. After that venture collapsed, Kleemeier joined the Department of Psychology at Washington University as a research professor, where he remained until his untimely death in 1966, a year after he had served as president of the Gerontological Society.

Kleemeier's major research in psychology fell into three domains: experimental abnormal psychology, flexibility measurement, and the psychology of aging. In "Age Changes in Psychomotor Capacity and Productivity," *Journal of Business,* 27 (1954): 146–55, he confirmed a finding by James E. Birren* and Jack Botwinick* that shortly before or around the fourth decade of human life, there is a consistent decline with advancing age in psychometric scores. In his contribution to the *Handbook of Aging and the Individual,* ed. James E. Birren (Chicago: University of Chicago Press, 1961), pp. 400–51, Kleemeier discussed in broad terms the relationship between "Behavior and the Organization of the Bodily and the External Environment." Building on ideas set forth in his "Environmental Settings and the Aging Process" (in *Psychological Aspects of Aging,* ed. John E. Anderson* (Washington, D.C.: American Psychological Association, 1956), pp. 105–16), Kleemeier suggested that "familiar age changes which occur in body, size, structure, and appearance become germane to the study of age-environment relationship." Sensory changes, particularly in vision and audition, require aids in compensating for age-acquired losses in modalities. Thermal and atmospheric conditions, moreover, often affect older persons more than younger ones.

In 1961, Oxford University Press published Kleemeier's edited collection, *Aging and Leisure.* The intellectual roots of the book can be traced to the work Kleemeier did for Anderson and Birren, which was extended in a conference sponsored by the Ford Foundation. The subtitle, "A Research Perspective into the Meaningful Use of Time," punctuates various contributors' foci on what older people did during non-working time and what meaning or significance they attributed to these activities. Kleemeier and his colleagues (such as Oscar J. Kaplan,* Margaret Gordon, and Fred Cottrell) were interested in establishing "basic" objectives and positing "elemental" questions.

In 1967, the Gerontological Society decided to rename the Searle Award, first awarded in 1965, the Kleemeier Award in recognition of his outstanding research in the field of gerontology. In 1969, the Society began alternating the award between the bio-medical and the social science/practice halves of the membership. The first five recipients were Nathan W. Shock,* James E. Birren,* Robert J. Havighurst,* Ewald W. Busse,* and Carl Eisdorfer.

NATHAN KOGAN. Nathan Kogan earned a doctorate from Harvard University in 1954. As a graduate and postdoctoral student in social psychology during the 1950s, Kogan was immersed in the research in attitudes toward ethnic and religious groups. An opportunity to join a gerontological research organization in Boston opened up for him the possibility of extending this type of research to older people. "The weakness of the Tuckman-Lorge corpus offered a further impetus to push ahead in this area," Kogan recalls.

Following the correction of what he saw as defects in the Tuckman-Lorge research, Kogan began a period of taking stock and assessing progress. His article, "Beliefs, Attitudes, and Stereotypes about Old People: A New Look at Some Old Issues," in *Research on Aging,* 1 (1979): 11–36, is indicative of his work during this period. See also his more recent "Person Perception," in *Encyclopedia of Aging,* ed. George Maddox* (New York: Springer, 1987).

Another aspect of Kogan's research has emerged from a focus on judgment and categorization. His latest work, done in collaboration with Montie Mills, has been a close examination of the basis for gender differences in age preferences and cognitions. See their recent paper, "Gender Influences on Age Cognitions and Preferences: Sociocultural or Sociobiological?" in *Psychology and Aging,* 7 (March 1992): 98–106. Kogan and Mills found that, while their studies were not conclusive, age is a more salient feature for men than for women when judging others, and that men exhibit a youth bias. These findings were interpreted as consistent with current theorizing in evolutionary psychology.

Kogan points out that Susan Sontag's concept of a "double standard of aging" has captured the attention of those interested in the relationship between gender and aging, but there have been few empirical studies. His article, "A Study of Age Categorization," *Journal of Gerontology,* 34 (1979): 358–67, was an initial effort in that direction. His latest work, again with Mills, offers a more extended test and examines the relative value of sociocultural and sociobiological interpretations.

In addition to this work, Kogan was one of the first to ask when children first become aware of age differences. See N. Kogan, J. W. Stephens, and F. A. Shelton, "Age Differences: A Developmental Study of Discriminability and Affective Response," *Journal of Abnormal and Social Psychology,* 62 (1961): 221–30. He also did early seminal studies on adult age differences in risk taking (with Michael Wallach), and integrated studies of age differences in creativity and cognitive style. More recently, he contributed a chapter on "Personality and Aging" to the third edition of the *Handbook of the Psychology of Aging,* eds. J. E. Birren* and K. W. Schaie* (San Diego: Academic Press, 1990).

Kogan is currently a professor and chairman of the Psychology Department at New York City's New School for Social Research.

MARVIN ROBERT KOLLER. Marvin Koller was born in 1919. He earned his B.S. in education from Kent State University in 1940, an M.S. in 1947 and Ph.D. in 1950 in sociology from Ohio State University. He was one of forty professors who in 1959 were trained at the University of California, Berkeley, under an National Institute of Mental Health grant in social gerontology. Wilma Donahue* served as the group's leader and mentor, along with Clark Tibbitts,* Robert Kleemeier,* and Ernest W. Burgess.*

Koller is primarily known for his pioneering book, titled *Social Gerontology,* which appeared in 1968 (New York: Random House). "This was an effort to reach the interested public in calling attention to the rapidly developing specialization known as social gerontology," he recalls. It was designed to be accessible to scholars and the public and to serve as an introduction to the large literature on aging. It was also intended to be the foundation of future efforts to serve the elderly.

In 1974, Koller published *Families, a Multigenerational Approach* (New York: McGraw-Hill), which discussed in detail the central place of families in connecting the heritages of past, present, and future generations. His approach stressed the symbolic linkages over the passage of time in which deceased generations continue to affect the living generations of the young, the middle-aged, and the elderly. In turn, the living generations hope to leave their symbolic estates to future generations.

Koller has also worked directly to enhance the lives of the elderly, and it is of this work that he seems most proud. He founded the Senior Guest Students program at Kent State University in 1974. The program provides classes to retired men and women on a free, non-credit basis. By 1980, this program was serving some 600 elders in classes throughout the university. It became the model for an Ohio state law mandating similar programs in state-supported schools. Not only has this program helped the senior students, but Koller reports, it has also been of great value to other students, faculty, and the administration. "The high cooperation I received made this program a great success and sources of much personal satisfaction," he says.

Koller "retired" in 1989 from Kent State University, having reached the state-mandated age of seventy as the year tenured professors were required to retire. As emeritus professor, however, Koller continued to teach until August 1994. Having brought an elderhostel class to Kent State in 1975 when this remarkable form of adult education first went "national," Koller returned to teaching an elderhostel class in the sociology of humor for Baldwin-Wallace College, Berea, Ohio, from 1990 through 1992. He followed this three-year summer series with humor classes at Kent State University in 1993 and 1994.

His text, *Humor and Society: Explorations in the Sociology of Humor* (Houston: Cap and Gown Press, 1988), was a "first" in terms of developing the specialty in the field of sociology. Koller continues to promote humor as a therapeutic tool as a lecturer for groups concerned with serving the elderly, patients, and those experiencing various forms of stress.

WILLIAM B. KOUNTZ. William Bryan Kountz was born in 1896 in Saxton, Missouri. After earning his M.D. from Washington University in 1926, he completed residencies in three St. Louis hospitals. He also joined the faculty of his alma mater, where he remained for the rest of his career. Kountz served as director of clinical services and as a member of the board of control of the division of gerontology. Concurrently he was a consulting physician to the Barnes, Lutheran, and several other St. Louis hospitals. At the St. Louis City Hospital, Kountz was instrumental in establishing a research unit for geriatrics.

During the course of his career Kountz published more than 100 scholarly papers. Best known for his endocrinological and circulatory studies, Kountz contributed to the American lectures in circulation, *Thyroid Function and Its Possible Role in Vascular Degeneration* (Springfield, Ill.: C. C. Thomas, 1951). There, he argued that too little attention had been paid to internal metabolism and blood supply of the blood vessel walls, which affect arterial functioning, which in turn affect nutrition and thus result in body degeneration.

Other contributions underscored his geriatric and gerontologic interests: "Alpha-2 Lipoprotein in Man and Its Relation to Myocardial Infarction," in *Proceedings of the Society of Experimental Biology and Medicine* (1959); "The Action of Chlorotrianisene with Androgen on Nitrogen Retention in Elderly People," *Journal of the American Geriatrics Society* (1959), and "Sex Hormone Replacement in the Aged: Experimental Variables of Time and Dosage," *Journal of Gerontology* (1961).

Kountz was president of the American Society for the Study of Arteriosclerosis in 1948–1949 and of the Gerontological Society in 1956. He was a member of the national advisory committee for the 1961 White House Conference on Aging. Active in many national professional bodies and as well as state and local associations, he became director of the St. Louis-based Gerontological Research Foundation in 1954. In 1960 he received the Willard O. Thompson Award from the American Geriatrics Society.

William Kountz died in 1962.

BRUCE S. KRISTAL. Bruce Kristal was born in Boston in 1965. He graduated from MIT in three years, studying cellular and molecular biology under Phillip A. Sharp. From 1986 to 1991, initially supported by a National Science Foundation Graduate Fellowship, Kristal pursued a Ph.D. in virology. He was a predoctoral fellow in the laboratory of James I. Mullins while working on his dissertation, "Multiple Roles of the Feline Leukemia Virus Envelope Glycoprotein."

Kristal anticipated doing AIDS research, but after a few years, he became interested in aging, following the advice of a mentor to look at large, important problems in biology. After considering his options, Kristal chose in 1991 to take postdoctoral training in the Department of Physiology at the University of Texas Health Science Center in San Antonio. His mentor is Byung Pal Yu.

Kristal's research has been supported by an NIH postdoctoral training fellowship and a Glenn Foundation Postdoctoral award. He also received an American Federal for Aging Research (AFAR) grant to underwrite his work on "oxidant-induced repression of mitochondrial transcription: testing the predictions of the free radical and free radical/glycation theories of aging."

As the title of his AFAR grant suggests, Kristal has been very interested in similarities in and differences between three biological theories of aging. The free Radical Theory of Aging, first proposed by Denham Harman in "Aging: A Theory Based On Free Radical And Radiation Chemistry," *Journal of Gerontology,* 11 (1956): 289–300, proposes that intracellular, free radical reactions damage cellular constituents. Glycation theories, in contrast, suggest that damage is extracellularly induced by non-enzymatic glycation. The Maillard model, which is related to the glycation theory, hypothesizes that the consequent modification of macromolecules is the primary cause of aging.

Kristal and his mentor, Yu, have conducted studies on the mitochondria that suggest that both extra- and intracellular models must be integrated because the mechanisms are actually linked: Free radicals increase glycation; glycation induces free radical-related damage. See B. S. Kristal and B. P. Yu, "An Emerging Hypothesis: Synergistic Induction of Aging by Free Radicals and Maillard Reactions," *Journal of Gerontology,* 47 (1992): B107-B114.

JOHN A. KROUT. John A. Krout fell into the study of gerontology through his interest in service utilization in rural areas. Shortly after completing his doctorate in sociology at Pennsylvania State University in 1977, a "serendipitous encounter" with a local aging agency turned his attention to the field. After fifteen years at the State University of New York in Fredonia, Krout now directs the newly formed Gerontology Institute at Ithaca College.

Although he was one of few scholars who did major research in the field of aging at Fredonia (historian William Graebner, who wrote *A History of Retirement* is also there), he turned his location into a virtue by focusing on rural issues. His first book, *The Aged in Rural America* (Westport, Conn.: Greenwood Press, 1986), initially received little attention from gerontologists, but it made his reputation in the field. His work on rural issues has looked at the characteristics of the rural elderly population, including familial support and health-related questions. He has also explored the rural long-term care system. His recent work on that subject, "Rural Area Agencies on Aging: An Overview of Activities and Policy Issues," can be found in the *Journal of Aging Studies,* 5 (1991): 404–24.

His second work, *Senior Centers in America* (Westport, Conn.: Greenwood, 1989), sparked relatively little interest at first, but it, too, has solidified his reputation as a solid researcher. He has recently published *Providing Community-Based Services to the Rural Elderly* (Beverly Hills, Calif.: Sage, 1994). The bulk of his research on senior centers comprises a series of national surveys on aspects of the aging services network that have been only marginally studied.

These have involved rural and urban service providers, including area agencies on aging, senior centers, and case management agencies.

He has attempted to refine the Andersen Framework of predicting service utilization in his "Utilization of Services by the Elderly," *Social Service Review* 58 (1984): 281–90; and "Correlates of Service Utilization Among the Rural Elderly," *The Gerontologist,* 23 (1983): 500–504.

All of Krout's research has been oriented toward field practice, and he has presented his findings directly to practitioners. This work has been recognized by several awards from the National Council on Aging in 1993, honoring his work on senior center research and professional leadership in rural aging issues. He has been a consultant to a number of Administration on Aging grants.

MARGARET E. (MAGGIE) KUHN. Margaret E. Kuhn was born in Buffalo, New York, in 1905. She graduated from the College of Women of Western Reserve University in 1926. Kuhn worked with the YWCA in Cleveland, Philadelphia, and New York, and served for two years with the General Alliance of Unitarian Women in Boston, and then for 22 years in the social action arm of the United Presbyterian Church (U.S.A.).

Kuhn's role in gerontology did not become evident, or at least radicalized, until she reached the age of sixty-five, when she was forced into mandatory retirement. Kuhn rebelled. In 1970, with five other people, she established the Consultation of Older and Younger Adults for Social Change. A year later the group changed its name to Gray Panthers. Thereafter, Kuhn and her allies attracted considerable media attention. Perhaps the Gray Panthers' most dramatic moment was its guerilla theater skits at the 1974 American Medical Association convention to protest the nation's health care industry.

In 1973, the Gray Panthers merged with Ralph Nader's Retired Professional Action Group, and it established a project fund to accept and allocate money for intergenerational projects. By 1985, the Gray Panthers had more than 120 chapters, or "networks" as they were called. Membership had grown to 60,000, roughly 25 percent of whom were under the age of thirty. The group enjoyed observer and consultative status at the United Nations. Kuhn shared the limelight with luminaries such as Betty Friedan and Robert N. Butler*; George Maddox* invited her to engage in friendly but serious debate at a Gerontological Society meeting. The "responsible contributions of old people are essential to the survival and well-being of society," Kuhn insisted in *Maggie Kuhn on Aging* (Boston: Beacon Press, 1977). "Old people have a large stake in this new community—in helping to create it and extend it." In her autobiography, *No Stone Unturned: The Life and Times of Maggie Kuhn* (Philadelphia: Gray Panthers, 1991), she emphasized the importance in late life of "having a goal: a passionate purpose which bears upon the public interest."

As Kuhn herself became "an elder of the tribe," as she is fond of calling older people, the Gray Panthers faced tough choices. Despite some successes, the members' commitment to a broad agenda of social justice issues presents a

200   LOUIS KUPLAN

constant challenge. Kuhn remains the best-known leader of the organization, but
has said, "I'm not leaving a successor but rather an effective organization for
justice and peace."

The 1978 edition of *World Almanac* named Kuhn one of "the twenty-five
most influential women in America." The *Ladies Home Journal* in 1983 also
saluted her contribution. In 1992, she was profiled by the Caring Institute in
Faces of Caring: A Search for the 100 Most Caring People in History. Two
years later, *Ms.* magazine saluted her as one of the "50 Faces of Feminism."

LOUIS KUPLAN. Louis Kuplan was born in New York City in 1906. He received his B.A. from the University of California, Los Angeles, in 1929 and
did graduate work at Berkeley in the 1930s. From 1934 to 1940, Kuplan was a
county director in the California Relief Administration. During the next three
years he was based in San Francisco, working as an administrative assistant in
the Farm Security Administration, which was followed by a two-year stint with
the city's Public Housing Authority.

Kuplan's entry into the aging network began in 1945, when he spent two
years as a public assistance analyst for the Social Security Administration. He
then became chief of the division of old-age security for the California Department of Social Welfare (1947–1951). The *Proceedings of the Governor's Conference on the Problems of the Aging* (Sacramento: State of California, October
1951) divided its reports into ten divisions with 22 sections. Recognizing that
issues concerning physical health and recreation were not unique to Californians,
as executive secretary of the California Interdepartmental Coordinating Committee on Aging (1950–1955) and then as executive secretary of the California
Citizens Advisory Committee on Aging (1955–1960), Kuplan assembled experts
and older citizens to issue reports that ensured that California was in the forefront of state-level initiatives during the 1950s. See, for instance, his "Health
Programs for California's Senior Citizens," *California Health,* 14 (1956): 1–4.

To focus attention on the elderly, Kuplan used the media. He was editor of
Maturity magazine from 1954 to 1960, and an editorial consultant for the San
Francisco-based Harvest Years Publishing Company (1960–1963). In "Building
a Philosophy towards Aging," an occasional paper on adult education (University of British Columbia: Department of University Extension, 1958), Kuplan
compared (mis)understanding about aging's technological, demographic, and social problems to the complex root structure of a California redwood.

From 1969 to 1978, he was moderator and producer of KRON-TV's program,
A Gift of Time. Kuplan also taught in the University of California extension
system and at Bay Area community colleges. From 1975 until his death, he also
served on the board of directors of the Food Advertising Service and the Catholic Committee on Aging, and on the board of Optimum Achievers Inc. (1981–
86).

Kuplan was founding president of the Western Gerontological Society, which
became the American Society on Aging, in 1955. The organization named him

Gerontologist of the Year (1957) and gave him a leadership award (1975). He was also president of the Gerontological Society in 1958–1959. A president of the International Association of Gerontology (1960–1963), Kuplan was made an honorary member of the gerontological and geriatric societies of Argentina and Chile. He also was honored by San Francisco and California organizations.

JAMES N. KVALE. Many have argued that, as the nation's population ages, the current health care system will prove unable to cope. Dr. James N. Kvale, who until recently, taught at the Youngstown, Ohio-based St. Elizabeth Hospital Medical Center, has proposed a solution to this problem, but efforts to publish his ideas have been frustrated.

"American health care is physician driven and technologically oriented," Kvale explains. "It is apparent as the demographic shift advances, that America will not have the resources to deal with these changes, hence the imperative to explore other models of health-care delivery." Kvale argues for an increased reliance on non-physician health care providers. A collaborative nurse-physician practice, with the nurse functioning in a markedly expanded role, could form part of a solution. "The translation of this concept into the American culture is a significant challenge," Kvale says.

This has been the solution of the World Health Organization for the provision of health care in developing nations. Working with Denise Eldemire of the University of West Indies in Jamaica, Kvale is comparing health service delivery for the elderly in Jamaica and the aged of Northeast Ohio. He is directing the Ohio-based portion of the research, a longitudinal survey of some 3,000 subjects. Working with survey researcher Jerry Buss, Kvale asks questions about health-service delivery.

Yet Kvale, who earned his M.D. from Howard University in 1963, counts teaching as his most significant contribution to the field. It is also the aspect of his work that is most gratifying.

It was a teacher, Andrew Achenbaum, that led Kvale into geriatrics. While caring for a large number of older people, Kvale said he realized "that I was not doing it well." A summer course at the University of Michigan exposed him to the multidisciplinary quality of aging and led the way into geriatric medicine.

L

PETER P. LAMY. Peter P. Lamy was among the first researchers to address rational drug use for and by the elderly in a consistent, ongoing manner. He earned his Ph.D in 1964 and first published on the topic in 1969. See P. P. Lamy, M. C. Delcher, and M. E. Kitler. "Therapeutics and the Geriatric Patient," *Hospital Form Management* 4(9), 13.

Lamy introduced the concept of primary, secondary, and tertiary aging and their interactions, as well as their effect on drug action. Having introduced the concept of geriatric pharmacotherapy, Lamy holds the first endowed chair in the subject. Pharmacotherapy is used to assess factors that can affect drug action, including pharmacodynamics, nutrition, and level of exercise. He has long advocated making the geriatric patient an active participant in his or her health care.

CALVIN A. LANG. Calvin Allen Lang, born in Portland, Oregon, in 1925, received his B.A. from Princeton University in 1947. He earned his Sc.D. in biochemistry and nutrition from the Johns Hopkins University School of Hygiene and Public Health in 1954. He has done extensive research on the biochemistry of aging, including much ground-breaking work.

One of Lang's early studies was the development of the yellow fever mosquito as a model of human aging. His studies included the biology, biochemistry, pharmacology, and nutrition of the mosquito in the laboratory. See, for example, C. A. Lang, H. Y. Lao, and D. J. Jefferson, "Protein and Nucleic Acid Changes During Growth and Aging in the Mosquito," *Biochemical Journal,* 95 (1965): 372–81; and C. A. Lang and J. K. Stephan, "Nicotinamide Adenine Dinucleotide Phosphate Enzymes in the Mosquito During Growth and Aging," *Biochemical Journal*, 102 (1967): 332–38. Moving from mosquitoes to mice, and collaborating with George Hazelton, Lang characterized the C57BL6/J mouse as an aging mammalian model. See their article, "Glutathione Contents of Tissues in the Aging Mouse," *Biochemical Journal*, 188 (1980): 25–30.

Currently, Lang's emphasis is on human subjects, especially quantitative profiles of glutathione, cysteine, homocysteine, and recently, their nitric oxide adducts. See C. A. Lang et al., "Low Blood Glutathione Levels in Healthy Aging Adults," *Journal of Laboratory Clinical Medicine*, 120 (1992): 720–25. As a whole, Lang's research has served to validate the use of aging models. He has insisted on rigorous control of biological and chronological ages, culture conditions, analytical methods, and statistical design and analysis.

This work led to the discovery and extensive characterization of "Gutathionc and Cysteine as Indexes of Aging and Health." Glutathione deficiency was a quantitative measure of the redox potential and the free radical theory of aging. Subsequent studies expanded the work with animal subjects to include human populations. Most important, Lang and his associates have been able to correct the GSH-cysteine deficiency to show a concomitant and significant enhancement of lifespan. See C. A. Lang, B. J. Mills, and W. Mastropaolo, "Glutathione Deficiency Occurs in 77% of Hospitalized Subjects of Various Ages," *The Gerontologist*, 30 (1990): 39A. Lang has collaborated principally with Belly Jane Mills, John P. Richie, Jr., Theresa Chen, Mara Julius, and especially Nathan W. Shock.* Shock's discussions encouraged his focus on aging, and Lang counts Shock as his mentor.

Lang is still an active, full-time professor with the Department of Biochemistry at the University of Louisville School of Medicine and also has adjunct appointments in the Departments of Pharmacology and Toxicology (University of Louisville) and in the Department of Nutrition, University of Kentucky. He is the first honorary professor at the Stedman Nutrition Center, Duke University Medical Center. He served as vice president of the Gerontological Society, south east director of Sigma Xi, and national lecturer of Sigma Xi.

NEOTA LARSON. Neota Larson was assistant chief of the Children's Bureau. In 1952, she joined the staff of the Old-Age and Survivors Insurance, which was renamed in 1963 as the Social Security Administration.

Larson focused on the need for health and welfare programs for the aged, disabled, widows, and children. She was instrumental in developing policies in the area of administrative guardianship and establishment of a full-scale system of accountability by administrative guardians (called representative payees) for beneficiaries who are unable to manage their own benefits. When Medicare was formed, Larson placed strong emphasis on the need to realize the potential of Medicare as an instrument to stimulate the development of health services.

She was chair of the Social Research, Planning, and Practice Section of the Gerontological Society of America.
Larson died in 1966.

PETER LASLETT. Peter Laslett is arguably one of Britain's foremost historians, though he would now describe himself as a historical sociologist. Karl Mannheim was his teacher, Sir Herbert Butterfield his mentor. A longtime fellow of Trinity College, Cambridge, Laslett was awarded a Litt.D. from Trinity in 1979. Before and after serving in the British Navy as an intelligence officer and in the BBC as a talks producer, Laslett concentrated on philosophical issues and political ideas. He recovered the papers and books of Sir Robert Filmer, the philosopher, and then the relevant portions of Filmer's much more famous critic, the philosopher John Locke, in particular the large remaining portion of Locke's library. His book, *Locke on Government,* established for Laslett a worldwide reputation in that field and is still in print after thirty-five years as the best-selling social science title of the Cambridge University Press.

In the 1950s Laslett founded and continues to edit the well-known series, *Philosophy, Politics and Society.* In the 1960s, with his colleagues E. A. Wrigley and R. S. Schofield, Laslett instituted the Cambridge Group for the History of Population and Social Structure. Some of their initial findings were published in the *World We Have Lost* (Scribner's, 1965, third edition in print from Macmillan, New York, 1992), which contrasted the small-scale, primarily rural and familial society in which Shakespeare, Cromwell, and Newton lived with the large-scale, industrial, and urban society of twentieth-century Britain. The book, provocative and exquisitely written, fanned interest in social and demographic history on both sides of the Atlantic and in many other countries. It is in print in seven or eight languages and has sold hundreds of thousands of copies. It was followed by definitive studies in the history of the household, of sexual nonconformism, of orphanhood, of social transfers, and many other topics in the field of historical sociology that Laslett has done much to open up.

Laslett's interest in aging evolved out of this work. (Other factors included his acquaintance with James E. Birren,* whom he met through his Cambridge colleague Alan Traviss Welford,* and an invitation to participate in a ''Human Values and Aging'' conference for historians and other experts in the humanities in the mid-1970s.) He was interested in applying historical sociology, especially issues surrounding the family, the household, and the demography of pre-industrial society, to the study of aging and the elderly. He focused on Western patterns but also engaged in comparative analyses with various other cultures and countries.

Like much of his earlier work, Laslett's studies of aging have been markedly revisionist. The elderly were not always respected in a world we have lost. Neither were they invariably given much position in the families of their children or their other kin. In the West, however, the collectivity of kin ties (in collaboration with the immediate family or others) and communal networks has always been a source of support for those too old to work. Much of this historical demography is summarized in two versions of an essay, ''Societal Development and Aging,'' which appeared in the 1976 and 1983 editions of the *Handbook of Aging and the Social Sciences,* eds. Robert H. Binstock* and Ethel Shanas* (New York: Van Nostrand Reinhold).

Laslett is something of a presence at the High Table of Trinity College, but he is also a radical with a bit of a flair for the popularization of scholarly work and ideas, something that has to be referred to his earlier experience as a producer at the BBC. In the 1960s and 1970s, he helped to pioneer distance teaching by the use of TV and radio in Britain, and took part in developing the British Open University, on which thirty-six national distance teaching universities were modeled worldwide.

In 1981 he joined with others in elaborating the British model of the University of the Third Age (U3A), which was actually started in his rooms in Trinity College. Organizations of this kind were first developed in France, but they have a very different identity in Britain, Australia and elsewhere, and one better calculated to mobilize the more intellectually inclined of those who come under the title of the young-old in the United States. As of 1994 there were well over 250 University of the Third Age in Britain, the largest organization of intellectually engaged elders so far to appear. His career as a theorist of aging and the life course owes much to European as well as to American scholars, and especially to Francoise Cribier* of Paris.

In 1989 Laslett produced his own account of age and aging in the contemporary world, developing out of the past and reaching forward into the future. This book, which includes an account of the theory and practice of the U3A, has the title *A Fresh Map of Life, the Emergence of the Third Age* (original edition London, Weidenfeld; published Harvard Press, 1991; Italian and German translations now available; another edition due from Macmillan in London in 1995). He has also become involved in the study of generational justices: See *Philosophy, Politics and Society VI: Justice Between Age Groups and Generations* (1985), in collaboration with James S. Fishkin, head of the Department of Government at the University of Texas at Austin. Though now nearing his 80s, Laslett has added to these subjects the study, at the Ageing Unit of the Cambridge Group, of the maximum length of life, collaborating with several other scholars also in their Third Age, for that purpose. He has been described in *The Times* of London as ''one of the founders of the 20th century.''

ALFRED H. LAWTON. Alfred Henry Lawton was born in Carson, Iowa, in 1916. He took his B.A. from Simpson College, which gave him an honorary D.Sc. in 1958. He then pursued his graduate and professional training at Northwestern, where he earned an M.S. (1939), B.M. (1940), M.D. (1941), and a Ph.D. in physiology (1943). From 1940 to 1941, Lawton was an intern at Passavant Memorial Hospital in Chicago; he was a resident the following year at the Henry Ford Hospital in Detroit. During the war, Lawton was attached to the U.S. Public Health Service.

After the war, Lawton served as an assistant professor of medical physiology and pharmacology at the University of Arkansas Medical School and as dean and professor of physiology and pharmacology at the medical school in North Dakota. From 1948 to 1951, he was chief of the research division at the central office of the Veterans Administration. For the next four years, Lawton served as a liaison member of the U.S. Public Health Service's council on arthritis and metabolic diseases.

During his Washington tour of duty, Lawton was an assistant clinical professor at George Washington University Medical School. From 1955 to 1962, he served as chief of intermediate services at the Bay Pines VA center. From 1962 to 1966, Lawton directed a study center for the National Institute of Child Health and Human Development. In 1966, he became assistant dean for academic affairs at the University of South Florida and later became acting vice president of academic affairs. In 1974 he became director of a VA Geriatric Research Education and Clinical Center in Bay Pines, Florida. Four years later, he became clinical professor of medicine at the University of Florida.

Despite his heavy administrative responsibilities, Lawton performed research on aging and chronic diseases. In addition to belonging to the American Association for the Advancement of Science and various physiological and pharmacological societies, Lawton was a member of the Gerontological Society. He served as president in 1973.

M. POWELL LAWTON. M. Powell Lawton was born in Atlanta in 1923, but raised in western Pennsylvania, where his father worked as an engineer in the steel industry. His college education at Haverford was interrupted by World War II; Lawton was a conscientious objector who worked in a mental hospital and participated as a guinea pig in an infectious-hepatitis experiment. After the war, he took an introductory psychology course at nearby Bryn Mawr College with Donald MacKinnon, who introduced Lawton to the work of his Harvard mentor Henry Murray and of Kurt Lewin. Lawton served as a VA trainee while pursuing his Ph.D. in clinical psychology at Columbia University's Teachers College. His thesis topic was "Stimulus Structure as Determinants of the Perceptual Response."

After receiving his degree in 1952, Lawton spent the next decade working in the Providence, Rhode Island, VA hospital and the Norristown, Pennsylvania State Hospital. In these facilities he extended his dissertation research, testing the extent to which a person's projective response to a stimulus was a function of both the subject's psychopathology and the gestalt quality of the stimulus. See "Stimulus Structure as a Determinant of the Perceptual Response," *Journal of Consulting Psychology,* 20 (1956): 351–55. That Lawton elected to conduct experiments in the midst of his clinical and administrative duties suggests three tensions that animated his career: the challenge of doing basic versus applied research; whether it made more sense to engage in theory-building or to generate empirical data; and, within these two tensions, whether the research should emphasize the significance of the person or the environment.

In 1963, Lawton switched to gero-psychology, when a full-time research position became available at the Philadelphia Geriatric Center (PGC). In making this career change, he was greatly influenced by Arthur Waldman, the center's innovative executive vice president who in 1960 initiated a range of support services for semi-independent older people in moderate-income housing on the grounds. (This is now called "congregate housing.") Waldman recognized that a high-quality, creative service institution could attract national attention in an emerging field if it supported intramural scientific research in gerontology. Lawton's initial task was to design a research program to evaluate the new environmental settings that PGC was developing. Rather than sit in his office devising theories, Lawton watched how older people used the space—hallways, lounges, laundry, lobby—at their disposal. Those in poorest health, he discovered, tended to interact mainly with others close by. Those healthy and active enough to move around sought out those who shared similar values, interests, and compatible personalities.

From this initial work, Lawton blazed a career that focused on environmental aspects of aging. He was not the first to recognize the importance of the environment to the aged: John Dewey, after all, had stressed this point in his Introduction to Edmund V. Cowdry's *Problems of Ageing* (Baltimore: Williams and Wilkins, 1939), and academics such as Robert Havighurst,* Otto Pollak, and Clark Tibbitts* had made it a central point in their respective theories of "social adjustment to old age" in the 1940s. But, with his colleague Lucille Nahemow, Lawton developed an ecological model that expressed graphically a multifaceted theoretic framework that related outcome to the interactions between persons and their environments. An important facet of the model was the "environmental docility hypothesis," which stated that environment became a stronger determinant of outcome as the competence of the person decreased. Lawton demonstrated the robustness of this hypothesis in congregate housing, institutions, and in neighborhoods. As in his report to the U.S. Department of Housing and Urban Development, with S. L. Hoover, *Annual Housing Survey: 1973. Housing Characteristics of Older Persons in the United States* (1979), Lawton's research has been very relevant to the practice of architecture, urban planning, and other forms of design. Some of this work influenced the directions taken in framing national housing policy, design guidelines for housing and institutions, and in designing services for elders living in planned housing.

Another impact of Lawton's work has been more episodic. Lawton has attempted to formulate a conception of overall quality of life that measures morale, instrumental activities of daily living, and other scales. On this, see his *Environment and Aging* (Monterey, Calif.: Brooks/Cole, 1980; Center for the Study of Aging, 1986). For a multidimensional view of the frail elders' quality of life, see his contribution to *The Concept and Measurement of Quality of Life in the*

Frail Elderly, eds. James E. Birren* et al. (New York: Academic Press, 1991). (Lawton considers Birren his role model, because his "originality is matched by the amazing diversity of his contributions to gerontology.")

The most complete statements of Lawton's views appear in his Kleemeier Award Lecture, "Environment and Other Determinants of Well-Being in Older People," *The Gerontologist,* 23 (1983): 349–57. In 1987, at age 64, Lawton was awarded a MERIT grant from the National Institute on Aging to pursue his work. This research and other recent projects involve the exploration of emotion in the lives of older people.

MORTON H. LEEDS. Morton H. Leeds, born in 1921, graduated from City College of New York with psychology honors in 1944. He earned an M.A. in 1948 and his Ph.D. in political sociology from the New School for Social Research in 1950.

As did many gerontologists, Leeds entered the field accidentally. Based on medical social work for the U.S. Army in India and public welfare work while he was at graduate school, the Sephardic Home for the Aged in New York offered him the position of director of social service. In 1953, he became director of the Borinstein Home for Aged in Indianapolis, where he stayed ten years. In 1954, he was named a fellow of the Gerontological Society.

Similar to many who entered the field in the 1950s, Leeds's thinking was conditioned significantly by the conferences he attended led by Wilma Donahue* and Clark Tibbitts* in Ann Arbor, Michigan. Herbert Shore* also served as a long-distance partner. "I met Herb Shore in Chicago, before he went to Dallas, discovered that we thought alike, and a functional partnership rapidly evolved," Leeds recalls.

Leeds pressed for keeping elderly residents in their communities. He obtained federal funds in the mid-1950s to create a community day center in connection with the Borinstein Home. The project received the Council of Jewish Federations and Welfare Funds' Shroder Award for creative community service.

Leeds has also made a number of important contributions to the institutional structure of geriatric care. He helped put together the Indiana State Commission on Aging in 1955, served as its first secretary for seven years, while running the Borinstein Home as well. In 1961, he published *The Aged, the Social Worker and the Community* (Cleveland: Howard Alien). The commission work led to a series of conferences and hearings around Indiana, and out of these materials emerged ten booklets and the book *Aging in Indiana* (Indianapolis: Bookwalters, 1959). He also led a vigorous campaign for Medicare around the state in the early 1960s. Building on these efforts, he compiled views on the institutional management of the elderly with Shore, and created the compilation *Geriatric Institutional Management* (New York: G.P. Putnam's, 1964).

Leeds also chaired the merger of the various Indiana associations into the National Association of Social Workers. He helped found and served as president of the Indiana Association of Philanthropic Homes for the Aged, the National Association of Jewish Homes and Hospitals for the Aged (serving as its first secretary, while Shore was president), and the American Association of Homes and Services for the Aging. He also attended the White House Conferences on Aging in 1961, 1971, and 1981.

Partly because of his active leadership in the Medicare campaign, Leeds became the first permanent chief of the direct loan programs for housing the elderly, at the federal level in HUD, 1962. Using his strong contacts in the philanthropic community, he sold the idea of federal financing and local sponsorship around the country in more than 1,000 speeches. This program now exceeds $9 billion in construction, and serves as the prototype for nongovernmentally sponsored elderly housing.

Leeds served as housing assistant for the elderly for a number of assistant secretaries in HUD in the 1970s. As a side interest, he presided over the Career Programming Institute, which guided more than 750 priests and nuns who had left the church to enter the civil sector. As one consequence, Leeds was asked to organize and direct an outplacement office when HUD dropped from 18,000 to 12,000 employees in the mid-1980s. He produced a series of specialized booklets on job process, and these led to nine years of work as director of the Washington office of an Ann Arbor-based, woman-owned outplacement firm.

For five of these years he hosted two local radio shows, "Jobs and People," and "Around Washington." For ten years he has taught at Marymount University, and for the past four years has counseled mature Russian emigre professionals on the American job process. Currently, he is working with the Elderly Housing Coalition in the various pre-conference activities leading up the White House Conference on Aging of 1995.

Leeds has written or edited ten books, more than ninety articles, booklets, or chapters of books, 125 stories, and more than 250 poems. Two of his books are in psychology, with Gardner Murphy, former chief psychologist at Menningers.

CYNTHIA L. LEIBSON. Cynthia L. Leibson of the Mayo Clinic is best known for her application of the Rochester Epidemiology Project to a number of aging-related questions. Specifically, she used this established data base to test the compression of morbidity hypothesis. See C. Leibson, David J. Ballard, Jack P. Whisnant, and L. Joseph Melton, "The Compression of Morbidity Hypothesis: Promise and Pitfalls of Using Record-Linked Data Bases to Assess Secular Trends in Morbidity and Mortality." *The Milbank Quarterly,* 70(1) 1992: 127–54.

In addition to her work with Ballard, Whisnant, and Melton, Leibson has collaborated with James Naessens and Mary Elizabeth Campion.

Leibson, who earned her Ph.D. in 1987 from the University of Colorado in Boulder, was attracted to gerontology by Edward Wilson's work in sociobiology. She has been intrigued by the question of the evolutionary advantage of senescence.

ANTHONY LENZER. Anthony Lenzer began his gerontological career in 1956, when he became executive secretary of the Michigan Legislative Advisory Council on Problems of Aging. His early career of studying and teaching about the elderly was shaped, as have been so many others, by the influence of Wilma T. Donahue,* whom Lenzer considers his mentor. After teaching at the University of Michigan School of Public Health, he moved to the University of Hawaii at Manoa in 1969. He received his doctorate in sociology from Michigan in 1970.

After teaching gerontology at the undergraduate and graduate levels for many years, he became interim director and director of the Center on Aging (1988–1993). The center presents gerontology in a "holistic and interdisciplinary" way to graduate and undergraduate students. With support from the Annenberg/CPB Project, the center developed a thirteen-part PBS series and college television course, "Growing Old in a New Age," first broadcast in August 1994. Lenzer served as executive producer for the series.

Narrated by Susan Stanberg of National Public Radio, "Growing Old in a New Age" shares the stories of more than 100 elderly Americans, combined with expert commentary from leading gerontologists. Its topics include the myths and realities of aging, learning and memory in the aged, societal and political aspects of aging, and love, intimacy, and sexuality. The series has aired on over ninety PBS stations, has been used as a credit course by over sixty colleges, and received national awards.

Lenzer has also been politically active in gerontological issues. He served as the first president of the Hawaii Pacific Gerontological Society; as a founding board member of Hospice Hawaii; and as a member of the boards of the State Commission on Aging and the Policy Advisory Board for Elderly Affairs. He is currently president-elect of AARP Chapter 60 in Honolulu.

Despite these accomplishments, Lenzer considers himself foremost an educator. "I would want to be remembered first as a teacher of gerontology," he says. "I would also hope to be remembered as one who helped develop and administer educational programs and projects in aging."

Lenzer retired from the University of Hawaii faculty in June 1994.

GARI LESNOFF-CARAVAGLIA. Gari Lesnoff-Caravaglia received her Ph.D. from the University of California at Los Angeles. There, she worked with George Kneller, who helped her "to appreciate the relationship between philosophy and existence." Carl Eisdorfer, who became one of Lesnoff-Caravaglia's role models, first attracted her to research on aging. Eisdorfer convinced her that aging was a "broad humane issue." She then studied human development at Harvard and worked with Ruth Weg at the University of Southern California's Andrus Gerontology Center.

Lesnoff-Caravaglia's interest in philosophy and religion was especially evident in the early stages of her career. In "Ethics and Gerontology," in *Gerontology in Higher Education: Developing Institutional and Community*

Strength, eds. Harvey Sterns et al. (Belmont, Calif.: Wadsworth Publishing, 1979), 101–107, she explored the ethical dimensions of human existence, particularly in the later years; she emphasized the moral importance of individual self-determination in the aging process.

Lesnoff-Caravaglia made a contribution to the humanities with her *Aging and the Human Condition* (New York: Human Sciences Press, 1982). Three years later, as part of the Frontiers in Aging series she edited for Human Sciences Press, she issued *Values, Ethics, and Aging.* ''The advantage of being an aging nation is that it causes us to examine all of our values and ethical positions,'' Lesnoff-Caravaglia noted in her introductory essay. ''We need to move away from the notion that mind and body are separate, and to stop looking at what is referred to as 'basic' needs as somehow antithetical to human enjoyment. For it is under the art of living that all other arts are subsumed.''

Lesnoff-Caravaglia has also engaged in several projects that enabled her to examine aging and institutional supports for the elderly from a cross-cultural perspective. She has conducted research in the former Soviet Union, Bulgaria, and Italy. Under a grant from the World Health Organization, she also studied the teaching of gerontology and geriatrics at European universities and medical centers. In a fascinating essay on ''The Black 'Granny' and the Soviet 'Babushka': Commonalities and Contrasts,'' in *Minority Aging: Sociological and Social Psychological Issues,* ed. Ron Manuel (Westport, Conn.: Greenwood Press, 1982), 109–14, Lesnoff-Caravaglia showed that both images connoted grandmothers' positive roles in rearing children and providing economic support. Yet both images also embody negative clusters of ideas, including the drag of the past.

Lesnoff-Caravaglia left her position as executive director of the Center on Aging at the University of Massachusetts Medical Center in Worcester to become director of the division of aging at Ohio University in Athens. She also directs the National Clearinghouse on Technology and Aging, which builds on her international network of researchers and applied gerontologists. There, she has been developing linkages between advances in technology and the needs and interests of the older population in wide-ranging areas such as home automation, ethics and health care, city planning, and gender differences. In addition to publishing *Aging in a Technological Society* (New York: Human Sciences Press, 1988), Lesnoff-Caravaglia has served as editor of the *International Journal of Technology & Aging.* She is convinced that linking technology and aging is ''one of the most significant issues on the gerontological horizon.''

WALTER N. LEUTZ. Walter N. Leutz earned an M.S.W. from the Columbia University School of Social Work in 1973, specializing in community organizing and planning. He completed his Ph.D. in 1981 at Brandeis University's Florence Heller Graduate School for Advanced Studies in Social Welfare. While a graduate student, he worked for the public assistance workers' union with the Lexington-based Massachusetts Labor Research Group. He remained to become an associate research professor at the Heller School's Bigel Institute for Health Policy.

Leutz has been instrumental in popularizing the concept of the Social Health Maintenance Organization on a national level. As director and principal investigator for the Social HMO Consortium, he has led a four-site, national demonstration of an integrated, prepaid health and long-term care system for the aged.

Much of Leutz's research has been congressionally mandated and federally supported. With funds from the Health Care Financing Administration, Leutz also directed the design of new Social HMO sites, including one to serve Medicare beneficiaries with End Stage Renal Disease. The Office of Technology Assessment supported his study of community care payment mechanisms, and a grant from the Administration on Aging is supporting a study of service planning guidelines and consumer autonomy in state long-term care systems.

"In developing health care programs for the aged, it is wrong to separate acute and chronic-care systems, because it is impossible to separate acute and chronic conditions and the needs that arise from them," Leutz argues. He has therefore sought to develop community care systems that combine the management of, and payment for, skilled and long-term care services in the home and community, as well as providing nursing home preadmission screening and short-term nursing home care.

For his most recent work, see Walter Leutz, et al., "Adding Long-Term Care to Medicare HMOs: Four Years of Social HMO Experience," *Journal of Aging and Social Policy* 4 (1992); Walter Leutz et al., "Variations in Care Planning in the Social/HMO: A Qualitative Study," *The Gerontologist* 29 (1989): 725–36; Walter Leutz, *Care for the Frail Aged: Developing Community Solutions* (New York: Auburn House, 1992); Walter Leutz, Merwyn Greenlick, and John Capitman, "Integrating Acute and Long-Term Care," *Health Affairs,* Fall (1994): 58–74.

DANIEL LEVITON. Daniel Leviton helped develop the field of death education for all age groups. His early publications include "Education for Death," September 1969. "The Need for Education on Death and Suicide," *Journal of School Health,* April 20, 1979; "Educating for Death or Death Becomes Less a Stranger," *Omega,* 6 (1975): 183–91; and "Thanatological Theory and My Dying Father," *Omega,* 17 (1987): 129–46.

Leviton also developed the Adult Health and Development Program (AHDP) at the University of Maryland. The AHDP was created in 1972 as a academic health education course and medical school elective in which students and others are trained to work on a one-to-one basis with older adults for nine Saturdays each semester. The AHDP's goals are to positively affect the health, well-being, physical and social activity, and health knowledge of its older adult members; to provide an environment for students and others to apply gerontological health theory and data; and to improve human relations by integrating a diverse group of young and older people as they work toward a common purpose.

Through a three-year U.S. Department of Education grant, the AHDP has spread to other colleges and universities in the United States and Israel. Members of this National Network for Intergenerational Health include: Northern Virginia Community College, Aurora College (Illinois), Bloomsburg State University (Pennsylvania), Nicholls State University (Louisiana), Gallaudet University (Washington, D.C.), and the University of Miami at Ohio. Sites that expect to have their AHDPs operational within a year include Banneker High School (Washington, D.C.), University of Delaware, SE Louisiana State University, Utica College (New York), Florida A & M University, Paine College (Georgia), and Clarke Atlanta University (Georgia). Over twelve colleges, universities, and high schools have requested the AHDP.

References include D. Leviton and L. Santa Maria, "The Adult Health and Development Program: Descriptive and Evaluative Data," *The Gerontologist,* 19 (1979): 534–43; "The Adult Health and Development Program: More than Just Fitness," in *Physical Activity, Aging and Sports, Vol. 2: Practice, Program and Policy,* eds. S. Harris, R. Harris, and W. Harris (Albany: Center for the Study of Aging, 1992); and "From Theory to Practice: The Adult Health and Development Program and Theories of Children's Love and Peace Behaviors," *Horrendous Death and Health: Toward Action* (New York: Hemisphere Publishing Corporation, 1991), 245–60.

A more global sense of death's relationship to health and well-being was also developed by Leviton, integrating thanatology and public health. Its goal is to remove or significantly reduce deaths caused by people who are motivated to kill others (as in homicides, war, terrorism, the direct result of racism or poverty, and genocide) or where that motivation is lacking (as the result of accidents, pollution, substance abuse, and directly as a result of racism or starvation). See D. Leviton, "Horrendous Death as a Stimulus to Intergenerational Health Protective Action and Global Well-Being," eds. S. Haberlein and H. Corals, *Proceedings of the 32nd ICHPER Anniversary World Congress* (Frostburg, Md.: Frostburg State University, 1990), 15–21; *Horrendous Death, Health, and Well-being,* ed. D. Leviton (New York: Hemisphere Publishing Corporation, 1991); *Horrendous Death and Health: Toward Action,* ed. D. Leviton (New York: Hemisphere Publishing Corporation, 1991); and "Toward Rapid and Significant Action," in *Horrendous Death and Health: Toward Action,* ed. D. Leviton (New York: Hemisphere, 1991), 261–83.

MYRNA I. LEWIS. Myrna Lewis, a Phi Beta Kappa graduate of the University of Minnesota, earned her M.S. at Columbia University's School of Social Work in 1965 and is currently a doctoral candidate at Columbia in social welfare. Early in her career she worked in the Minneapolis and St. Paul county welfare departments, the Community Service Society of New York City, the Veterans Administration Hospital in New York City, and for a community mental health center in Washington, D.C. Later she became a psychotherapist in private practice working with women entering the profession in the 1970s. Following a move to New York City in 1982, Ms. Lewis has been an assistant professor at the Mount Sinai School of Medicine, with special focus on the bio/psycho/social problems of older women.

Ms. Lewis has always combined a concern for the poor and disadvantaged, an interest in the use of power and privilege, and the development of broad public policy—especially in the area of mental health. In 1973 she joined forces with Dr. Robert Butler, then a psychiatrist in private practice, in writing a book, *Aging and Mental Health* (St. Louis: C.V. Mosby, 1975), which was designed to bring together psychosocial and biomedical approaches to the mental health problems of older persons. The work broke new ground in stressing the impact of ageism, sexism, and poverty on the elderly. The book's subtitle, *Positive Psychosocial Approaches*, expressed the authors' desire to introduce a positive approach within a broad psychosocial framework. The work was also interventionist in character, concerned with the ways that employment opportunities and volunteering affected wellbeing, yet it also dealt with psychoactive medications and psycotherapeutic efforts to prevent and treat mental illnesses. Each author added ideas from his/her earlier work, with Lewis, for example, emphasizing "responsible dependency"—the idea that the patients must play an important role in defining preventative and pro-active approaches to their own care. Empowerment, Lewis contends, must take precedence over the traditionally passive role of the patient or "illness victim."

In the fourth edition (1991) of *Aging and Mental Health*, Butler and Lewis have teamed up with a third co-author, Dr. Trey Sunderland, chief of Geriatric Psychopharmacology at the National Institute of Mental Health.

Aging for women has been a major theme in Lewis' efforts. As a lecturer, consultant, advisory board member and general advocate, she has given hundreds of lectures and media presentations and has written numerous publications and articles, book chapters, and the like on various aspects of women's lives as they grow older. She also served on the United Nations non-governmental organization (NGO) Committee on Aging, emphasizing the issues of older women worldwide.

Male gender issues have also been of interest to Lewis. She began an experimental psychotherapy practice with male CEO's and company presidents in New York City. This has enabled her to study the nature and disposition of power and the extent to which such men may lose touch with the personal and family aspects of life due to absorption in work and power over their life course. She has developed unique and effective interventions for men in these circumstances.

In 1976, Ms. Lewis co-authored (with Robert N. Butler, M.D.) a book, *Love and Sex After Sixty*, dealing with the ageist attitude toward sexuality in later life and offering practical solutions. This book is now in its third edition (1993).

Ms. Lewis also writes a monthly psychology column for women and men over age 50 in *New Choices Magazine*.

LESLIE L. LIBOW. Leslie Libow earned his M.D. at Chicago Medical School in 1958. In the early 1960s, Libow was working at the National Institutes of Health. He specialized in internal medicine for a longitudinal, interdisciplinary study of healthy human aging undertaken by James E. Birren,* Louis Sokoloff, Robert N. Butler,* Marion Yarrow, and Samuel Greenhouse. The final report, *Human Aging,* co-written with Frederick T. Sherman, M.D., was published in two volumes (Bethesda, Md.: National Institutes of Health, 1963). Robert Butler in particular became Libow's teacher, attracting his interest to the field of aging.

Libow's major accomplishments lie not primarily in bench science, but in advancing the field of geriatric medicine. While convinced that all physicians should grasp the body of knowledge, skills, and attitude appropriate to care for the elderly, Libow believed that geriatrics entailed more than just taking care of older persons, just as pediatrics involved, but hardly was limited to, taking care of children. At a time in which the U.S. medical establishment was opposed to recognizing geriatrics as a specialized area of health care, Libow embraced the concept and then tried to demonstrate the wisdom of his then unorthodox approach.

At two sites between 1964 and 1982, including New York's Jewish Home and Hospital for the Aged, Libow developed the principles and established the rules for operating the nation's first two academic nursing homes. He hoped to demonstrate that the way to ensure quality care in the nursing home is through cultivating an atmosphere of excellence linked to teaching, research, and program innovation, all of which Libow believed would enhance staff skill, morale, and patient care. The first twenty-five to thirty geriatric specialists in the United States received their training in these two pioneering teaching programs. Prior to the late 1970s, these were in fact the only places where physicians could obtain formalized training with a fellowship- or residency-approved program. Libow has described his efforts in ''A Geriatric Medical Residency Program: A Four-Year Experience,'' *Annals of Internal Medicine,* 85 (1976): 641–47; and in his Donald P. Kent Memorial Lecture before the Gerontological Society, published as ''Geriatric Medicine and the Nursing Home: a Mechanism for Mutual Excellence,'' *The Gerontologist,* 23 (1982): 134–44. In addition, Libow published a major geriatric text, *The Core of Geriatric Medicine: A Guide for Students and Practitioners* (St. Louis: Mosby, 1981).

Thus, by the late 1970s, when debates arose in Congress and within the medical establishment concerning the viability and desirability of underwriting fellowship and residency opportunities in geriatrics, Libow's programs already existed. Advocates such as Robert N. Butler* could point to them as models that demonstrated that there was much to teach and that there were many doctors who wanted to obtain training in geriatrics. Since 1982, Libow and Butler have been colleagues at the Mount Sinai School of Medicine. In addition to serving as chief of geriatric medicine at the Jewish Home and Hospital for the Aged, Libow is also Greenwall Professor of Medicine at Mount Sinai.

All senior medical students at Mount Sinai experience an obligatory four-week clerkship in geriatric medicine, a major portion of which is at the Jewish Home and Hospital for Aging (JHHA) and its related programs. Thus far, more than 1,200 senior medical students, approximately fifty fellows in geriatrics, and more than 100 geriatric nurse practitioners have been training in this program. Libow has established a Center on Ethics and Long Term Care at JHHA, co-directed by Ellen Olson, M.D., and coordinated by Eileen Chichin, D.S.W.

A national Restraint Minimization program supported by the Commonwealth Fund, with co-principal investigator, Richard R. Neufeld, M.D., has reduced restraint use from 41 percent before beginning the program to an average of 4 percent at present.

PHOEBE S. LIEBIG. Phoebe S. Liebig was born in Cambridge, Massachusetts, in 1933, the third daughter of Marshall Stone, a Harvard mathematician, and Emmy Stone, a watercolorist. She attended the University of Chicago Laboratory School and Radcliffe College and received both her bachelor's and master's degrees in political science from the University of California at Los Angeles.

Liebig was first attracted to the field by working with James E. Birren,* and she traces her political gerontology roots to Neal R. Cutler,* Robert Hudson, and William Lammers. She has done extensive comparative work on state and federal policies as they apply to the aged. Her studies of state policies have focused on public employee and state teacher pension systems, housing, and long-term care. See, for example, her *A Basic Guide to State Teachers Retirement Systems* (Washington, D.C.: AARP, 1987); P. Liebig and W. Lammers, *California Policy Choices for Long-Term Care* (Los Angeles: Andrus Gerontology Center, 1990): and P. Liebig, "State Units on Aging and Housing for the Elderly, Current Roles and Future Implications," *Journal of Housing for the Elderly* (1995).

She has also considered the effects of federalism on aging policy, demonstrating the need for coordination among housing, health and social services departments by two or more levels of government. See her "State Health Policies, Federalism and the Elderly," *Publius: The Journal of Federalism,* 20 (1990): 131–48; P. Liebig and W. Lammers, "Federalism and Suitable Housing for the Frail Elderly—A Comparison of Policies in Canada and the United States," *Housing Policy Debate* 4 (1993): 199–237; P. Liebig, "Federalism and Suitable Housing for Frail Elders: A Comparison of Policies in Four Nations," in *Housing Frail Elders: International Policies, Perspectives, and Prospects,* eds. J. Pynoos and P. Liebig (Baltimore, Md.: Johns Hopkins Press, 1995); and P. Liebig, "Decentralization, Aging Policy and the Age of Clinton," *Journal of Aging and Social Policy,* 6 (1994): 9–26.

In addition, she has studied older-worker pension and benefit policies. See her "Three Legged Stool of Retirement Income," in *Retirement Preparation,* ed. Helen Dennis* (Lexington, Mass.: D.C. Heath, 1994); "Retirement Health Benefits," *Pension Briefings* (1987); and "Factors Affecting the Development of Employer-Sponsored Eldercare Programs: Implications for Employed Caregivers," *Journal of Women and Aging,* 5 (1993): 59–78.

Liebig counts her studies of administrative professionalism as among her most important work. By measuring the use of external advisers and investment portfolio managers, she examined the level of professionalism in state-pension management in her dissertation, which focused on disclosure by the fifty public employee retirement systems. Her broader aim continues to be an examination of the attributes of state-level agency effectiveness. Her yardsticks include budget levels and sources, types of training for staff, leadership, use of external consultants, adherence to legislation and other standards, and interorganizational relations/networks. Her current research is focused on State Units on Aging (SUAs), as well as Area Agencies on Aging, and their efforts in combining housing and long-term care, and on the assistive technology efforts of state-level rehabilitation agencies and SUAs.

She has advanced the teaching of gerontology by developing new courses of study at the Los Angeles-based University of Southern California, where she completed her doctorate in public administration in 1983. These courses cover corporate policies and aging, the economic foundations of aging policy, federalism and aging policy, and the politics of aging. She has also helped develop a Ph.D. in gerontology and a policy internship on aging. For undergraduates, Liebig is currently part of a group that is developing a multidisciplinary text encompassing the biology, psychology, sociology, politics and humanities of aging.

Liebig was the first holder of the Hanson Family Assistant Professorship and is a Fellow of the Gerontological Society of America. Active in several gerontological, political science, and public administration professional societies, she most recently has served as president of the California Council on Gerontology and Geriatrics, a statewide educational consortium.

CHARLES F. LONGINO, JR. Charles F. Longino, Jr. earned his Ph.D. in sociology from the University of North Carolina at Chapel Hill in 1967, but his real introduction to the field of aging occurred during a postdoctoral fellowship he held through the Midwest Council for Social Research on Aging from 1974 to 1976. The work and personalities of Gordon F. Streib* and M. Powell Lawton* made "strong and indelible impressions . . . that have endured throughout [his] career." Warren Peterson, Jack Siegler, and Harold Orbach nominated Longino for the postdoctoral fellowship and then guided his gerontological education, which included showing him how to write research applications. Other luminaries—Donald Cowgill, Helena Lopata,* Erdman Palmore,* and Irving Rosow*—also served as mentors. So did Ed Powers, who was an earlier postdoctoral student in the Midwest Council, and Susan R. Sherman,* who provided Longino with a clear model of retirement community research. When Longino served on NIH's Human Development and Aging Study Section, Vern L. Bengtson* and M. Powell Lawton were major role models.

Longino is probably best known for his efforts to guide the research area of retirement migration securely into the demography of aging as an active subfield.

218 CHARLES F. LONGINO, JR.

His research team was the first to study the detailed patterns of state-to-state migration over the past four decades, beginning with the 1960 U.S. Census, and to analyze the characteristics of older migrants in those streams. No doubt the big surprise in this endeavor has been the identification of counterstreams of older people returning home from popular destinations to places where they had spent much of their earlier lives. Longino explored such migration back to the state of birth, focusing on patterns between metropolitan and non-metropolitan areas. Joining forces with Victor W. Marshall,* Richard Tucker, and Larry Mullins, Longino has also studied international seasonal migration, focusing on older Canadians wintering in Florida.

Eugene Litwak and Longino developed a theoretical model for understanding the probabilities of geographical mobility using a life-course perspective. They argue that moves soon after retirement, when couples are still intact and retirement income is at its highest, are different in many respects from moves later in life when moderate levels of disability tend to motivate residential change to be closer to family members (second type moves). These, in turn, differ from institutional moves toward the end of life (third type moves). The Litwak-Longino model, now widely cited in the migration literature, appeared in "Migration Patterns among the Elderly: A Developmental Perspective," *The Gerontologist*, 27 (1987): 266–72.

Using data from the Longitudinal Study on Aging, Longino has been able to pinpoint features of the second type of elderly migration, which heretofore has been less widely documented in the literature. See (with colleagues J. E. Bradsher, D. J. Jackson, and R. S. Zimmerman in various order), "The Second Move: Health and Geographic Mobility," *Journal of Gerontology: Social Sciences*, 46 (1991): S218–S224; "Environmental Adjustments to Declining Functional Ability: Residential Mobility and Living Arrangements," *Research on Aging*, 13 (1991): 289–309; and "Interpersonal and Economic Resources as Mediators of the Effects of Health Decline on the Geographic Mobility of the Elderly," *Aging and Health*, 5 (1993): 35–57. Longino's 1995 book, *Retirement Migration in America: 1970–1990* summarizes his life work on this topic.

Longino currently is developing a multidisciplinary center on aging, with strong ties to the medical school at Wake Forest University. His 1995 book, *That Old Age Challenge to the Biomedical Model: Paradigm Strain and Health Policy*, with co-author John Murphy, reflects his current interests.

HELENA ZNANIECKA LOPATA. The daughter of Florian Znaniecki, one of the nation's foremost sociologists, Helena Znaniecka Lopata was born in 1925 in Poznan, Poland, and came to the United States during World War II as a refugee. She concentrated on three subjects—sociology, psychology, and philosophy—at the University of Illinois (B.A., 1946). She took an M.A. in philosophy and sociology at Illinois a year later, and then earned her Ph.D. at the University of Chicago in 1954. After spending four years (1965–1969) at Roosevelt University, she became a professor of sociology at Loyola University of Chicago in 1969, where she has remained. (Loyola named her "faculty member of the year" in 1975.)

Since 1972, Lopata also has served as director of the Center for the Comparative Study of Social Roles. Her interest in aging develops from, and typically sustains, her interest in the sociology of women, work, and social roles.

Lopata began doing interviews on women in the suburbs for a study that eventually became a best-selling book, *Occupation: Housewife* (New York: Oxford University Press, 1971). In the course of that research, she obtained funding from the Administration on Aging (1968–1971) to study "Widowhood: Changes in Roles and Role Clusters." This research became the basis for *Widowhood in an American City* (New York: Schenkman, General Learning Press, 1973), a monograph that was the first major contemporary scientific study of widowhood and remains influential, conceptually and empirically, for researchers on aging interested in this topic.

Lopata's interest in the status, networks, and place of widows in society has expanded over time. In 1979 she issued *Women as Widows: Support Systems* (New York: Elsevier-North, 1979). Building on research she did with a team under contract with the Social Security Administration, Lopata published, with Henry Brehm, *Dependent Wives and Widows: From Social Problem to Federal Policy* (New York: Praeger, 1986). In 1985, she organized a round table on "Widowhood: International Perspectives" for the 13th Congress of the International Association of Gerontology. A Fulbright grant two years later took her to India to study widows' support systems in New Delhi and seven other cities. This study culminated in a two-volume work, *Widows*; Volume 1 deals with the Middle East, Asia, and the Pacific, while Volume 2 focuses on North America (Durham, N.C.: Duke University Press, 1987). Also of interest to social gerontologists is her recent *Circles and Settings: Role Changes of American Women* (Albany, N.Y.: State University of New York Press, 1993), which traces the life course of changes in these roles. Forthcoming is *Current Widowhood: Myths and Realities* (New York: Guilford Press).

Unlike many of gerontology's best-known figures, who concentrate primarily on aging-related issues, Lopata has simultaneously pursued issues along theoretical lines not directly relevant to gerontology. For instance, she published *Polish Americans: Status Competition in an Ethnic Community* (Englewood Hills, N.J.: Prentice-Hall, 1976), and *Polish Americans* (Greenwich, Conn.: JAI Press, 1978). She has published, in both English and Polish, studies that reflect interests that she shares with her father. See her "Polish American Families," in *Ethnic Families in America*, eds. Charles H. Mindel and Robert V. Habenstein (New York: Elsevier, 1981), 17–42; and "Euro-Ethnic Families and Housing in Urban America," in *Civil Rights Issues of Euro-Ethnic Americans in the United States*, ed. U.S. Commission on Civil Rights (Washington, D.C.: Goverment Printing Office, 1980). Lopata has also edited a series of volumes on *Current Research on Occupations and Professions*, including a volume with David

Maines on *Friendship* (Westport, Conn.: JAI Press, 1990), and widely reprinted articles on loneliness, which stem from her interest in social roles.

Lopata's professional commitments reflect her wide interests. In addition to chairing the Social and Behavioral Section of the Gerontological Society of America and participating in World Congresses of Gerontology in Budapest, Acapulco, New York, Jerusalem, and Tokyo, she has served as president of the Midwest Council for Social Research on Aging, the Illinois and Midwest Sociological Societies, the Society for the Study of Social Problems, and Sociologists for Women in Society. Lopata has been very active in the Polish Academy of Arts and Sciences in America, as well as various city, state, and regional service groups. She chaired a technical committee on age integration and the family for the 1981 White House Conference on Aging and served on the board of overseers (1978–1983) of the Wellesley College Women's Research Center.

Lopata received the Distinguished Scholar Award from the Society for the Study of Social Roles in 1989, the Burgess Award from the National Council on Family Relations in 1990, and the Distinguished Scholar Award of the Aging Section of the American Sociological Association in 1992.

LOUIS LOWY. Louis Lowy, born in 1920, received his diploma at the age of eighteen from the Pedagogic Academy in Prague. While teaching modern foreign languages, he studied philosophy at Charles University. The Nazis incarcerated Lowy from 1941 to 1945; he spent time in several concentration camps, including Terezin and Auschwitz. Immediately after the war, Lowy served as a welfare worker and administrator for the United Nations Relief and Rehabilitation Administration.

Upon arriving in the United States, Lowy became a social group worker in Boston's Hecht Neighborhood House. For the next few years, while earning his B.S. in education (1949) and M.S.W. (1951) from Boston University, he held posts with the Quincy Jewish Community Center and Boston Children's Services. From 1951 to 1955, Lowy supervised programs for older adults at the Bridgeport, Connecticut, Jewish Community Center. He then returned to Boston, directing the Golden Age Council of Greater Boston (1955–1957), coordinating community day camps for the Jewish Community Center of Greater Boston. From 1958 to 1965, he directed the international community service and welfare specialist program of the National Assembly for Social Policy and Development under the auspices of the U.S. Department of State. In 1957, Lowy also assumed an appointment as an assistant professor of social work at Boston University. As he rose through the ranks, he found time to earn a Ph.D. from Harvard's School of Education. His dissertation topic was "Self and Role Clarification during Social Work Training: Study of Incorporation of a Professional Role."

Lowy spent his entire academic career at Boston University. He became a full professor in 1966. In 1974, with Dr. Marott Sinex, his collaborator on several health care projects, he founded the university's Gerontology Center, which formalized arrangements established in a council Lowy had helped to launch nine years earlier. In addition to playing an active role at Boston University, Lowy frequently traveled to Germany, Switzerland, Austria, and other European countries to consult on social welfare matters and curriculum development. He was also active in community affairs, serving as associate commissioner of Boston's Commission for the Aged (1969–1972) and as a member of the advisory council of the Commonwealth of Massachusetts's Department of Elder Affairs.

Over the course of his career, Lowy wrote nearly two dozen books, half in German. Most dealt with broad topics in social work. Most U.S. researchers in aging are familiar with his efforts to bridge theory and practice in social work. See, for instance, his two chapters on the "Role of Social Gerontology in the Development of Social Services" and "A Social Work Practice Perspective in Regard to Theoretical Models," both in *Research, Planning, and Action*, eds. Donald P. Kent,* Robert Kastenbaum,* and Sylvia Sherwood* (New York: Behavioral Publications, 1973).

"Social work is *sanctioned* by society as a field of practice and as a profession," he noted in "Social Work and Aging," in *The Science and Practice of Gerontology*, eds. Nancy Osgood and Ann H. L. Sontz (Westport, Conn.: Greenwood Press, 1988). That said, he noted that the informal system is still the main source of social assistance, providing at least 80 percent of the health and social services received by the elderly. Hence, he wrote, "social work with the aging makes use of specialized knowledge about aging and the aged but deploys generic methods and skills in performing social work tasks incumbent upon the practitioner in working with older persons."

Lowy, who died in 1991, was active in the Gerontological Society, serving as chairman of what was then called the Social Welfare section in 1966 and 1967. He was founding president of the Massachusetts Association of Gerontology. Boston University gave him its Distinguished Alumni Award (1966) and staged a gala seventieth birthday celebration for him. In 1979, the Gerontology Center established the Louis Lowy Certificate in Gerontological Studies and a decade later created the Louis Lowy Fund for Gerontology and Social Welfare Policy.

M

WILLIAM deB. MacNIDER. William deBerniere MacNider was born in Chapel Hill, North Carolina, in 1881. He earned his M.D. from the University of North Carolina in 1903, and later received honorary degrees from Davidson College, the Medical College of Virginia, Western Reserve, and the University of Chicago.

MacNider spent his entire medical career at the University of North Carolina. From 1902 to 1905, he was a clinician; for the next thirteen years he was a professor of pharmacology. In 1918, he was promoted to a Kenan Professorship and became the University's Kenan Research Professor in 1924. MacNider was dean of the medical school from 1937 to 1940.

MacNider is primarily remembered for his research on the pharmacology of the kidney. He studied nephritis, the acid-base equilibrium of the blood in liver, and the development of acquired resistance of fixed tissue cells after injury to the liver and kidney. Late in his career, he developed an interest in processes of aging. His contribution to Edmund Vincent Cowdry's* *Problems of Ageing* (Baltimore: Williams and Wilkins, 1939), titled "Aging Processes Considered in Relation to Tissue Susceptibility and Resistance," stressed the considerable variations in cell susceptibility and by cell resistance "which give to the downward progress of the curve, representing aging, an irregular course." As cell adaptation became more tenuous, he noted, an organism's capacity to function diminished.

MacNider won the Sibbs Prize for medical research (1930) and a medal from the Southern Medical Association three years later. He died in 1951.

GEORGE MADDOX. George Maddox earned his Ph.D. in sociology at Michigan State University in 1956. He never had formal training in gerontology in
college or in graduate school. His dissertation was about alcohol use among
adolescents. For the first fifteen years of his career, in fact, most of his
publications dealt with "normal" and "abnormal" aspects of people's response
to alcohol, and their risk for manifesting pathological behavior.

After three years as professor of sociology at Millsap College in Jackson,
Mississippi (1956–1959), Maddox came to Duke, where he has spent most of
his career. He began as a Russell Sage Postdoctoral Fellow in Medical Sociology. Gerontology was not on his research agenda; his first projects in Durham
dealt with teen-age drinking and adult obesity. But Maddox's growing interest
in the interactions between biomedical and psychosocial factors, and an invitation to analyze the first wave of participants in Duke's Longitudinal Study of
Normal Aging, brought him into the field. He began to exchange ideas with
Carl Eisdorfer, Walter Obrist, and Morton Bogdonoff; these three men, in turn,
were working with Ewald W. Busse* in developing a gerontology center in the
medical school at Duke. Maddox claims that, in retrospect, his most effective
teachers were his own students, including Dan G. Blazer,* Linda K. George,*
and Richard Campbell.*

Maddox used his 1985 Kleemeier Lecture, published in *The Gerontologist,*
27 (1987): 557–64 as "Aging Differently," to summarize most of his important
intellectual contributions to gerontology. First and foremost, Maddox has underscored the importance of specifying the extent and types of differentiation in
the processes of aging and in the experiences of the elderly. "The acceptance
of the maxim, 'Existence precedes essence,' is not a license for sociocultural
reductionism," Maddox declared. "The game is to specify correctly and measure adequately an appropriately complex biosocial model of human adaptation
over the life course." Thus, he emphasized the importance of cross-cohort analyses, cross-cultural studies, and stipulating salient variations by race, gender,
and socioeconomic status. "Societies are natural experiments in the effects of
differential allocation of social resources over the life course," he wrote.

Just as Maddox's entry into gerontology was oblique, so, too, his interest in
exploring the modifiability of aging through purposive intervention was unexpected. By his account, it occurred between 1968 and 1972, years marked by a
Public Health Service postdoctoral fellowship to study the British health service
and his appointment as director of the Duke Center on Aging and Human Development. Responding to an invitation from the federal government to explore
"alternatives to institutionalization for the vulnerable elderly," Maddox and his
colleagues developed the Older Americans Resources and Services (OARS) program at Duke, described in "Interventions and Outcomes: Notes on Designing
and Implementing an Experiment in Health Care," *International Journal of
Epidemiology,* 1 (1972): 339–45.

Maddox has been quite interested in the effects of caregiving for elders by
women in the work force and, more broadly, by the differential effects of work,

work settings, and career experiences on the timing and significance of retirement, and gender differences in income security. He also has returned to his earlier interest in alcoholism, see his *The Nature and Extent of Alcohol Problems among the Elderly* (New York: Springer, 1986).

Maddox's emphasis on the variations within the aged population serves as an intellectual brief for combining basic research and policy science under the rubric of gerontology. "Some public policy initiatives demonstrably may have beneficial effects for older adults in aging societies," he declared in his Kleemeier Lecture. "Social scientists can play a useful role in clarifying the implications of alternate choices." Thus, investigators must design their samples and cohort-sequenced longitudinal observations to take account of a differentiated older population. Multidisciplinarity, in Maddox's view, is not just a good idea, but an essential condition for understanding aging itself. Yet Maddox's definitions of "science" and "practice" in gerontology go far beyond the usual demands of free inquiry in the scientific enterprise or in reaffirming the need to satisfy public confidence that researchers on aging are indeed credible. Maddox considers science a "public enterprise" that requires consensus among scientists regarding the evaluation of evidence and a commitment of public resources to scientific research perceived to be beneficial to society.

Maddox's broad definition of the gerontological realm has perforce propelled him out of the classroom and beyond data analysis to endorse a more "activist" stance for researchers on aging than is expressed by most of his colleagues. He is committed to studying the heterogeneity of late life from as many perspectives as possible. Yet, as he wrote (with his former student Richard T. Campbell) in the lead article of the second edition of the *Handbook of Aging and the Social Sciences* (New York: Van Nostrand Reinhold, 1987), Maddox is blunt about the fact that "the social scientific study of aging needs, but currently lacks, widely shared paradigms that would provide a common conceptualization of issues, standard measurements, and clearly defined agendas for the systematic testing of hypotheses derived from theory."

Believing that "differentiation" is *the* (or, at least, a prime) quality of late life, Maddox contends that gerontologists, in their capacities as practitioners and scientists, must overcome their skepticism about applied research and seize the real possibility for modifying the conditions of aging. "We do not know the limits of modifiability of aging processes and the experience of aging," he says. "We do know that if we want to understand aging processes and the experience of aging, we can learn from trying to change them when the observed outcomes are unacceptable." This possibility gives gerontologists a practical incentive for engaging in policy research and advocacy.

Accordingly, more than most U.S. social scientists interested in aging, Maddox has played a critical role in developing a social and behavioral research agenda on aging. A founding member of the National Institute on Aging Advisory Council in 1975, Maddox recommended the appointment of Robert N. Butler* to be the NIA's first director. With Bernice L. Neugarten,* who remains one of his role models, Maddox wrote the behavioral and social sciences section of *Our Future Selves* (Bethesda, Md.: National Institutes of Health, 1977), which summarized the best consensual thinking about significant theoretical and methodological issues in aging. In preparing their report, Neugarten and Maddox relied heavily on ideas set forth by authors in the first edition of Robert H. Binstock* and Ethel Shanas's* *Handbook of Aging and Social Sciences* (New York: Van Nostrand Reinhold, 1976), and James E. Birren* and K. Warner Schaie's* *Handbook of the Psychology of Aging* (New York: Van Nostrand Reinhold, 1977).

Maddox remained active in shaping NIA priorities. He has consistently stressed the need to increase the total funds available for basic research, and when efforts were made to reduce the share (consistently about 15 percent) of the budget for social and behavioral research, he argued the case for the status quo ante. Maddox was a pivotal figure when NIA invited the Institute of Medicine to produce a multidisciplinary national research agenda for the 1990s. With Leonard Poon, he chaired a fifteen-member Liaison Group of emerging and established scholars in the behavioral and social sciences. In *Extending Life, Enhancing Life* (Washington, D.C.: National Academy Press, 1991) and *Disability in America: Toward a National Agenda for Prevention* (Washington, D.C.: National Academy Press, 1991), Maddox and his colleagues emphasized three areas in the social-behavioral domain: (1) the dynamic interaction of persons and social contexts, including the macroscopic effects of the societal allocation of resources in a broad range of ''ordinary'' social milieu; (2) differential aging, including the long-term decline in functional competence and increased disability; and (3) purposeful interventions for at-risk and high-risk older adults in the workplace and in their living arrangements. (See Maddox's ''Social and Behavioral Research on Ageing: An Agenda for the United States,'' *Ageing and Society,* 14 (March 1994): 97–107.)

Maddox's commitment to multidisciplinary research endeavor and science as a public enterprise has been evident in his work at Duke and on the national scene. One of the field's most respected peer reviewers in the sociology of aging, Maddox nonetheless has spent much of his career collaborating with psychiatrists and demographers. Having learned much of his administrative skills from Busse and Eisdorfer, Maddox directed the Center for Aging from 1972 to 1982 and then chaired Duke's All-University Council on Aging for the next decade. He also is professor of medical sociology and director of Duke's World Health Organization/Pan American Health Organization Collaborating Research Center on Aging. He currently directs the Duke Aging Center's Long Term Care Resources Program and its Leadership in Aging Program.

Maddox has been active in the Gerontological Society of America, serving as president in 1978. He was secretary general of the International Association of Gerontology (1981–1989). Maddox served as editor-in-chief of the first edition of the well-received *Encyclopedia on Aging* (New York: Springer Publishing, 1987), and its second edition (1995). He received in 1983 the Sandox

International Prize for Longitudinal Research on Aging. Two years later, in addition to winning the Kleemeier Research Award, Maddox was given the American Sociological Association's Distinguished Contribution in Aging Award. In 1992, he received the GSA's Distinguished Mentorship Award from the Behavioral and Social Sciences Section.

KEVIN JOHN MAHONEY. Kevin John Mahoney earned his master's degree in social work at the University of Connecticut in 1972 and his Ph.D. from the University of Wisconsin in Madison in 1978. He was attracted to the field by Helena Z. Lopata's *work on widowhood. His teachers included Vivian Wood, Mary Wylie, Virginia Little, and Robert Morris,* and his dissertation was on the "effects of forced coordination on organizational interrelationships and services to clients."

Like many in the field, Mahoney has tried to bridge the gap between research and practice. This is most evident in his studies of the structure and financing of long-term care facilities. He has advocated linking private insurance and Medicaid to fund long-term care.

In addition to publishing in academic journals, Mahoney has conducted research for legislators. See, for example, his "Meeting the Challenge: Organizational and Policy Imperatives for Long-Term Care in Florida," which was prepared for the State of Florida Department of Health. With the assistance of Max Rothman, Mahoney conducted this three-volume study while affiliated with the Southeast Florida Center on Aging at Florida International University in 1987.

His collaborators include Terrie Wetle,* Carol Ansten, Robert Applebaum, and Fred Seidl.

Mahoney is currently affiliated with the State of Connecticut Office of Policy and Management.

TAKASHI MAKINODAN. Takashi Makinodan was born in Hilo, Hawaii, in 1925. He received his B.S. at the University of Hawaii in 1948. He then studied at the University of Wisconsin, where he earned his M.S. in 1950. While working as an assistant in serology, Makinodan completed his Ph.D. on the Madison campus, combining his interests in zoology and biological chemistry.

Makinodan began his career as a research associate in immunohematology at the Mount Sinai Medical Research Foundation in Illinois (1953–1954). After holding a fellowship from the National Institutes of Health the following year, he served as a biologist at the Oak Ridge National Laboratories (1955–1957). Makinodan then became head of Oak Ridge's immunology group for the next fifteen years. Concurrently, he held a senior National Science Foundation Fellowship (1961); from 1968 to 1972, he also was a professor in the Graduate School of Biomedical Sciences at the University of Tennessee, and he directed the training program of the National Institute of Child Health and Human Development. From 1971 to 1973, he served on the National Science Foundation's advisory panel governing regulatory biology programs. From 1972 to 1976, Makinodan was chief of the cellular and comparative physiology branch of the Gerontology Research Center of NIH. Since 1976, he has been director of the Geriatric Research, Education and Clinical Center (GRECC) at the Wadsworth Veterans Administration Medical Center in Los Angeles.

Makinodan's research focuses on radiation immunology, the mechanisms of antibody formation, and the aging of the immune system. He has published basic texts in the field, such as *Immunology and Aging* (New York: Plenum Press, 1977), and the *CRC Handbook of Immunology in Aging* (Boca Raton, Fla.: CRC Press, 1981). He typically tries to show why the immune system provides an excellent model for studies of the cellular and molecular etiology of aging, the pathogenesis of aging, and various approaches for improving the quality of life in the termination phases.

In 1988, the Gerontological Society recognized Makinodan's research accomplishments by honoring him with the Kleemeier Award.

KYRIAKOS S. MARKIDES. Kyriakos S. Markides earned his Ph.D. from Louisiana State University in 1976. Rather than being attracted to research on aging by a mentor or teacher, Markides's curiosity was piqued by studies published by Reuben Hill and Vern L. Bengtson.*

Markides, who is a key investigator at the University of Texas Medical Branch, Galveston, is primarily known for developing a program of research on elderly Mexican-Americans. This included a three-wave longitudinal sutdy (1976, 1980, and 1984), as well as a three-generation study of Mexican-Americans conducted in 1981–1982, which was followed up in 1992–1993. He is now principal investigator of a five-year epidemiological study of the health of 3,050 elderly Mexican-Americans from five Southwestern states. On the basis of his work, Markides developed the notion of "selective survival." See K. Markides and R. Machalek, "Selective Survival, Aging, and Society," *Archives of Gerontology and Geriatrics,* 3 (1984): 207–22.

More broadly, Markides has tried to show the significance of ethnicity as a demographic characteristic, social factor, and cultural construct in explicating the relationship between health and aging. He has tried to give shape and direction to the fields of ethnicity and aging and to minority aging. See, for example, K. Markides and C. Mindel, *Aging and Ethnicity* (Beverly Hills, Calif.: Sage, 1984). Markides was also founding editor of the *Journal of Aging and Health* (1989 to the present).

Neal Krause, David Lee, and Jeffrey S. Levin have been Markides's closest collaborators to date.

ELIZABETH W. MARKSON. Elizabeth W. Markson was a French major at Bryn Mawr. She did postgraduate study through the Committee on Communication at the University of Chicago, where she worked with Carl Rogers. Markson's M.A. and Ph.D. in sociology are from Yale, where she worked primarily with Robert N. Wilson. Her dissertation, written as Elizabeth Casper, is "Parents, Spouses, and the Chronically Ill."

Markson became interested in gerontology in 1967, when she began to work with Elaine Cumming, whose work on disengagement theory had attracted considerable attention a few years earlier. For the next five years, she worked closely with Elaine and John Cumming, M.D. With John Cumming, Markson called attention to the advantages and problems associated with deinstitutionalization of chronic (usually elderly) mental patients. This work led to one of her earliest papers, "A Hiding Place to Die," which first appeared in *Trans-Action/Society* (November/December 1971), and was widely reprinted. There, she excoriated the ways in which impaired elderly people were categorized and warehoused.

Markson held appointments at SUNY Albany (1967–1976), while she held various research and administrative positions in the New York State Departments of Mental Hygiene and Social Services. She then moved to Boston, where she directed the Massachusetts's research and evaluation division in the Department of Mental Health. Markson taught at Northeastern University (1976–1977), and Wellesley (1976–1980), before becoming affiliated with Boston University (BU). In 1979, she was appointed a research associate professor in BU's Sociology Department, and a year later, an adjunct associate professor in the Department of Socio-Medical Sciences and Community Medicine. After serving six years as director of social research in BU's gerontology center, Markson became the unit's associate director in 1985. In 1994, she was appointed a professor in the Department of Sociomedical Sciences and Community Medicine. She is also research professor in the Department of Medicine and adjunct professor of sociology. In addition, she has worked as a faculty member at the Kantor Family Institute in Cambridge, where she had done postgraduate training in family therapy.

Perhaps Markson's most important contribution has been to call attention to gender-related differences in aging. Her *Older Women* (Lexington, Mass.: Lexington Books, 1983) was cited as one of the 1984 "Books of the Year" by the *American Journal of Nursing*. With Beth Hess,* who has been her primary collaborator, Markson has published four editions of *Growing Old in America. (New Brunswick, N.J.: Transactions)* since 1980. Hess and Markson, with Peter Stein, have also produced five editions of *Sociology* (New York: Harper and Row). With support from the AARP Andrus Foundation, Markson has also developed gender-specific risk profiles for nursing home placement: *Social, Functional, and Medical Predictors of Institutionalization: Development of a Risk Profile from the Framingham Study* (New York: Springer 1991).

In addition to support from AARP, Markson has been both a recipient and a reviewer for the Administration on Aging and for private foundations interested in health care. She is currently principal investigator of an NIA interdisciplinarpy training grant.

Markson has also been very active in regional professional associations. She served as president of the Massachusetts Sociological Association (1977–1978) and the Northeastern Gerontological Society (1992–1993) and worked on the publications committee of the Gerontological Society of America (1987–1989), serving as book editor of *The Gerontologist* (1983–1986).

VICTOR W. MARSHALL. Victor W. Marshall's interest in gerontology was self-generated. Although he studied with Donald Spence, their intellectual discussions focused on sociology rather than aging. Marshall believed that he could easily gather appropriate data for a doctoral thesis by using a sample of older people. He earned his Ph.D. in sociology from Princeton University in 1973. His mentors, in addition to Spence, were Richard Kalish, Robert Kastenbaum,* Leonard D. Cain, and Walter M. Beattie, Jr.* He often collaborates with Vern L. Bengtson* and Charles F. Longino, Jr.*

Marshall's early work focused on the sociology of aging and dying. See, for instance, his *Last Chapters: The Sociology of Aging and Dying* (San Francisco: Brooks/Cole, 1990), and his essay, "Aging and Dying," with J. Levy in the third edition of the *Handbook of Aging and the Social Sciences,* eds. Robert H. Binstock* and Linda K. George* (New York: Academic Press, 1990). Marshall operationalized the concept of an "awareness of finitude," an idea introduced by J. Munnichs. See his essay, "A Sociological Perspective on Aging and Dying," in *Later Life: The Social Psychology of Aging,* ed. Victor W. Marshall (Beverly Hills, Calif.: Sage, 1986).

More generally, Marshall's work as a theorist has emphasized the interpretive and political economy approaches to aging. This perspective is notable in his collection of essays in *Later Life,* which often refine the views set forth by his U.S. and British colleagues. The notion of a "generational cohort," for instance, which Marshall acknowledges is "controversial," draws on such classics as Mannheim and Marx. The phrase refers to "a cohort which experiences qualitatively different historical events from those of adjacent cohorts." See Victor Marshall, "Generations, Age Groups, and Cohorts: Conceptual Distinctions," *Canadian Journal on Aging,* 2 (1983): 51–62.

As the first Canadian sociologist to supervise students in aging (Carolyn Rosenthal and Anne Martin Matthews are among his trainees), Marshall served as a founding member of the Canadian Association on Gerontology; he was a key member of the executive board for fourteen of the organization's first twenty years. Marshall also edited the *Canadian Journal on Aging* for five years. He edited the first Canadian text in aging, *Aging in Canada: Social Perspectives* (Don Mills, Ontario: Fitzhenry & Whiteside, 1980; second edition, 1987). He currently directs the Centre for Studies of Aging at the University of Toronto.

With Neena Lane Chappell* (University of Manitoba), Anne Martin Matthews (University of Guelph), and Fergus Craik (University of Toronto), Marshall was instrumental in launching CARNET (The Canadian Aging Research Network) in 1990. CARNET brings together roughly 160 researchers in the social and behavioral sciences across Canada. Four CARNET research groups have been established to analyze products and services for the elderly, work and eldercare, cognitive functioning, and issues of an aging work force. In addition to serving as director of CARNET, Marshall leads the research group on the aging work force. This research is designed to promote independence and productivity for Canada's aging population. His current research interests focus on work and aging and theory development.

GEORGE M. MARTIN. George M. Martin earned his M.D. at the University of Washington in Seattle. During residency training, his primary teachers were two members of the University of Chicago's Department of Pathology, Eleanor Humphreys and Robert W. Wissler. Martin has spent most of his career in his alma mater's Department of Pathology.

Martin's interest in research on aging was sparked by a year he spent as a Fellow in Guido Pontecorvo's laboratory in the Genetics Department at Glasgow University in 1961. There, he used cultures of human cells to develop methods for the genetic analysis of the donors of those cells. For an example of this work (on the parasexual cycle), see his article in *Science,* 166 (1969): 761. Martin's experiments were frustrated by the striking limitations of the replicative potential of individual clones of cells. The reasons for this phenomenon were made evident in the now-famous paper by Leonard Hayflick* and Paul Moorhead on the serial cultivation of human diploid cell strains (1961). Hayflick and Moorhead documented and quantified the limited replicative lifespans of such cells. Intrigued by their research, Martin entered the field of aging to determine whether this limitation was some sort of correctable artifact of the cell culture or was a fact of considerable biological significance.

Over the next three decades, Martin's research emphasized individual variations in patterns of human aging. He confirmed and extended experimental support for the limited replicative lifespan of cultivated human somatic cells. He developed conceptual and experimental evidence for the phenomena of clonal attenuation, clonal selection, clonal succession, and terminal differentiation during the decline of somatic cells' proliferative potential. See his articles in the *American Journal of Pathology,* 74 (1974): 137; *Advances in Experimental Medical Biology,* 53 (1974): 67; and *Cytogenetic Cell Genetics,* 30 (1981): 108. In a 1973 *Lancet* article, Martin was one of the first to propose a relationship between clonal senescence and atherogenesis.

Martin conducted the first investigations of relationships of dominance and recessivity in in vitro senescence using heterokaryons. See his papers in the *Proceedings of the National Academy of Science,* 71 (1974): 2231; and the *Journal of Cell Biology,* 64 (1975): 551; and of synkaryons between diploid cells in *Cytogenetic Cell Genetics,* 21 (1978): 282. He characterized Werner's syndrome (adult progeria) as a mutator phenotype in ibid., 30 (1981): 92; and *Human Genetics,* 84 (1990): 249. Martin investigated various somatic mutational theories of aging, emphasizing the importance of chromosomal lesions. A highlight of these various studies on genetics and aging has been the evidence for genetic heterogeneity in familial Alzheimer's Disease, especially the discovery of a common form of familial Alzheimer's Disease that maps to chromosome 14. See his articles in *Science,* 241 (1988): 1507; *Science* 258 (1992): 668; and the *American Journal of Human Genetics,* 48 (1991): 563; and 49 (1991): 511.

One common thread ties together this research. Martin has used the concepts and methods of genetics to analyze gerontological mechanisms. In particular, his research has highlighted the great potential of spontaneous genetic variation in man for elucidating such mechanisms. These studies provided estimates of the proportion of the human genome modulating specific aspects of the senescent phenotype, and introduced the concept of both segmental and unimodal progeroid syndromes of man.

EDWARD J. MASORO. Edward J. Masoro, born in Oakland, California, in 1924, received his A.B. from the University of California at Berkeley in 1947. Studying under Leslie Bennett, Masoro received his Ph.D. from the same institution three years later. He was attracted to gerontology by the work done by Clive McCay* and his collaborators at Cornell. In the first edition of Edmund V. Cowdry's *Problems of Ageing* (Baltimore, Md.: Wilkins and Williams, 1939), McCay had shown that dietary restriction prolonged the life of rats.

The characterization of the dietary restriction rodent model as a tool for the study of basic aging processes has been Masoro's most important contribution to the advancement of gerontology. He was greatly influenced by the animal models for investigating human senescence articulated by Bennett Cohen, who ran the animal laboratories at the University of Michigan. Masoro summarized his studies, largely at the University of Texas Health Science Center in San Antonio, where he headed a major gerontological lab, in "Food Restriction in Rodents: An Evaluation of Its Role in the Study of Aging," *Journal of Gerontology: Biological Sciences,* 43 (1988): B59–B64. There, he reviewed the evidence for retardation of the aging processes by food restriction in terms of longevity, age changes in physiological processes, and age-associated diseases. The positive effects seem to be due to the caloric restriction per se, not to the elimination of a specific nutrient or a toxic contaminant in the diet. Research now should focus on mechanisms, Masoro contends, because this will create a data base that will elucidate "primary aging processes" and suggest ways to development interventions in human aging.

The most important concept that Masoro introduced was the role of the characteristics of fuel use as opposed to its rate. Masoro (with I. Shimoikawa and B. P Yu) proposed this concept in "Retardation of the Aging Processes in Rats by Food Restriction," *Annals of the New York Academy of Science,* 621 (1991): 337–52.

Masoro's major contribution to gerontology has been to provide compelling evidence for the important role of animal models in meeting the gerontological challenge of the twenty-first century. This subject provided the theme for Masoro's 1991 Kleemeier Lecture, which was published as "The Role of Animal

Models in Meeting the Gerontologic Challenge of the 21st Century'' in *The Gerontologist*, 32 (1992): 627–33. Masoro claimed that ''the development of biological gerontology has lagged far behind that of most other areas of biology'' because philosopher-scientists ''did not test their hypotheses using animal models or other alternatives.'' Although he has been attacked personally for his use of rodents in his experiments on dietary restriction, Masoro claims that animal models will yield the data necessary to determine which interventions will inhibit primary aging processes and/or enhance broadly protective ones. He also elaborated his claims in delivering the 1992 Bennett Cohen Memorial Lecture at the University of Michigan.

Masoro's primary mentors were I. Lyon Chaikoff and David Rapport. In addition to Cohen, Masoro considers Sidney Weinhouse, who directed the Fels Institute in Philadelphia, to be a role model. Masoro's primary collaborators have been Byung Pal Yu, Helen Bertrand, and Roger McCarter.

Masoro served as president of the Gerontological Society in 1995–1996.

CLIVE M. McCAY. Clive M. McCay was born in Winamac, Indiana, in 1898. He received his B.A. from the University of Illinois (1920), his M.S. from Iowa State College (1923), and his Ph.D. in biological chemistry from the University of California in 1925. He did postgraduate work at Yale under L. B. Mendel, holding a National Research Fellowship (1925–1927), and spent a year at Oxford (1935–1936).

After holding assistantships at Texas Agricultural and Mechanical College, Iowa, and Berkeley, he became an assistant professor of animal husbandry at Cornell in 1927. He became a professor of nutrition at Cornell in 1934.

Unlike most contributors to *Problems of Ageing*, ed. Edmund Vincent Cowdry* (Baltimore: Williams and Wilkins, 1939), McCay was already primarily identified for his research in gerontology when that volume was planned. Indeed, his interest in nutrition and aging began at Yale, with brook trout and then rats. His contribution to *Problems*, ''Chemical Aspects of Ageing,'' dealt mainly with growth rates, lifespan, nutrition, and chemical composition. His interest in dogs and teeth was very evident. In the middle of his essay, McCay turned to the issue of dietary restriction in old age as a way of prolonging life—a research topic for which he is mainly remembered. He introduced the topic by quoting Thomas Cogan in *The Haven of Health* (1596): ''For the diet of youth is not convenient for old age nor contrariwise.''

Most of McCay's work was based on protein levels in rats, but he also extended his analysis to studies of the decline in basal metabolism in humans. ''The life span can be greatly extended by manipulating the diet,'' McCay concluded in *Problems of Ageing*. ''The field of nutrition probably affords the most promising line of attack.'' Some students of the field believe that McCay's findings may be the *only* research on the biology of aging that represents a genuine, original contribution by a gerontologist.

McCay directed more than thirty graduate students and wrote over 150 scientific papers.

McCay died in 1967, of a stroke, having retired four years.

IVAN NORMAN MENSH. After graduating from George Washington University (B.A., 1940; M.A., 1942), Ivan Norman Mensh served as an analyst for the National Institutes of Health in Bethesda, Maryland, from 1941 until 1943. He joined the U.S. Naval Reserve and was in the Third Fleet in the South Pacific until 1945. He worked for the Navy as a psychologist (1945–1946), and then at Northwestern University, where he served as a research assistant in a Navy research unit until 1947. He completed his Ph.D. in psychology at Northwestern in 1948. Later, Mensh reactivated his Navy connection, serving as an adviser to the Surgeon General of the Navy from 1964 to 1967 and as a consultant to the U.S. Navy Health Research Center from 1961 to 1974.

His first faculty appointment upon finishing his degree in 1948 began at Washington University School of Medicine in St. Louis. He started as an instructor in medical psychology in the Department of Neuropsychiatry and rose to professor, heading the Medical Psychology program at Washington University's School of Medicine, a position he held until 1958. Mensh credits his students with drawing him into the field of gerontology; the first three dissertations he directed were studies in aging. He also credits the pioneering work of Edmund Vincent Cowdry* in geriatrics and John E. Kirk with attracting him to the field.

From St. Louis, Mensh moved to Los Angeles, where he led UCLA's Division of Medical Psychology at the medical school. He has served in a wide range of professional capacities, including consultant to the Veterans Administration from 1953 to date. He has been an active member of the American Psychological Association, serving on a number of boards and committees since 1951, particularly in its Division of Maturity and Old Age.

Mensh has done important work in the clinical assessment and psychological treatment of the elderly. Most of his research and teaching has focused on stress and coping. His most recent work, "A Study of a Stress Questionnaire: The Later Years," *International Journal of Aging & Human Development,* 16 (1983): 201–207, is indicative of his style. The research surveyed a sample of sixty-two elderly patients hospitalized for neurobehavioral diagnosis and treatment. It concluded that the degree of impact of various stresses must be sought out systematically if they are to be understood. He has contributed reviews of gerontology in Victor Corsini's *Encyclopedia of Psychology* (Washington, D.C.: American Psychological Association, 1987, 1994).

His essays under two headings in the latest edition are "Gerontology: Action Research, Behavioral Changes in Aging, Behavioral Intervention, Family Crises, Forgetting, Geriatric Psychology, Memory, Memory Disorders, Panic Disorders, and Supportive Care," and "Therapies for Institutionalized Psychiatric Aged

Patients: Behavior Changes in Aging, Gerontology, Life Span Development, Psychotherapy, Sociopsychophysiology, and Somatopsychic.''

ELIE METCHNIKOFF. Elie Metchnikoff, born in 1845 in the steppes of Russia, was the youngest of five children. His father, a general in the Imperial Army, was a modest landowner; his mother was the daughter of a Jewish writer. Elie was a precocious but sickly child with a mercurial temper. Dissuaded by his mother from pursuing medicine, he embarked on a career in zoology. By the age of twenty, ''Quicksilver'' (his family nickname) had already published his first scientific articles, written several combative book reviews, and refuted the criticism of a prominent German physiologist.

In 1865, Metchnikoff began to collaborate with another Russian zoologist on a study of germ layers in invertebrate embryos. By comparing the growth to maturity of two closely related turbellarians, he demonstrated that recapitulations of particular developmental patterns in lower forms of life occur in radically different ways. Thus, he was interested early on in the relationships among growth, development, and maturity.

Metchnikoff's experiments in the 1860s and 1870s showed his classical training. ''Makers of generalizations should proceed very slowly,'' he wrote, ''passing only by the smallest stages from particular facts . . . to attain principles neither vague nor ambiguous, but clear and exact and that would not be denied by nature herself.'' Unlike many peers, whose scientific views were being transformed by Darwin's ideas, Metchnikoff initially had reservations about the theory of natural selection. In the first stage of his career, he systematically investigated particular variations in development within species (such as medusas and sponges) in order to discover ''disharmonies'' both among parts of an organism and between a species and its environment. His studies of digestion revealed no underlying unity; disharmonies presented themselves over the life course. ''Development,'' Metchnikoff wrote in 1871, ''appears to be a more general phenomenon than progress.''

The second stage of Metchnikoff's career began in 1882, when he moved his lab to Messina, Italy, to escape political turmoil in Russia and to recuperate from an illness. ''A new thought suddenly flashed across my brain,'' he wrote. As he toiled in his lab, Metchnikoff noticed that a splinter introduced into starfish larvae would provoke reactions between parasites and phagocytes (that is, devouring cells), similar to the process in humans. ''Thus it was in Messina that the great event of my scientific life took place,'' Metchnikoff recalled decades later. ''A zoologist until then, I suddenly became a pathologist. I entered a new road in which my later activity was to be exerted.''

For the next twenty-five years, Metchnikoff refined and defended his phagocytic theory. Expertise he had acquired through studies of embryology, parasitology, and digestion prepared him well for his foray into the domains of comparative pathology and medicine. Rudolph Virchow, whose cell theories had revolutionized pathology, and Louis Pasteur, the eminent chemist and microbiologist, immediately heralded the Russian's discoveries. Metchnikoff's phag-ocytic theory was recognized to have implications for scientists working in microbiology, pathology, embryology, evolutionary biology, and biological chemistry. Here, truly, was a pathfinder working at the cutting edge of science.

In 1888, Metchnikoff relocated to the newly founded Pasteur Institute, where he remained for the rest of his life. "In Paris I succeeded at last in practicing pure Science apart from all politics or any public function," he wrote. Yet by 1905, when Metchnikoff attempted to rebut critics by publishing his 591-page *Immunity in Infective Diseases,* his phagocytic theory was already in eclipse. This theory became the basis for his research on old age. Just as Metchnikoff was well prepared to blaze the frontiers of immunology because of the questions he had pursued in his studies of zoology and embryology, so, too, his investi-gations of immunity prompted the metaphors and theories he would elaborate as he embarked on research in aging. "A veritable battle rages in the innermost recesses of our body," he wrote.[1] Phagocytes, he posited, turned hair white; "senile atrophy" resulted from disappearing nerve cells. Building upon and extending the logic of earlier inquiries, Metchnikoff attributed the "principal phenomena of old age" to the action of macrophages, microbes that collected in the digestive system.

Metchnikoff's theory of aging squarely challenged ideas advanced by con-temporary European scientists. He did not hide his contempt for panaceas pro-moted by journalists, quacks, and charlatans. He treated scholarly publications harshly, too. Metchnikoff rejected works hypothesizing that tissues and organs invariably degenerated in old age. He demolished various studies of comparative longevity and "natural death" in reptiles, birds, mammals, and humans. He dismissed August Weismann's theory that the proliferation of certain cells cul-minates in a given organism's death.[2] Rather than concede the inevitability of decay and degeneration with advancing years, Metchnikoff thought that someday a "normal," "physiological old age" could be attained by humans. The ravages of age, he felt certain, could be reversed: Metchnikoff cited evi-dence that phagocytes devouring blood corpuscles in a clot could undo the effects of paralysis in cases of apoplexy. The strategy, then, was to find ways in accordance with his theory to ward off infectious diseases in late life.

Metchnikoff acknowledged that pathologists, embryologists, cytologists, and clinicians had not figured out why people grew weaker as they aged. Science surely did not yet advance efforts to attain a healthful old age. Nonetheless, he offered an "elixir of life" that promised some benefits. Eating yogurt, he claimed, killed noxious "macrophags." In both *The Nature of Man* (1903) and *The Prolongation of Life* (1908), he offered a biochemical paean to the powers of sour milk. He noted the extreme longevity enjoyed by yogurt-loving Bulgar-ians. That he himself had reached age seventy demonstrated the importance of "hygiene," plain living, and daily ingestion of yogurt. Not everyone was im-pressed. Some physicians and scientists derided the old man as "the modern

Ponce de Leon searching for the Fountain of Immortal Youth and finding it in the Milky Whey."[3]

Elie Metchnikoff's work on longevity was well publicized in the United States. He prepared a long essay on "old age" for the 1904–1905 Smithsonian Annual Report. Popularized accounts of his research appeared in *McClure's* and *Cosmopolitan,* and an American journalist hailed Metchnikoff as one of the *Major Prophets of To-Day* (1914).

Metchnikoff died in 1916.

NOTES

1. Metchnikoff, *Nature of Life* (New York: Scribner's, 1908), p. 239; A. I. Tauber and L. Chernyak, "Metchnikoff and a Theory of Medicine, *Journal of the Royal Society of Medicine,* 82 (December 1989): 699–701.

2. Metchnikoff, *Prolongation,* pp. 36, 53, 118; "Old Age," p. 538.

3. Slosson, *Major Prophets* (New York: Longmans, 1913), p. 175. For more on yogurt, see *Prolongation,* pp. 168–78; *Nature,* pp. 248–57; Olga Metchnikoff, *Life,* p. 251; Sir Ray Lankester, *Science from an Easy Chair* (New York: Macmillan Company, 1911), 43. For a contemporary interpretation, see Debra Jan Bibel, "Elie Metchnikoff's Bacillus of Long Life," *ASM News,* 54 (1988): 661–65.

STEVEN H. MILES. Steven H. Miles, born in 1950, majored in biology and psychology at St. Olaf College and earned his M.D. at the University of Minnesota in 1976. After a year of postgraduate work on medical ethics at the United Theological Seminary, he spent five years as a resident in internal medicine at the Hennepin County Medical Center. In 1981–1982, Miles was chief medical officer for 45,000 refugees in twenty-three camps on the Thai-Cambodian border under the aegis of the United Nations. From 1982 to 1986, he was an assistant professor of medicine at his alma mater, University of Minnesota, and affiliated with the local VA Geriatric Research, Education and Clinical Care program. After spending three years at the University of Chicago's medical school, where he was associate director of the Center for Clinical Medical Ethics, Miles became head of the Division of Geriatrics and Extended Care at the Hennepin County Medical Center and associate professor of geriatrics and bioethics at the University of Minnesota.

Miles's experiences in a Cambodian refugee camp gave him a perspective on the excesses of the U.S. health care system. A self-acknowledged "autodidact," Miles prefers to be known as a clinician rather than an ethicist—one "able to clearly and effectively hear and speak about patients' needs from their health care system." Thus, he claims that his patients have been his most important teachers: They have shown how to construct meaning out of tragic choices.

Miles's counseling approach has been greatly influenced by his reading of Otto Rank. From Bernice L. Neugarten* and Christine Cassel at the University of Chicago, and from Rosalie L. Kane* at Minnesota he came to respect the diversity in the details of older people's lives. Because so much of Miles's work is at the interstices of policymaking, global and local politics, and phenomenology, it is pertinent to note that he has gained insight from the novels and plays of Toni Morrison, Tennessee Williams, Flannery O'Connor, and Aleksandr Solzhenitsyn, and educators such as Ivan Illich, Michael Harrington, Paulo Friere, Mulford Sibley, and Stephen Toulmin.

Miles has published many reviews, abstracts, editorials and articles on various aspects of decisions to forgo treatment and other ethical issues. His major contribution, however, has been to develop the conceptual process of deciding to forgo life-sustaining treatment. Although no-code orders had been discussed in the mid-1970s, his paper (with Dr. Ronald Crawford and A. Schultz), "The Do-Not-Resuscitate Order in a Teaching Hospital," *Annals of Internal Medicine,* 96 (1982): 600–604, was the first to use the term "DNR" and to suggest a nationally emulated policy framework and counseling duties. Miles refined his ideas in several journals, culminating in two articles—"Advanced Directives to Limit Treatment," *Journal of the American Geriatrics Society,* 35 (1987): 74–76; and "Resuscitating the Nursing Home Resident," *Journal of the American Geriatrics Society,* 38 (1990): 1037–38. These articles set national standards, codified in his work with Chicago colleagues, *Institutional Protocols for Decisions about Life-Sustaining Treatments* (Washington, D.C.: Office of Technology Assessment, 1988).

Miles's recent work has focused on emerging medical legal controversies, especially dealing with the concept of "futility." He was involved in the Wangle case, a landmark in the futility debate. The deeper significance of practical day-to-day issues concern him; see, for instance, his "Choices about Food and Water: The Emerging Ethical and Legal Standard of Care," in *Geriatric Nutrition,* ed. J. E. Morley et al., (New York: Raven Press, 1990). He explored possible gender biases in right-to-die legal decisions.

A Henry J. Kaiser Foundation Faculty Scholar in General Internal Medicine since 1987, Miles has been active in health care reform as a member of President Clinton's Health Care Reform Task Force on Bioethics and in various organizations in his state.

WALTER R. MILES. Walter R. Miles was born in Silverleaf, North Dakota, in 1885. He received his undergraduate training at Pacific College (B.A., 1906), and earned his M.A. (1910) and Ph.D. (1913) in psychology from the University of Iowa. After spending a year at Wesleyan, Miles became a research psychologist in the Nutrition Lab at the Carnegie Institution in Washington, D.C. (1914–1922). He then moved to Stanford University, where he was a professor of experimental psychology. In 1931, after spending a year as a research associate in Yale's Institute for Human Relations, Miles became a professor of psychology at Yale University.

Miles early on made his name doing research on personality measurements and abnormal states. Unlike most contributors to Edmund V. Cowdry's* *Prob-

lems of Ageing (Baltimore: Williams and Wilkins, 1939), Miles had staked out his interest in old age and maturity. With C. C. Miles he already had published an important article, "The Correlation of Intelligence Scores and Chronological Age from Early to Late Maturity," in the *American Journal of Psychology*, 44 (1935): 44–78. That same year, he published "Age in Human Society" in C. Murchison's *Handbook of Social Psychology* (Worcester, Mass.: Clark University Press, 1935), which served as a prototype for the Cowdry volume.

Miles's entry in Murchison's *Handbook*, "Psychological Aspects of Ageing," summarized his work on measurements of psychological traits of normal maturity and old age, focusing on perception and age, the influence of age on speed and accuracy in learning and memory, intelligence and age, age and interests, the effect of age on drive, motivation, and achievement, the relationship between age and certain personality traits, and the subjectivity of time. Miles acknowledged that "the psychological factors of ageing include and depend upon a completely demonstrated physiological regression," yet in light of the variability of human response, there seemed to be no age barrier for productivity. Indeed, prefiguring a major theme of subsequent investigators, Miles asserted that "the more the behavior product involves experience and considered judgment, the more resistant it is to the psychophysiological age deterioration. . . . This is the characteristic prerogative and contribution of well preserved age."

Miles died in 1978.

RICHARD A. MILLER. Richard Miller, born in 1949, was a *summa cum laude* graduate of Haverford College who earned his Ph.D. in human genetics at Yale University in 1976, and his M.D. from Yale a year later. His most significant teachers were Frank H. Ruddle and Osias Stutman, who was his sponsor at Sloan Kettering Institute from 1980 to 1982. Though he notes with regret that he has not had any mentors, he considers Caleb Finch and Edward J. Masoro* two gerontologists who have served as role models.

After several years at Boston University, Miller came to the University of Michigan in Ann Arbor, where he has appointments in the Department of Pathology, the Institute of Gerontology, the local VA, and serves as associate director of research for the Division of Geriatrics.

Miller was attracted to research in aging "before [he] knew of any good work in this field." The specific questions that captured and has retained his interest are the general ones of why older animals fall apart, and why this happens at different rates in different species. Miller jumped from genetics into immunology to find a system that he hypothesized would be less complicated than the whole animal—yet still complex enough to reveal biochemical and genetic "facts" about aging that could be tested in other models of age-related change.

Representative of an early phase of his work was a paper (with his teacher Osias Stutman), "Decline, in Aging Mice, of the Anti-Tnp Cytotoxic T Cell Response Attributable to Lost of Lyt-2', II-2 Producing Helper Cell Function," in the *European Journal of Immunology*, 11 (1981): 751–56. This paper, and five related ones, showed a loss with age in the ability of T lymphocytes in mice and humans to make the growth factor Interleukin-2 (IL-2). Using the tools of modern cellular immunology, Miller was able to determine how functional loss could be attributed to alterations in specific subsets of T cells.

Three years later, in "Age-Associated Decline in Precursor Frequencies for Different T Cell-Mediated Reactions with Preservation of Helper or Cytotoxic Effect per Precursor Cell" in the *Journal of Immunology,* 132 (1984): 64–68, Miller suggested a "mosaic" theory of the aging immune system in which some, but not all, of the cells present in the aging animal were seen as defective. He asserted that aging not only led to losses in production of IL-2, but that other losses resulted from this factor. This paper, in turn, prompted a further refinement. In "Decline, with Age, in the Proportion of Mouse T Cells that Express IL-2 Receptors after Mitogen Stimulation," *Mechanisms of Aging and Development,* 33 (1986): 312–33, Miller and H. Vie showed that the loss of production of IL-2 also inhibited the number of cells that could develop receptors for this factor.

In a series of papers published between 1987 and 1989, Miller and his lab showed that defects in the ability of T cells to generate calcium occurred very early in the activation process; that calcium is involved in the age-sensitive step(s); and that alterations in the T cells' ability to resist changes in calcium signals were probably responsible for the functional problem. Recent work, such as his "Diminished Calcium Signal Generation in Subsets of T Lymphocytes that Predominate in Old Mice," *Journal of Gerontology: Biological Sciences,* 45 (1990): B87–B93, ties together the "calcium defect" with the "mosaic" nature of the aging immune system. Memory cells that increase with aging, Miller found, have diminished calcium signals, compared with the "naive" T cells that decline in aging mice.

Taken together, Miller's work has helped to introduce the idea that changes in the function of an age-sensitive tissue or organ may be caused by changes in the relative proportions of its constitutive cell types. Although both young and old mice have T cells of the naive and memory types, an increase with age in the proportion of the latter cell type seems to account for some of the differences in age-specific immune responses. Hence, further study of differences between T cell subsets and very early events in T cell activation is likely to yield interesting new findings.

In the 1990s, Miller began to take an active role in Gerontological Society activities, chairing the Biological Sciences Section and doing editorial work. Like Richard C. Adelman,* he has been successful in translating concepts in the biological sciences into plain English so that non-specialists can grasp their importance. Miller's early penchant for boundary-crossing is also evident in his willingness to think about cross-species comparisons of theoretical ideas and the need to compare biochemical hypotheses across organ systems. As head of the University of Michigan's animal colony for geriatricians and gerontologists, Miller has been keen to use genetically heterogeneous rodents for robust tests of hypotheses on aging.

LINDA S. MITTENESS. Medical anthropologist Linda Mitteness received her B.A. *summa cum laude* in child psychology from the University of Minnesota in 1973 and her Ph.D. from Pennsylvania State University's Human Development and Family studies program in 1979. She was a National Institute on Aging trainee at Penn State in the mid-1970s. Mitteness was drawn to the field of gerontology by Paul B. Baltes* and John Nesselroade. She refers to Nesselroade as her model for the "ideal academic," one who combines methodological rigor with a "respect for the complexity of life."

Mitteness made her way to San Francisco and joined the faculty of the University of California. As an associate professor at UCSF's medical anthropology program since 1987, Mitteness educates physicians and other health professionals about the cultural logic of their patients' behavior. Initially, she did collaborative work with Corinne Nydegger on issues surrounding the timing of fatherhood.

Turning to the aged in 1982, Mitteness began a study of the relatively widespread problem of urinary incontinence. The project, supported by the NIA and nearing completion, has allowed her over the past decade to document the underreporting and inappropriate acceptance of urinary incontinence as irremedial, despite the availability of effective treatment. "If effective interventions are to be designed to reduce the negative consequences of urinary incontinence among the elderly, then an understanding of the strategies currently used by elderly people to manage the problem is sorely needed," Mitteness reported in "The Management of Urinary Incontinence by Community-Living Elderly," *The Gerontologist,* 27 (April 1987): 185–93.

Part of a large study of illness management in the elderly, the incontinence research exemplifies Mitteness's ethnographic approach to medical social science research. Her method involves intensive observation and interviews with a relatively small sample of individuals. Mitteness and her colleagues want to know how older people decide whether urinary incontinence is an "illness" or a normal part of aging. The question allows the researcher to understand the social, psychological, and emotional context of patients, not merely their contact with health care servers. This mode of inquiry has led her to focus on multiple chronic conditions and the management of the dilemmas created by more than one health problem.

Mitteness has called for an integrated anthropological approach to life course studies in Western society. "Until psychologists and anthropologists begin to consider the life span as an integrated whole when they develop their middle range theory, the fundamental premise of a life-span approach remains unimplemented and impossible to evaluate," wrote Mitteness in 1985.

Along with her research and teaching, Mitteness has served as president of the Association for Anthropology and Gerontology (1990–1991) and a consultant to the NIH and CDC. She has actively pursued public service, donating her expertise to church organizations in the San Francisco area. Her recent work can be found in *Journal of Aging Studies* (Fall 1994), *Medical Anthropology Quarterly* (Summer 1995). She has been interim chairwoman of the Medical Anthropology Graduate Program at UCSF since 1992.

DAVID O. MOBERG. David O. Moberg, born in 1922, earned his B.A. from Seattle Pacific College. He earned his M.A. at the University of Washington in 1949, and a Ph.D. in sociology at the University of Minnesota in 1952. No single person attracted him to the field of aging, though F. Stuart Chapin and others at Minnesota permitted him to write seminar papers in the area of gerontology, even though no courses were offered on the subject. Rather, Moberg's interest was sparked by his growing awareness of demographic trends and social issues related to aging. As he became aware of work in the field, Moberg found papers and books by sociologists pioneering in gerontology to be particularly useful. The title of his doctoral dissertation, ''Religion and Personal Adjustment in Old Age,'' not only signaled Moberg's major intellectual interest but also underscored his desire to link his work with the prevailing social-scientific paradigms of the day.

Although Paul Maves was the first scholar to focus on the connections between religion and aging, David Moberg probably did more than any other scholar of his cohort to stimulate interest in the elderly's religious dimensions, and more specifically, to the spiritual well-being of the aged in later years. His first book, *The Church and the Older Person* (Grand Rapids, Mich.: Eerdman's, 1962; rev. edn., 1977), co-written with Robert M. Gray, became an oft-cited work; Ernest W. Burgess* wrote a foreword. Moberg then grappled with the theoretical points of convergence and divergence between existential and empirical realities; see, for instance, ''The Encounter of Scientific and Religious Values Pertinent to Man's Spiritual Nature,'' *Sociological Analysis,* 28 (1967): 22–23. Building on his expertise, Moberg prepared a background paper for the 1971 White House Conference on Aging, issued as *Spiritual Well-Being: Background and Issues.* This led to Moberg's playing a major role, from 1973 to 1988, in the formation and development of the National Interfaith Coalition on Aging. From this he spun off additional lectures, workshops, research, and articles, all of which Moberg used to keep the concept of ''spiritual well-being'' in the forefront of attention.

Although others—such as Craig Ellison and Raymond Paloutzian, who built on Moberg's work, and Jeffrey Levin—have constructed more widely used instruments to measure spiritual well-being, Moberg's theoretical and practical papers remain major stimuli, in part because they embrace both the religious and existential dimensions of their subject matter. See, for instance, his ''Subjective Measures of Spiritual Well-Being,'' in *Review of Religious Research,* 25 (1984): 351–64, and his edited collection, *Spiritual Well-Being: Sociological Perspectives* (Washington, D.C.: University Press of America, 1979). See also his chapter on "Religion and Aging" in *Gerontology: Perspectives and Issues,* ed. Kenneth F. Ferraro* (New York: Springer, 1990), 179–205.

After teaching at the University of Washington and Bethel College (1949–1968), Moberg became a professor of sociology at Marquette University. He has been a visiting professor at several seminaries and was president of the Religious Research Association. He currently is co-editor of *Research in the Social Scientific Study of Religion,* published annually by JAI Press.

Indeed, in introducing Moberg's article in *Spiritual Maturity in Later Years* (New York: Haworth, 1990), theologian James Seeber refers to him as the "godfather of the religion and aging research field."

HARRY R. MOODY. Philosopher and ethicist H. R. "Rick" Moody was born February 20, 1945. He graduated *magna cum laude* from Yale University in 1967, where he was elected Phi Beta Kappa. After doing graduate work in the history of consciousness program at the University of California in Santa Cruz, he moved to Columbia University, where he was appointed a faculty fellow (1969–1971). In 1973, Moody received a Ph.D. from Columbia in medieval philosophy, specializing in mysticism and comparative religion. He subsequently worked for two years managing employee education programs for the Citicorp Foundation and taught philosophy at New York University's School of Continuing Education. Since 1974, he has been at Hunter College's Brookdale Center on Aging.

Moody's interests lie in ethics and social values as they relate to the role of the elderly in society. Beginning with teaching in senior centers in 1971, he has brought his philosophical training to bear on a number of policy issues though his administrative positions. From 1980 until 1984, Moody co-directed the National Policy Center on Education, Leisure, and Continuing Opportunities for Older Persons, sponsored by the U.S. Administration on Aging (National Council on the Aging). He was the principal consultant for policy issues to the New York Center for Policy on Aging (supported by the New York Community Trust) from 1986 until 1989.

With Rose Dobrof,* Moody has been a major figure at the Brookdale Center on Aging of Hunter College. Since its founding in 1975, the center, with a staff of fifty and a budget of more than $3 million, has grown into the largest gerontology academic research facility in the New York metropolitan area.

Moody's first important gerontological book, *Abundance of Life: Human Development Policies for an Aging Society* (New York: Columbia University, 1988), addressed a range of topics from "old age in the welfare state," and "ideology and gerontology," to "retraining older workers." His subsequent effort is the first single-author monograph on bioethics and aging, *Ethics in an Aging Society* (Baltimore: Johns Hopkins University Press, 1992), which elaborated ethical issues surrounding suicide, Alzheimer's Disease, autonomy in long-term care, and intergenerational justice. These interests reflect his activities in the field of bioethics; Moody is an adjunct associate of the Hastings Center.

Aging: Concepts and Controversies (Thousand Oaks, Calif.: Pine Forge Press, 1994), his attempt to bring newcomers to the field, has found a large market.

Moody has served as a reviewer for the *Journal of Gerontological Social Work* (since 1982), and for *The Gerontologist* (since 1980). He has been on the editorial board of *Educational Gerontology* (1976–1984), and currently serves on the board of the journal *Generations*. He also co-edits, with Thomas R. Cole,* the *Aging and the Human Spirit Newsletter*. This scholarly periodical, published by the University of Texas Medical Branch (Galveston), includes book reviews and articles on religion and aging, and reports of research on comparative religion, humanistic psychology, and lifespan development. He has been a member of the board of directors of Elderhostel since 1982 and in 1994 was elected chairman of the board.

VINCENT MOR. Vincent Mor was attracted to gerontology by Sylvia Sherwood,* onetime director of the Department of Social Gerontological Research at the Hebrew Rehabilitation Center for Aged. Sherwood's work evaluated the impact of social intervention programs on poor, elderly populations in the late 1960s and early 1970s. It has been on Sherwood career, claims Mor, that he has modeled his. In addition to Sherwood, Mor counts David Greer and Sidney Katz as mentors. Greer introduced him to research in medicine and geriatrics, while Katz "taught me the value of big ideas, and the importance of pursuing to those ideas, regardless of the vagaries of funding," says Mor.

All three remain collaborators for Mor. Together with Katz, Mor developed a construct of primary prevention of functional decline. Their paper, "Risk of Functional Decline Among Well Elders," *Journal of Clinical Epidemiology,* 42 (1989): 895–904, examines the relationship between discretionary activity and the probability of future loss of physical functioning among the young elderly who are free of impairments. A second significant area of Mor's research has been a nationwide evaluation of the impact of hospice services on the costs and clinical outcomes of terminal cancer patients. He found that the elders utilizing hospice services are very different from those with traditional long-term care services, and that the two services are not interchangeable for the elderly. See Mor's paper from the Thirteenth Congress of the International Association of Gerontology, "Hospice and the Elderly: Insights from the National Hospice Study," in *Aging: The Universal Human Experience,* eds. G. L. Maddox* and E. W. Busse* (New York: Springer, 1987), 479–92.

Mor has also studied age bias in the treatment of cancer patients in Rhode Island. His research found that despite the capability of older individuals to physiologically withstand chemotherapy and radiation therapy, they were "systematically not offered those services by a variety of practitioners." These studies are summarized in *Cancer in the Elderly: Approaches to Early Detection and Treatment,* eds. R. Yanick and J. W. Yates (New York: Springer, 1990), 127–46.

Mor was part of the research team that developed and then evaluated the resilient assessment instrument mandated in the nursing home reform act. In 1994, he was awarded a MERIT award to study the influence of organizational factors on various outcomes that residents experience.

JAMES N. MORGAN. James N. Morgan probably does not consider himself a researcher on aging, although he has presented papers at a few Gerontological Society meetings over the course of his long and distinguished career and he has co-written papers on the economics of old-age poverty. Morgan merits inclusion in this volume, however, because he was the principal architect of a survey that has been an invaluable source of information for social scientists and policy analysts concerned about trends in the economics of aging. Born in 1918, Morgan has technically attained emeritus status, but he is still active.

Morgan earned his B.A. from Northwestern University in 1939 and his Ph.D. from Harvard University in 1947. His principal teacher was Nobel laureate Wassily Leontief. Morgan's own aging-related work began around 1954, when as a rising star at the Institute of Social Research at the University of Michigan, he began tracking the economic status of Americans by age. His interests were encouraged by his mentor, George Katona. In *Income and Wealth in the United States* (New York: McGraw-Hill, 1962), which he co-wrote with Martin David, Wilbur Cohen,* and Harvey Brazer, Morgan estimated that 48 percent of all families headed by a man or woman over the age was sixty-five in 1959 was a potential welfare recipient. In contrast, only one in four of all U.S. families was similarly at risk. Morgan's findings independently confirmed an analysis by the Social Security Administration, which reported that 35.2 percent of all older Americans had inadequate incomes that year. Such findings provided a statistical underpinning for federal interventions during the Great Society.

In 1968, Morgan led the team of economists and social scientists at the Institute for Social Research (ISR), located at the University of Michigan, that launched the Panel Study for Income Dynamics (PSID). They were interested in doing more than counting casualties as the nation's commitment to waging a "War on Poverty" waned. Starting with a sample of 5,000 families, heavily weighted to capture patterns of diversity among minorities and other low-income households, researchers have tracked changes in marital status, income, occupation, economic and geographic mobility, and other behavioral and attitudinal characteristics of members of the original households. As a result, this data set is arguably the richest and most carefully documented of its kind in the United States. Insofar as survivors are now nearly three decades older than when they first were surveyed, the data set has become a gerontological instrument. Some respondents are now in the ranks of the old-old, many have experienced retirement and widowhood. Those leaving to form other families are followed, so there are many two-generation pairs and divorced pairs.

Thus, it is not surprising that in the ninth volume of analyses emanating from the PSID survey, *Five Thousand American Families—Patterns of Economic Progress* (Ann Arbor, Mich.: Institute for Social Research, 1981), Morgan should have contributed an essay on "Antecedents and Consequences of Retirement." To underscore his wide-ranging interests, the subjects of his other contributions to the collection should be noted: persistence and change in economic status and the role of changing family composition; intertemporal variability in income; trends in non-money income through do-it-yourself activities; trends in residential property taxes; tests of wage trade-off hypotheses; and child care. After reviewing the scholarly literature on timing and reasons for retirement, Morgan turned to the PSID data. Although the impact of Social Security on people's decisions was not clear, there was strong evidence that workers wanted to retire.

Elsewhere, Morgan has addressed conceptual and methodological problems of measuring the economic status of the aged. With ISR colleagues Regula Herzog, Robert Kahn, James S. Jackson,* and Toni C. Antonucci,* Morgan examined "Age Differences in Productive Activities," *Journal of Gerontology: Social Sciences,* 44 (1989): S129–S138. The group showed that women and men spend about equal time in productive activities, though women spend more of it overall in unpaid work. Participation rates and average hours spent, however, are "age sensitive," influenced by age and cohort factors.

Morgan and Regula Herzog explored ways of valuing unpaid productive activity in "Age and Gender Differences in the Value of Productive Activities: Four Different Approaches," *Research on Aging,* 14 (1992): 169–98. This essay illustrates a larger theme: Morgan is convinced that the usual measures of economic status are imprecise and biased for the aged. They are imprecise, he believes, because of the significant variability among individuals, and this variability increases with age; they are biased because they do not take account of all of the elderly's assets. See his "Equity Considerations and Means-Tested Benefits," *Journal of Policy Analysis and Management,* 12 (1993): 773–78. Morgan has also challenged the growing myth about intergenerational conflict, which feels the need to ensure that each generation "gets its money back" from Social Security.

ROBERT MORRIS. Robert Morris was born in Akron, Ohio, in 1910. He received his B.A. in economics and sociology in 1931 from the University of Akron and an Ms.Sc. from Case Western Reserve University's School of Applied Social Sciences in 1935. His early career in social work involved casework, supervision, and administration in several non-profit and public agencies, working with families, children, and patients in VA hospitals. In 1948, Morris became a social planning consultant with the National Council of Jewish Federations, working on the coordination of health and social services agencies and on the organization of social services. While thus employed, he earned his D.S.W. from Columbia University's School of Social Work in 1959.

Morris's early consulting involved helping community planning groups confront the changes in medical and social services induced by changes in public funding and in medical technology especially effecting the elderly. Illustrative was an analysis for the Jewish Federation of Chicago, which led to the development of one of the earliest comprehensive programs to provide a full range of services for all the elderly in a defined area of a major city—all through a single agency with a simplified, single access to whatever was needed, from housing and home care to social programs and transportation. Similarly, chairing a community study of several institutions in Boston prompted the creation of the Hebrew Rehabilitation Centre which, by joining efforts of a teaching hospital and a home for the aged, led to a multifunction center combining various types of residential services, a chronic disease hospital, and a major geriatric research facility.

In the 1950s, Morris secured an early U.S. Public Health demonstration in research grants to study a wide range of community, social, and health services and the ways communities structured them to meet the growing needs of the chronically ill. Leading public health practitioners participated in the study, which led to the publication of an influential report on "The Community Plans for Its Chronically Ill and Aged." A companion study of community planning was widely used in dealing with principles involved in trying to rationalize community services via coordination.

In 1959, Morris was invited to join with Charles Schottland to establish at Brandeis the Florence Heller Graduate School for Social Welfare Policy, the first to offer doctoral study only for careers in social policy in social welfare. There, Morris became director of the Levinson Policy Institute (later absorbed by the Health Policy Institute at Brandeis). With the encouragement of Ollie A. Randall,* then consultant on aging for the Ford Foundation, Morris concentrated much attention on gerontological issues, as Kirstein Professor of Social Planning. An early study of gerontology planning efforts in major cities led to publication of the text *Feasible Planning for Social Change,* co-written with Robert H. Binstock* and Martin Rein, which was in print for over twenty years.

The Levinson Policy Institute initiated demonstrations to enlarge the scope of home- and community-based care for the elderly and disabled in several states, including Massachusetts, Wisconsin, and New York, and extended consultation and information to other organizations in Connecticut, Virginia, Arizona, and elsewhere. A score of substudies disseminated information about various aspects of home care. In 1970, a report prepared for the U.S. Senate Special Committee on Aging was published, stressing alternatives to institutional care. Out of these varied initiatives, Morris and his institute colleagues, especially Francis G. Caro,* developed the concept of a Social and Health Maintenance Organization (S/HMO), which could deliver both medical and social support services through a single managed care system, a single provider, financed by insurance methods (an early effort to cover social supports by insurance protection).

After Morris retired from Brandeis, the successor Health Policy Institute secured Health Care Finance Administration support for four demonstrations sites (later enlarged to eight). A competing model also developed by the institute, the

Personal Care Organization, was field tested in Wisconsin, and influenced the state adoption of its community-based care (COP) program.

While interested in linking social care components with medical systems, at home and in the workplace, Morris was simultaneously testing the parallel development of social support systems in their own right. See, for instance, his 1961 report to the New York City Council of Jewish Federations, "The Community Plans for Its Chronically Ill and Aged"; "Status of Non-Profit Homes for the Aged," in *Geriatric Institutional Management,* eds. M. Leeds,* and H. Shore* (New York: G.P. Putnam's Sons, 1964); and "Chronic Illness and Disability," in the *Encyclopedia of Social Work,* 15th edn. (Washington, D.C.: National Association of Social Workers, 1965). His 1971 report to the Gerontological Society, "The Relationship Between Social and Health Benefits: Linkage Through a Personal Care Organization," is a related but separate policy initiative.

The gist of Morris's Senate testimony is captured in "Alternatives to Nursing Home Care," issued by the U.S. Senate Special Committee on Aging, 1971; and with Larry Diamond and Leonard Gruenberg, in "Elder Care for the 1980's: Health and Social Service in One Prepaid Health Maintenance System," *The Gerontologist,* 23 (1983): 148–54; and his "Long-Term Care Issues: Identifying Problems and Potential Solutions," in *Reforming the Long-Term Care System* (Lexington, Mass.: Lexington Books, 1981).

Morris developed his gerontology work in the larger framework of a systematic planning base for organizing all social services through theory-building and designing curricula to train people interested in policymaking including, but not limited to, the aged. See, for instance, "Basic Factors in Planning the Coordination of Health Services," first published in the *American Journal of Public Health,* 81 (1961) and then issued as a monograph by the U.S. Public Health Service. "The Interrelationships of Social Welfare Theory, Practice, and Research," in *Relationship of Development and Aging,* ed. James E. Birren* (Springfield, Ill.: C. C. Thomas, 1963), anticipated themes in his classic text, with Robert H. Binstock* and Martin Rein, *Feasible Planning for Social Change* (New York: Columbia University Press, 1966). This book was one of the first to make sense of the largely scattered local and state efforts to organize welfare programs for the elderly.

Morris has been richly honored for his accomplishments. He served as president of the Gerontological Society (1966–1967), received its Kent Award twenty years later, and in 1993 its Maxwell Pollack Award. A fellow of the American Association for the Advancement of Science and of the American Public Health Association, Morris has received an honorary degree from Brandeis (the school from which he retired in 1979), and has been honored by a variety of civic and philanthropic organizations.

A strong advocate of "productive aging," Morris accepted an appointment as the Cardinal Medeiros Visiting Lecturer and Senior Fellow at the University of Massachusetts in Boston, in 1983. Four years later, he became co-editor of the *Journal of Aging and Social Policy.* He continues consulting and writing in Maryland, and teaches in the Boston area and in Florida.

MALCOLM H. MORRISON. Born in Boston in 1944, Malcolm H. Morrison earned his B.Sc. in 1965 from McGill University in Montreal, an M.A. in sociology (1967) from Boston University, and an M.P.A. (with a certificate in gerontology) from the University of Michigan in 1968. For his Ph.D. from Brandeis University in 1974, he wrote about the saving decisions of current workers and their perceptions of retirement-income planning. Morrison's interest in research on aging was sparked by reading the *Handbook of Social Gerontology* (Chicago: University of Chicago Press, 1961), which was edited by Clark Tibbitts,* and by his opportunity to work with Wilma Donahue* in Ann Arbor under one of the first training programs funded by the U.S. Administration on Aging. At Brandeis, Morrison was greatly influenced by Robert H. Binstock,* James H. Schulz,* and David Gil.

Morrison's intellectual work has concentrated in the areas of labor-force participation and retirement behavior. In his early career, he concentrated on investigating the factors that influence retirement decisions. These included the availability of public and private pensions benefits, employer retirement policies, and personal preferences. Much of this work is summarized in the *Economics of Aging: The Future of Retirement,* a collection he edited (New York: Van Nostrand Reinhold, 1982). He observed in a manner that reveals his proclivity to seek out all of the major factors that affect the big picture:

It is clear that a continuation of current retirement policies will result in very serious economic and social consequences for our society. The combination of demographic changes, high rates of inflation, efforts to control rising costs of retirement benefits, the early retirement trend, and the interrelated effects of current pension system functioning, however, will clearly result in significant changes in retirement policies and programs in the years ahead. The extent to which such policies [to provide for partial retirement and more broadly, to encourage more flexible retirement programs and work life approaches] can be developed and adopted is determined to a great degree by the information provided to public policy makers, particularly members of Congress and professional specialists in government agencies which administer retirement related programs.

Here was an insider addressing insiders.

From the 1970s through the mid-1980s, Morrison held successively more important government posts. From 1972 until 1979 he worked for the Social Security Administration. He was chief of the research support staff in the U.S. Department of Labor's Employment Standards Administration (1979–1983), and the department's representative to the 1981 White House Conference on Aging and to the United Nations World Assembly on Aging a year later. In this capacity, he directed several major national studies to examine the consequences of abolishing mandatory retirement (and, in the wake of the 1983 Social Security Act amendments, to raising the "official" retirement age) for employers and employees. Particularly notable was his report to Congress on the "Projected Consequences of Raising and Eliminating the Mandatory Retirement Age in the United States." Building on his earlier work, he also stressed the need for flexible retirement options and for developing specific strategies for business and industry to use. See, for instance, his "Retirement and Human Resource Planning for the Aging Workforce," in *Personnel Administration* (1984).

While in government, Morrison was permitted to work on projects in the private sector. He held adjunct appointments at Johns Hopkins and George Washington universities and was affiliated (1983–1985) with the Wharton School at the University of Pennsylvania and its Rehabilitation Research and Training Center in Aging. Stanley J. and Elaine M. Brody,* Ray Marshall, and Jack Habib served as important role models in this regard.

From 1983 to 1986, Morrison played an active role in the Carnegie Corporation's aging-society project. In his contribution to *Our Aging Society,* eds. Alan Pifer and Lydia Bronte (New York: W. W. Norton, 1986), "Work and Retirement in an Older Society," Morrison underscored his signal contribution to gerontology, the need to view productivity and work as reasonable goals for older persons in an aging society: "Only then will the definition of "retirement" gradually change, will public and private policies be modified to bring about a society that offers innovative alternatives for work and retirement, and will there be major enhancement of the roles and responsibilities of older persons."

From 1985 to 1990, Morrison returned to Social Security. Frustrated with public service during the Reagan-Bush years, he took a position in the private sector with the National Association of Rehabilitation Facilities. As director of research and program development, Morrison began to focus on the employment opportunities of those in poor health or with physical impairments. Representative of this work is his report, "Employment of Older Workers with a Disability: Attitudes and Legal Issues," for the National Rehabilitation Association in 1991.

JAMES A. MORTIMER. James A. Mortimer, born in 1944, received his B.A. *magna cum laude* from Tufts University in 1965. He earned his Ph.D. in computer and communication sciences from the University of Michigan in 1970, specializing in neurophysiology and cognitive psychology. There he studied information theory with Anatol Rapoport and systems theory with John Holland. His interest in brain modeling and function is reflected in his dissertation, "A Cellular Model of Mammalian Cerebellar Cortex." Following his Ph.D., Mortimer became a staff fellow at the National Institutes of Health, where he employed new techniques of single-cell recording to investigate the neurophysiological basis for movement. Moving to Minnesota in 1973, he began a long-term research program on Parkinson's Disease in collaboration with David

Webster, a clinical neurologist. His interest in gerontology and dementia grew out of this program and his early graduate training in cognitive psychology. Since 1977, Mortimer has been the associate director for research at the Geriatric Research, Education and Clinical Center in Minneapolis, a program he helped establish.

Mortimer has offered gerontology a threshold model of brain disorders to explain the increasing frequency of dementia and movement disorders with chronological age. His first expression of this concept was in a chapter, "Epidemiologic Aspects of Alzheimer's Disease," in *The Aging Nervous System* (New York: Praeger, 1980). The model was subsequently developed in *The Aging Motor System* (New York: Praeger, 1982) which he co-edited; in "Do Psychosocial Risk Factors Contribute to Alzheimer's Disease?" a chapter of *Etiology of Dementia of Alzheimer's Type* (Chichester: John Wiley & Sons, 1988); in "Education and Other Socioeconomic Determinants of Dementia and Alzheimer's Disease," *Neurology*, 4 (1993): S39–S44; and in "What Are the Risk Factors for Dementia?" in *Dementia and Normal Aging* (Cambridge: Cambridge University Press, 1994). The model has influenced such theoreticians as Paul Satz of UCLA. It also has had an impact on the design of several etiologic studies of dementia, including a study of dementia in aging twins. Mortimer credits Sir Martin Both and Alan T. Welford* with having the most important influences on its development.

The threshold model proposes that age-related dementia and movement disorders result from crossing a threshold of brain reserve. It has several testable implications. For example, it implies that the amount of neurocognitive reserve capacity available early in the life course can be used to predict the risk of dementia in late life. This implication is currently being tested in several studies. Results from these studies indicate that low linguistic ability in youth and small brain size are very strong predictors of the risk of cognitive impairment in old age.

Mortimer is an associate professor of neurology and epidemiology at the University of Minnesota, and conducts collaborative research with investigators at several universities and research centers. Among his many collaborators are Margaret Gatz,* Helena Chui, and Eugene Sobel of the University of Southern California, David Snowdon of the University of Kentucky, Amy Graves of the University of Washington, and Denis Gauvreau of the University of Montreal. Mortimer is listed in *American Men and Women in Science.*

GEORGE C. MYERS. George C. Myers received his Ph.D. at the University of Washington in Seattle in 1963. Although one of his teachers, Phillip M. Hauser, was one of the first social scientists after World War II to propose studying the nature and consequences of population aging, it was the work of Jean Bourgeois-Piochet who first stimulated Myers's interests in this area. The world-renowned French demographer had been the anonymous author of the landmark 1956

United Nations volume on *The Aging of Populations and Its Economic and Social Implications.*

Myers's main contribution to the advancement of gerontology has been the systematic statement of the dimensions of the field that has come to be known as the demography of aging. A field that contained only a handful of scholars in the early 1980s, it now is recognized as an important area of research and training in both gerontology and demography. The field has grown nationally, as evidenced by the creation of an institute-wide Office of the Demography of Aging within the U.S. National Institute on Aging, and internationally, by such organizations as the Committee for International Cooperation in National Research (CICRED) in its International Program on Population Aging. Myers has contributed to such efforts in terms of conceptual developments and the formulation of research programs on topics dealing with population aging.

For instance, in the second (1985) and third (New York: Academic Press, 1990) editions of the *Handbook of Aging and the Social Sciences,* Myers tried to encapsulate the long-term dynamics of population aging, especially its heterogeneous composition and ever-changing subgroups, by treating it as a special case of "population momentum." A second major concept in his work, "population metabolism," builds from a theme the demographer Gini introduced more than 65 years ago, and which makes an explicit analogy with the biological/physiological idea of the building up and tearing down of protoplasm: "A consideration of population metabolism for the aged population calls attention to the increments and decrements over time that modify its size and composition" ("The Demography of Aging," in *Handbook of Aging and the Social Sciences,* eds. Robert H. Binstock* and Linda George,* third edn. (New York: Academic Press, 1990), 31–32.) "Population diversity," the third concept Myers employs, draws attention to the relative distribution of socio-demographic characteristics among disaggregated subsets of the population. Delineating these three theoretical concepts has made the demography of aging more accessible to researchers.

Myers has also been concerned with the importance of declining mortality at advanced ages in altering the composition of the elderly population, especially in terms of the oldest-old and the sex imbalance among older persons. Related to these trends have been important changes in family/household structures and the creation of new societal demands on long-term care for older persons. Myers is mindful of the public policy implications of these issues. Thus, he has called for an expanded data base to permit "interactive projections" that will include consideration of the demographics of aging, that is, the consequences of future population changes associated with population aging. As his own field of vision broadens, his interests more closely complement those of two people he considers his role models, Kingsley Davis and Ethel Shanas.*

Myers is director of Duke University's Center for Demographic Studies, which he founded nearly twenty-five years ago. Among his students who have gained widespread reputations are Kenneth G. Manton and Beth J. Soldo. Within the National Institute on Aging, Myers has served on the Aging Review Committee and is currently a member of the National Advisory Council. Currently chairman of the Gerontological Society's Publications Committee, Myers served as editor-in-chief of the *Journal of Gerontology* at the time of its transition to four separate journals. He then became the first editor of the *Journal of Gerontology: Social Sciences.* In that capacity, Myers endeavored to broaden the journal's focus to represent more appropriately the range of social sciences included. He reached out especially to economists, geographers, and anthropologists.

JOHN MYLES. John Myles earned both a bachelor of arts and bachelor of philosophy degree from the University of Ottawa in 1965, and a bachelor of theology degree three years later from Gregorian University in Rome. He then pursued graduate studies in sociology, earning his M.A. from Carleton University in 1970 and his Ph.D. from the University of Wisconsin.

From 1971 to 1973, Myles served as a foreign service officer for the government of Canada. In 1976, he joined the faculty of Carleton, becoming a professor of sociology and anthropology in 1985. He served as a visiting scholar in the Department of Sociology at Harvard and as a research associate in its Centre for European Studies (1980–1981), and was a fellow of the Center for Advanced Studies in the Behavioral Sciences at Stanford in 1992. Myles then joined the faculty of Florida State University, where he serves as professor of sociology and director of the Pepper Institute on Aging and Public Policy. He currently serves as an adjunct professor of sociology at the University of Alberta and a research fellow at the Caledon Institute for Social Policy.

In the late 1980s, Myles began to write on the sociology of aging. See, for instance, his "Institutionalization and Sick Role Identification among the Elderly," *American Sociologial Review,* 43 (1978): 508–21; "Institutionalization and Disengagement among the Elderly," *Canadian Review of Sociology and Anthropology,* 16 (1979): 171–82; and "The Aged, the State, and the Structure of Inequality," in *Structured Inequality in Canada,* eds. John Harp and John Hofley (Toronto: Prentice-Hall, 1980).

His first book, *Old Age in the Welfare State: The Political Economy of Public Pensions* (Boston: Little, Brown, 1984; rev. edn., Lawrence, Kan.: University Press of Kansas, 1989), gave his thinking wide exposure in the United States. In it, one sees Myles's critical application of sociological theories (notably, issues surrounding structured inequality and institutional conundra at the interstices of politics, economics, and the social order) as well as his familiarity with the literature on the welfare state in Britain, Europe, and North America. Myles claimed, on the basis of his comparative analyses, that the welfare state in advanced industrial nations was in essence an old-age welfare state.

Over the next decade, Myles edited several volumes that refined his earlier ideas. See, for instance, his *States, Labor Markets, and the Future of Old Age Policy* (Philadelphia: Temple University Press, 1991), which he edited. Jill

Quadagno and he produced a special issue of the *Canadian Review of Sociology and Anthropology,* which he edited as *Comparative Macrosociology: Political Economy Perspectives.* With James H. Schulz* he prepared a cross-cultural analysis of "Old Age Pensions: A Comparative Perspective" for the third edition of the *Handbook of Aging and Social Sciences,* eds. Robert H. Binstock* and Linda K. George* (New York: Academic Press, 1990). His essay on "Social Security and Support of the Aged: The Western Experience," which originally appeared in the *Journal of Aging Studies* (1988), was reprinted in *Aging China: Family, Economics, and Government Policies in Transition,* eds. James Schulz and Deborah Davis Friedman (Washington, D.C.: Gerontological Society of America, 1987); and in *Aging, Self, and Community,* eds. Jaber F. Gubrium* and Kathy Charmaz (Greenwich, Conn.: JAI Press, 1992).

Myles also continued to write about Canadian social policies that affected other age groups. See his monograph with Garnett Picot and Ted Wannell, *Wages and Jobs in the 1980s: Changing Youth Wages and the Declining Middle* (Ottawa: Statistics Canada, 1989). Lately, Myles has focused on the structures and ideologies of post-industrialism. See his study, with Wallace Clement, *Relations of Ruling: Class and Gender in Postindustrial Societies* (Montreal: Mc-Gill-Queens University Press, 1994).

Myles was given the Distinguished Scholar Award by the American Sociological Association's section on aging in 1991. He became a member of the National Academy of Social Insurance two years later.

Myles has been listed in the Canadian *Who's Who* since 1991.

N

IGNATZ LEO NASCHER. Ignatz Leo Nascher, born in Vienna in 1863, was brought to the United States as an infant. He entered City College in New York and then transferred to Columbia, where he earned a pharmacy degree (1882) and his M.D. (1885). He published his first article on "A Young Living Fetus" in 1889 in the *Medical Record of New York*. The early years of his career, however, were mainly spent practicing medicine.[1]

In 1909, Nascher published in the same journal an article he titled "Geriatrics." Not only did he coin a new medical subspecialty, but in the process he made two assertions about old age that he would embellish for the rest of his life. First, Nascher claimed that "senility is a distinct period of life, . . . a physiological entity as much so as the period of childhood." And if pediatrics deserved to receive special attention, then it followed that geriatrics should be considered as a "special branch of medicine."[2] Nascher wrote *Geriatrics: The Diseases of Old Age and Their Treatment, Including Physiological Old Age, Home and Institutional Care, and Medico-Legal Relations* (Philadelphia: P. Blakiston's, 1914).

Nascher acknowledged his debts to past masters. *Geriatrics,* he claimed, was conceived as an update to the 1881 English translation of Charcot's *Lessons on the Diseases of Old Age*. He also cited the work of eighteenth- and nineteenth-century French, German, British, and (the few) American medical investigators who were doing geriatric research even if it was not so named. Nascher's claim that "all anatomical and physiological standards are based upon averages" manifestly harked back to Quetelet, an early 19th century statistican. His fascination with "problems that are intimately bound up in the grand mystery of life and death'' paralleled Metchnikoff's.*[3] Nascher accepted some of the underlying assumptions of the Nobel laureate's phagocytic theory, but he doubted that microbes were responsible for death in old age. ''A radical theory,'' he noted, ''should have a more substantial basis than plausible argument.''[4]

Nascher's views on senescence appear closer to embryologist Charles Segwick Minot and cytologist Charles Manning Child to the extent that he hypothesized that ''in the evolution of tissue cells the late cells differ from the earlier ones.''[5] Nascher reckoned that his new medical specialty had a better chance of garnering support if it was grounded in theories that were current and not too unorthodox.

Unlike many of his contemporaries, Nascher eschewed monocausal theories of senescence: ''There is undoubtedly a determining factor which is the subject of the various theories that have been advanced, but there are in addition contributing factors, causative and resultant, which hasten the senile processes.''[6] Rather than look upon old age as a malady, Nascher claimed that disease in late life was a ''pathological process in a normally degenerating body.'' Most of *Geriatrics* is devoted to identifying symptoms of thirty-seven primary senile diseases, twenty-one secondary senile diseases, thirty-three ''preferential'' diseases (not including eighteen different forms of carcinoma), twenty-seven modified diseases, and fifty-six diseases uninfluenced by advancing years. Nonetheless, Nascher's intent was to contrast ''senility'' and ''senile pathology.'' Old age, in his opinion, was not a pathological state of maturity but a distinct, ''normal'' physiological stage of life. Caring for the aged required a distinctive approach: ''My object . . . is to call attention to the primary indications in diseases in senility, which should be not to cure the disease but to prevent death. In maturity incidental complications and the questions of diet are secondary to the treatment of the pathological condition. In senility they are of primary importance.''[7] Traditional empiricism and a good bedside manner, Nascher believed, were as valuable in distinguishing pathological and physiological processes of aging as the scalpel and microscope.

However old-fashioned Nascher's description of a geriatrician may seem, his prescription for the specialty was truly forward-looking. ''As interest in the dependent child led to the scientific study of child welfare,'' he reasoned, ''so might an interest in the dependent aged lead to the scientific study of senility, of the needs and wants, the peculiarities and infirmities, the happiness and welfare of the aged.''[8] Nascher realized the field needed to be organized along lines that had proven successful in launching other specialties. Mindful of age-specific parallels, he invited A. Jacobi, M.D., the father of American pediatrics, to write the introduction to *Geriatrics.* (The analogy was not altogether persuasive intellectually, as Nascher fully acknowledged. The welfare of children aroused sympathy; ''the idea of economic worthlessness,'' he admitted, ''instills a spirit of irritability if not positive enmity against the helplessness of the aged.''[9] But the pediatric precedent, he figured, was the best available to him.)

In 1915, Nascher founded the New York Geriatrics Society. Two years later, he inaugurated a feature in the *Medical Review of Reviews.* The department's heading called him "the Father of Geriatrics."[10] Because he anticipated that geriatrics would thrive were it perceived primarily as a medical specialty, Nascher made his appeals mostly to fellow physicians. Nonetheless, like other gerontologic pioneers, he insisted that relevant social statistics be gathered. Social aspects of aging mattered to him.

Nascher's interest in medical sociology actually predated his commitment to geriatrics. His second publication (1908) was an article on prostitution. A year later he published *The Wretches of Povertyville: A Sociological Study of the Bowery,* in which he made passing references to characters such as "Duddy Ward" and "Old Shakespeare." By contrasting the living conditions and life-styles of the poor with "a rational ideal in the sociological aspect of our city," Nascher declared his allegiance to the reformist camp. With others he shared the Progressive hope that "scientific philanthropy and rational laws will take the place of the useless and pseudo-charities and inconsistent discretionary statutes now dealing with the wretches."[11]

No longer content to emphasize the need for clinical studies of the elderly, he embarked on a social survey of old-age poverty. "There is probably no class of dependents where welfare has been more completely neglected, who have received less scientific study and care, than the aged," Nascher told a National Conference of Social Work in 1917. "The child dependent has the world for its guardian; the aged dependent is disowned by his own."[12] Nascher's call to study and remedy the causes of old-age dependency was pioneering in America. Landmark investigations of old-age poverty social-insurance legislation in Britain, it is worth noting, had preceded U.S. initiatives by a quarter of a century. Indeed, before the 1920s, only Lee Welling Squier's *Old Age Dependency in the United States* (1912) and a 1915 Massachusetts *Report on Old Age Pensions, Annuities, and Insurance* came close to matching in scope and detail Charles Booth's 1984 classic, *The Aged Poor in England and Wales.* "In the United States," declared social reformer William Dwight Bliss Porter, "the old-age problem is not yet so serious."[13]

Despite his efforts to mobilize interest in a variety of circles, Nascher's advocacy of geriatrics had limited impact. Some shared the distinction he made between "pathological" and "physiological" causes of death in late life.[14] A few clinicians shared some of his interests in bench science, social research, and advocacy, but none so fully integrated them in their careers. Nascher's contributions were honored by his students, and they are duly recorded in histories of aging. Still, an important part of the legacy is that Nascher's pioneering ideas and organizations met with considerable resistance. He had difficulty finding a firm willing to publish *Geriatrics,* and things did not get easier over time. Nascher admitted that he was the only full-time geriatrician as late as 1926.[15]

Nascher was a "prophet" in every sense of the word when he died in 1944.

NOTES

1. Joseph T. Freeman, "Nascher: Excerpts from His Life, Letters, and Works," *The Gerontologist,* 1 (March 1961): 17–26.

2. I. L. Nascher, M.D., "Geriatrics," *New York Medical Journal,* 90 (1909): 358. Virtually the same themes are elaborated in "Practical Geriatrics," *Medical Council,* 22 (1917): 33–36.

3. I. L. Nascher, *Geriatrics* (Philadelphia: P. Blakiston's Son & Co., 1916 [1914]), v (2nd edn. preface) and vii-x (1st edn. preface). See also, Henning Kirk, "Geriatric Medicine and the Categorisation of Old Age," *Ageing and Society,* 12 (1992): 499–514.

4. I. L. Nascher, "Tissue Cell Evolution," *New York Medical Journal,* 92 (1910): 918.

5. I. L. Nascher, "Why Old Age Ends in Death," *Medical Review of Reviews,* 25 (1919): 291. Child and Manning from different perspectives held that old age resulted from cumulative changes in the properties of cells and tissues as an organism matured. See C.S. Minot, *Problem of Age* (New York: Harper, 1919): 249 and Charles Manning Child, *Senescence and Rejuvenescence* (Chicago: University of Chicago Press, 1915), 58, 271, 301, 309, 459, 465.

6. Nascher, *Geriatrics,* pp. 47–48.

7. I. L. Nascher, "The Treatment of Disease in Senility," *Medical Record of New York,* 76 (1909): 990.

8. I. L. Nascher, "The Neglect of the Aged," *Medical Record, New York,* 86 (1914): 457.

9. Point and from quotation in Carole Haber, "Geriatrics: A Specialty in Search of Specialists," in *Old Age in a Bureaucratic Society,* ed. David D. Van Tassel and Peter N. Stearns (Westport, Conn.: Greenwood Press, 1986), 77.

10. I. L. Nascher, "Salutatory," *Medical Review of Reviews,* 23 (1917): 29.

11. I. L. Nascher, *The Wretches of Povertyville* (Chicago: Jos. J. Lanzit, 1909), pp. 298–99. See Chap. 4 for some of his characterizations of the old.

12. I. L. Nascher, "The Institutional Care of the Aged," *Proceedings of the National Conference of Social Work* (Chicago: The Conference, 1917), 350–56.

13. I. L. Nascher, "The Institutional Care of the Aged," *Proceedings of the National Conference of Social Work* (Chicago: The Conference, 1917), 350–56.

14. William Dwight Porter Bliss, "Old Age Pensions," *The Encyclopedia of Social Reform* (New York: Funk and Wagnalls, 1897), 952–54. See also, William Graebner, *A History of Retirement* (New York: Yale University Press, 1980); and Brian Gratton, *Urban Elders* (Philadelphia: Temple University Press, 1985). For more on British trends, see Martin Bulmer, *Social Science and Social Policy* (London: Allen & Unwin, 1986), 224–26.

15. I. L. Nascher, "A History of Geriatrics," *Medical Review of Reviews,* 32 (1926): 283; Barclay Moon Newman, "Geriatrics," *Scientific American,* 163 (1940): 190.

BERNICE L. NEUGARTEN. Bernice L. Neugarten was born in 1916 in Nebraska. She began her studies at the University of Chicago at the age of seventeen. Neugarten concentrated in English and French literature as an undergraduate, where she studied with the writer Thornton Wilder and physiologist Anton Carlson. After earning an M.A. in educational psychology, Neugarten accepted an assistantship in the newly formed Committee on Child Development, which included Alison Davis, Helen Koch, Robert Redfield, W. Lloyd Warner, and Robert J. Havighurst.* Neugarten's dissertation dealt with the influence of social class on friendships among adolescents and children in Morris, Illinois, a community made famous as "Jonesville" and "Elmtown" by Warner and Havighurst. Although not the first to earn a doctorate through this interdisciplinary committee, Neugarten does take some pride in having been the first person to complete a Ph.D. after the group was renamed the Committee on Human Development, to reflect its broadening interest in studying the human lifespan, relying especially on the tools of sociology and psychology.

Neugarten chose to remain in Hyde Park because she married a European-born lawyer, Fritz, who owned a business in the area. She then spent eight years "out" of the academy, raising two children, doing part-time research and writing, and getting involved in local politics. Neugarten pursued psychological themes—such as personality changes in adolescence and a cross-cultural analysis of the moral and emotional development of children in six Native American tribes—and sociological issues that extended her earlier research. Later, in connection with the Kansas City Studies of Adult Life, she co-wrote with Richard P. Coleman, *Social Status in the City* (San Francisco: Jossey-Bass, 1971), which dealt with social class structure.

While Neugarten early on displayed extraordinary intellectual curiosity and rigor, as well as a penchant for crossing academic boundaries, in retrospect it seems almost serendipitous that she should have made her international reputation by concentrating on adult development and aging. It just so happened that the Committee on Human Development needed someone to teach its course on "Maturity and Old Age," and Neugarten was available. After reading what little was available (Erik Erikson's work was especially influential), Neugarten reorganized materials, renaming the course Adult Development and Aging. At the same time she was invited to join the research team studying middle-aged and aging persons in Kansas City. In 1960, Neugarten went on the tenure track. Four years later, she became the first scholar awarded full-time tenure in the Committee on Human Development. Neugarten became a full professor in 1968, and committee chairwoman the following year. Including her student days, Neugarten spent more than three decades on the Chicago campus.

Neugarten may have spent most of her life in one place, but her intellectual interests proved far-ranging. She has written or (co)edited at least eight books, more than 150 articles, and has given countless scientific and public lectures. "My pattern of research has been to open new topic areas rather than to follow a single line of inquiry; to use sometimes qualitative, sometimes quantitative methods; to prefer exploration to replication—in short, to map out some of the landscape of what had earlier been the neglected territory of the second half of life," she says.

Three characteristics nonetheless are evident throughout her research and writing. First, she has always been willing to cross intellectual boundaries. Working largely at the interstices of sociology and psychology at a time in which "social psychology" was flourishing, Neugarten really does not fit into any of the familiar camps. She did little survey research; engaging in symbolic interaction was not her interpretive mode. Rather, she followed ideas that intrigued her, adapting methods as she went along. This research style led to a second trait: Neugarten delighted in challenging, if not defying, the conventional wisdom about adult development and aging expressed by her contemporaries. Time after time she was ahead of the curve. Neugarten was one of the first researchers on aging to stress the importance of gender; she recognized the importance of societal aging before most of her peers. Third, while she was comfortable with theorists and did not hesitate to point out flaws in their constructs and empirical analyses, Neugarten had a very practical side. "So what?" was one of her favorite questions. She wanted scholars to make connections, to limn the big picture; she was interested in applying knowledge to address the needs and challenges of men and women adapting to fundamental changes in their midst. Neugarten carried on that process of critical inquiry that John Dewey had instilled at the University of Chicago at the turn of the century.

Three collections published in the 1960s underscore her perduring interest in the diversity of older people and fascination with changes in cohort-based, cultural, and historically grounded age- and sex-specific roles. In her *Personality in Middle and Late Life* (New York: Atherton Press, 1964), Neugarten and associates offered the first systematic studies of personality changes in late adulthood. Her work thus stands in stark contrast to those who stress basic continuities from childhood through maturity. Her *Middle Age and Aging: A Reader in Social Psychology* (Chicago: University of Chicago, 1968) became one of the most widely adopted anthologies in psychology and gerontology courses. Major attention was given to social scientific theories of aging; to work, retirement, and leisure; and to differences in culture.

Besides making a new field accessible to a wide readership, *Middle Age and Aging* also served as a vehicle for some of the work on personality done by Neugarten, her colleagues, and her students with the Kansas City data. In an even-handed way, she criticized the "disengagement theory" set forth by William Henry and Elaine Cumming—colleagues who had relied on the same data set. "The aging individual may or may not disengage from the pattern of role activities that characterize him in middle age," she wrote in an essay with Havighurst and Sheldon S. Tobin.* "It is highly doubtful, however, that he ever disengages from the values of the society. . . . It is even more doubtful that the aging individual ever disengages from the personality pattern that has so long been the self."

In one of her most frequently cited pieces in the same volume, "Age Norms, Age Constraints, and Adult Socialization" (written with Joan W. Moore and John C. Lowe), Neugarten noted that Americans of different ages generally agreed that there were certain ages at which it was appropriate to leave home, marry, and retire. Yet, as societal cues changed, and as different subsets of the age structure experienced the same life events in dissimilar ways, various subgroups were beginning to express divergent expectations about age-appropriate behavior: "Under these circumstances," Neugarten said, "there is likely to be a blurring of distinctions between what the respondent himself regards as right and what he thinks other people would 'naturally' regard as right." In addition to class variations, Neugarten underscored the importance of gender differences.

In the 1970s, Neugarten refined these concepts, providing readers with key phrases that quickly developed a life of their own. Her notion of increasing numbers of people being "off time" at various points of their adult development led her to speculate that people have internal "social clocks." In her 1976 Master Lectures on Developmental Psychology before the American Psychological Association, she stressed that it is the unexpected events—the premature death of a spouse or a child, forced retirement due to disability—that caused people great stress, over and beyond the discomfort they experienced in the face of anticipated transitions. And as a way to underscore the diversity to be found in the older population, Neugarten stated that the distinction between "a green old age" and "senectitude" invoked since Classical times no longer encapsulated the realities of growing old in postwar society. Instead, she contrasted the needs and capacities of the "young-old" from that minority of "old-old" people who needed special care and support. Neugarten's point in "Age Groups in American Society and the Rise of the Young-Old," *Annals of the American Academy of Political and Social Science,* 415 (1974): 187–98, was to stress that one generic age-based policy would not suffice. To her great dismay and annoyance, however, many reified Neugarten's distinction, affixing chronological boundaries (fifty-five to seventy-five and over seventy-five, respectively) that contradicted her increasing sense that years of life were a valid predictor of adult behavior.

In addition to her outpouring of papers and books, and service on various study sections and advisory panels for the National Institutes on Health and the U.S. Office of Education, Neugarten also was in charge of the committee's training program. Over the course of two decades, with support from the National Institute of Mental Health, the National Institute on Child Health and Human Development, and (after 1975) the National Institute on Aging, she trained more than eighty doctoral students in adult development and aging. (Scores more would be added to this number if master's degree students and colleagues' students were included.) Neugarten took particular pride in recruiting and mentoring housewives who decided in midlife to embark upon an academic career. Neugarten's sensitivity to women's issues was evident when she was asked to serve as the first chairwoman of the Committee on Women of the University of Chicago.

In the mid-1970s, Neugarten became increasingly fascinated with the relevance of gerontology to policymaking. With Robert J. Havighurst, she produced *Social Policy, Social Ethics, and the Aging Society* (Chicago: University of

Chicago Press, 1976) and *Extending the Human Life Span: Social Policy and Social Ethics* (Chicago: University of Chicago Press, 1977), reports prepared for the National Science Foundation. Neugarten drew not only on her colleagues at Chicago, but also on federal officials, legal scholars, and humanists. A broad forum was necessary. She also was a principal contributor to a special edition of *The Gerontologist*, 15 (February 1975) on aging in the year 2000. "If our institutions are to be more successful in the next few decades," Neugarten wrote in the introduction to *The Gerontologist*, "scholarly efforts should now be undertaken to forecast, as best we can, the likely demographic and social developments, to anticipate the problems of aging and the aging society that lie ahead, then to decide what types of information are needed for formulating politics that will be future-oriented."

Neugarten quickly was given an opportunity to direct such a policy-relevant research agenda. She was appointed to the fifteen-member Federal Council on Aging for a three-year term in 1980. She also was named deputy director of the 1981 White House Conference on Aging. After eighteen months of work, however, Neugarten was dismissed from the latter post by members of the Reagan administration who wanted to control the issues under consideration. Taking early retirement at the University of Chicago, Neugarten then moved her base of operations to Northwestern University, where she helped to launch a doctoral program on Human Development and Social Policy in the School of Education.

In the 1980s, Neugarten continued to publish provocative essays that inspired (and irritated) scholars and students from a broad range of disciplines and professions. In *Age or Need?* (Beverly Hills, Calif.: Sage, 1982), for instance, she noted that "the public debate is becoming more heated around the issues of how to enhance the welfare of the growing population of older people in this country in ways constructive to the whole society." The distinction between policies for aged individuals and policies for an aging society was critical to her at a time in which much age-based legislation seemed less relevant than at its time of enactment, or even quite counterproductive to the best interests of a country mired in stagflation. As a member of the steering committee of a Carnegie Corporation study, Neugarten (with her daughter Dail) contributed an essay on the "Changing Meanings of Age in the Aging Society" in *Our Aging Society*, eds. Alan Pifer and Lydia Bronte (New York: Norton, 1986) that built on her earlier thesis: "Perhaps the most constructive ways of adapting to an aging society will emerge by focusing, not on age at all, but on more relevant dimensions of human needs, human competencies, and human diversity."

Neugarten's manifold accomplishments have hardly gone unnoticed. The recipient of several honorary degrees, she was the first social scientist specializing in aging to be elected a Fellow of the American Academy of Arts and Sciences. She won the Gerontological Society's Kleemeier Award (1971), the American Psychological Foundation Distinguished Teaching Award (1975), the Brookdale Award (1982), and the Sandoz Prize (1987), among other prestigious honors. The Committee on Human Development in 1982 held a two-day symposium to mark the fourth decade of her accomplishments to the study of adult life. Events that might have been the culmination of other people's career—such as the decision she made during her presidency to relocate the Gerontological Society from St. Louis to Washington, D.C., to enhance its visibility; her editorship of *Human Development*, the *Journal of Gerontology*, and *Psychology and Aging*—pale in comparison with other achievements.

In 1988, Neugarten returned to the University of Chicago to serve as Rothschild Distinguished Scholar at the Center on Aging, Health, and Society.

Note: Unlike many other prominent figures in gerontology, Bernice Neugarten's biography has been recounted elsewhere. See, for instance, the entry by Nancy K. Schlossberg and Lillian E. Troll* in *Women in Psychology: A Bio-Bibliographic Sourcebook,* eds. Agnes N. O'Connell and Nancy Felipe Russo (Westport, Conn.: Greenwood Press, 1990), 256–65, and Neugarten's own reflections, "The Aging Society and My Academic Life," in *Sociological Lives,* ed. Matilda White Riley* (Beverly Hills, Calif.: Sage, 1989), 91–106.

ROBERT J. NEWCOMER. Robert J. Newcomer was born in 1943. He earned a master's degree in city planning from the University of Southern California in 1971 and completed a Ph.D. there in 1975. An initial (and continuing) concern has been housing for the elderly and such issues as the influence of design and services on consumer decision-making, and the effect of public and private policies on the supply of housing.

Louis Gelwicks, an architect, recruited Newcomer to the field of gerontology; the pair collaborated on a report entitled "Planning Housing Environments for the Elderly" for the Washington, D.C. based National Council on Aging in 1974. Newcomer has also worked extensively with M. Powell Lawton* and Thomas Byerts, producing two collections: *Community Planning for an Aging Society* (Stroudsberg, Pa.: Dowden, Hutchinson, and Ross, 1976), and *Housing an Aging Society* (New York: Van Nostrand Reinhold, 1986). His recent housing work extends these concerns by examining the relationships between financing, design, and levels of care. See, for example, R. J. Newcomer and S. Preston, "Relationships Between Acute Care and Nursing Unit Use in Two Continuing Care Retirement Communities," *Research on Aging,* 16 (1994): 280–300; and R. J. Newcomer and L. Grant, "Residential Care Facilities: Understanding their Role and Improving their Effectiveness," in *Aging in Place: Supporting the Frail Elderly in Residential Environments,* ed. D. Tilson (Glenview, Ill.: Scott, Foresman, 1990).

A second focus of work has been specific service delivery and/or financing structures. This work includes a project named the Evaluation of the Medicare Social Health Maintenance Organization Demonstration (spanning the period 1985–1991 and conducted in collaboration with Charlene Harrington), and an evaluation of a national Alzheimer's case management demonstration program (ongoing from 1989 to 1996 and conducted in collaboration with Patrick Fox).

This work encompasses acute care and chronic care delivery, financing, and regulatory systems, the points of interrelationship across these systems, and the interrelationship between delivery systems and residential settings. The S/HMO project has resulted in fifteen published journal articles and two book chapters. See for example, R. J. Newcomer, C. Harrington,* and S. Preston, "Health Plan Satisfaction among S/HMO Members and Disenrollees, and Medicare Beneficiaries in Fee for Service Care," in *HMOs and Other Health Care Systems for the Elderly,* ed. H. Luft (Melrose Park, Ill.: Health Administration Press, 1994); and K. G. Manton, R. Newcomer, J. Vertrees, G. Lowrimore, and C. Harrington, "Social/Health Maintenance Organization and Fee-for-Service Health Outcomes Over Time," *Health Care Financing Review,* 15 (1993): 173–202.

The third cluster of work is an outgrowth of Newcomer's experience in state- and community-level planning. Much of his early research was in the area of state and local government interrelationships, and community delivery systems, in which he collaborated with Carroll E. Estes* on two books: C. E. Estes and R. Newcomer, *Fiscal Austerity and Aging: Shifting Governmental Responsibility for the Elderly* (Beverly Hills, Calif.: Sage Publications, 1983); C. Harrington, R. Newcomer, and C. Estes, *Long Term Care of the Elderly: Public Policy Issues* (Beverly Hills, Calif.: Sage Publications, 1985). His most recent work, in collaboration with A. E. Benjamin and Dorothy Rice, explores approaches for organizing health and social indicators of community systems (that is, supply and entry control) and relating these with service need prevalence. This work builds on the rapidly developing fields of quality assurance and total quality management, and health plan "score cards."

Newcomer currently serves as professor and vice-chairman of the Department of Social and Behavioral Sciences, University of California at San Francisco.

LINDA S. NOELKER. In 1968, Linda S. Noelker received a call from George Rosenberg asking if she were interested in graduate work at Case Western Reserve University's Sociology Department as a gerontology trainee. "I had no idea what gerontology was, but he said not to worry," Noelker recalls. Her well-timed entry into gerontology coincided with the debate about disengagement and activity theories and the publication of key works in aging such as Irving Rosow's* *Social Integration of the Aged* (New York: Free Press, 1967) and Ethel Shanas's* *Old People in Three Industrial Societies* (New York: Atherton Press, 1968).

Noelker earned her M.A. from Case Western in 1971 and her doctorate in 1975. Her early postgraduate work explored innovative home health aide programs for the elderly. She conducted her research as project director of The Interdependent Home Health Care Project, funded by the Cleveland Foundation, at the Margaret Blenkner Research Center of the Cleveland-based Benjamin Rose Institute. Her dissertation research was an investigation of intimate relationships among nursing home residents and staff, and she has returned to this subject in her latest research.

In addition to the Cleveland Foundation, which continues to support her recent research, Noelker has been supported by the Administration on Aging, the Retirement Research Foundation, and the National Institute of Mental Health. She has explored the impact of in-home care on the families of impaired elderly, the interface between informal and formal helpers, and the relationship between nursing home residents and nursing assistants.

Noelker has continued her connection with the Margaret Blenkner Research Center, serving as the center's director since 1985. She is also an adjunct professor of sociology at Case Western Reserve University and Kent State University. The overall goal of her research has been to develop conceptual models that explain how informal and informal assistance is used by frail older persons. See, for example, Linda S. Noelker and David M. Bass, ''Home Care for Elderly Persons: Linkages Between Formal and Informal Caregivers,'' *Journal of Gerontology*, 44 (1989): S63–S70; and D. M. Bass and L. S. Noelker, ''The Influence of Family Caregivers on Elder's Use of In-Home Services: An Expanded Conceptual Framework,'' *Journal of Health and Social Behavior*, 28 (1987): 184–96. This work underscores the importance of including varied characteristics of informal helping networks and primary caregivers as predictors of the elderly's formal service use. It also attempts to assess the effects of perceptions of care management on their patterns of use.

Throughout her career, Noelker has noticed the deep and personal commitment of gerontologists to the field. Many trace this commitment to a close, loving relationship with an older relative in early life. She also appreciates the effort of gerontology's founders and ''well-published'' professionals to mentor the next generation.

O

MORRIS A. OKUN. Morris A. Okun was born in 1949 in New York. He attended Brooklyn College, where he majored in psychology. He then earned a Ph.D. in educational psychology from Pennsylvania State in 1975. Okun went on to postdoctoral work at Duke University's Center for the Study of Aging and Human Development before starting his continuing association with Arizona State University in 1976. Moving through the ranks of Arizona's Department of Psychology in Education, he became a full professor in 1985. In 1989, Okun became director of the Adult Development and Aging program and joined the Psychology Department.

Okun teaches actively and has so far directed thirteen doctoral dissertations. He notes proudly that 60 percent of his publications since 1980 have been co-written with current or former doctoral students. In addition to his students, Okun has collaborated with Irene C. Siegler and Linda K. George,* both of Duke University, and William A. Stock, who is also at Arizona State.

Research on risk taking—prompted by Jack Botwinick's* investigations into cautiousness as a function of age—led to one of Okun's most important intellectual contributions to gerontology early in his career. Through experimental research on behavioral risk taking, Okun was able to clarify the erroneous conclusion that older people are generally more cautious than younger people. By showing that age differences in risk taking are actually situation-specific, he introduced a new paradigm to the field. The research also refined the concept of cautiousness, separating risk-avoidance strategies from those employed to manage risk once it has been engaged. For his most recent work on the subject,

266 WILLIAM E. ORIOL

see M. A. Okun, W. A. Stock, and R. W. Ceurvorst, "Risk Taking Through the Adult Life Span," *Experimental Aging Research,* 6 (1980): 463–73.

During the 1980s, Okun's work focused on using meld-analysis to summarize current research on life satisfaction. In the process, he has created a standard for quantitative research syntheses in gerontology. See M. A. Okun, R. W. Olding, and C. M. G. Cohn, "A Meld-Analysis of Subjective Well-Being Interventions among Elders," *Psychological Bulletin,* 108 (1990): 257–66.

Okun's more recent research, in collaboration with Nancy Eisenberg, examines issues of motivation and emotional regulation among senior volunteers; see N. Eisenberg and M. A. Okun, "The Relations of Dispositional Regulation and Emotionality to Elders' Empathy-Related Responding and Affect While Volunteering," *Journal of Personality* (in press).

In addition to his teaching and research, Okun served as an editorial board member of the *Journal of Gerontology* from 1982 until 1985. In 1986, he assumed his current post on the editorial board of the *International Journal of Aging in Human Development.* Okun has also worked actively with the American Psychological Association's Division 20, including a period as membership chairman, and as chairman of the education committee guidebook, *Doctoral Opportunities for Specialization in the Psychology of Aging.*

WILLIAM E. ORIOL. William E. Oriol was born in West New York, New Jersey, in 1927. After serving in the Army from 1945 to 1948, he earned his B.A. from New York University in 1951. For the next six years, he worked on the Bergen (N.J.) *Evening Record.* In 1959, Oriol became press secretary to Senator Harrison A. Williams (D-NJ). Four years later, he joined the professional staff of the recently established U.S. Senate Special Committee on Aging. Oriol served as staff director for the body from 1967 to 1975. Since leaving Capitol Hill, Oriol has worked with Wilma Donahue in establishing the International Center for Social Gerontology, and he has held several positions with the National Council on the Aging.

In addition to teaching at the Andrus Gerontology Center, Oriol has contributed several chapters to gerontology books and articles to professional journals. For instance, in "Work and Retirement: Visible Issues at the U.N. World Assembly on Aging," *Aging and Work,* 7 (1984): 13–20, Oriol discussed recommendations made at that 1982 gathering. He argued that greater attention needed to be paid to older-worker issues in both industrialized and lesser developed nations. Regional issues also commanded attention.

Oriol received the Gerontological Society's Donald Kent award in 1979. In his speech, printed as " 'Modern' Age and Public Policy," *The Gerontologist,* 21 (February 1981): 35–45, Oriol tried to put the results of the 1980 election into broader perspective. He saw the decade from 1965 to 1975 as a period of consolidation in federal policymaking. Despite progress, including the erosion of ageism, more advances nonetheless had to be made.

MARCIA G. ORY. Marcia G. Ory received her Ph.D. from Purdue University in 1976, where she worked with Richard Kerckhoff. Ory earned her M.P.H. from the Johns Hopkins University five years later, working primarily with Evelyn Goldberg and Pearl German. Her interest in research on aging was sparked by Nancy Anderson (Eutis), a sociologist at the University of Minnesota, while Ory was in Minneapolis on a postdoctoral fellowship with Reuben Hill. At the time Anderson was looking at long-term care and aging.

Ory's main interests and areas of research include aging, health, and behavior; gender differences in health and longevity; and the implications of the AIDS epidemic for middle-aged and older populations. With Matilda White Riley,* Hubert Warner, and Ronald P. Abeles,* her senior colleagues at the National Institute on Aging, she has edited several volumes. See, for instance, *Aging, Health, and Behavior,* eds. Marcia Ory, Ronald P. Abeles and Paula Darby Lipman (Beverly Hills, Calif.: Sage Publications, 1992); this volume has helped identify and stimulate research in behavioral geriatrics at the federal level. See also, Marcia Ory and Hubert Warner, *Gender, Health, and Longevity* (New York: Springer Publications, 1990); and *AIDS in an Aging Society: What We Need to Know,* eds. Matilda W. Riley, Marcia Ory, and Diane Zablotsky (New York: Springer, 1989). Ory is also beginning a new initiative on health and menopause.

In a volume edited with Kathleen Bond, a social science analyst at NIA, Ory edited *Aging and Health Care: Social Science and Policy Perspectives* (New York: Routledge, 1989). This volume evolved out of work done independently and collaboratively at the National Institute on Aging as well as the National Center for Health Services Research. In their introductory essay, Ory and Bond state their operating assumptions. Like Riley, whose influence is evident throughout, Ory and Bond acknowledge the heterogeneity of the aged population and affirm that aging is a life-long process that occurs in specific social contexts. In particular, Ory notes her work with Marie Haug,* published in "Issues in Elderly Patient-Provider Interactions," *Research on Aging,* 9 (1987): 3–44, in which she reported that an older person's previous experiences with the health care system and health care providers affect his or her subsequent attitudes and behavior. Accordingly, she argues, "interventions for healthy older persons should be designed to enhance or maintain high levels of health and functioning." This means, among other things, not always making sharp distinctions between formal and informal care, and taking a broad approach rather than the segmental interventions appropriate for younger people. Ory and Haug then identify research gaps in the area of aging and health.

Ory's own distinctive contribution to the research literature has been to specify health and behavior linkages in old age. She has helped refine psychosocial geriatrics research. In particular, Ory has stimulated research on special-care units for people with dementia. This has involved the stewardship of national, multisite initiatives to evaluate the impact of special-care units on people with dementia, their families, and health care professionals.

Ory currently is chief of the Social Science Research on Aging in the Behavioral and Social Science Research Program at the National Institute on Aging. Ory is very active in such professional organizations as the American Public Health Association, American Sociological Association, and Gerontological Society of America, and serves on several national task forces and advisory boards dealing with aging and health issues. Ory currently directs the NIA collaborative Studies on Special Care Units for Alzheimer's Disease.

NANCY J. OSGOOD. Nancy J. Osgood earned her Ph.D. in sociology and certificate in gerontology from Syracuse University in 1979. She began her research in the shadow of Irving Rosow's* social integration theory of aging. Testing Rosow's thesis, Osgood conducted a study of social integration in three Sunbelt planned retirement communities. The study, originally her dissertation and later published as *Senior Settlers Social Integration in Retirement Communities* (New York: Praeger, 1982), emphasized the importance of environment to older individuals.

Her more recent research has focused specifically on suicide in the elderly. Osgood's four books on the subject—including the latest, *Suicide in Later Life: Recognizing the Warning Signs* (Lexington, Mass.: Lexington Books, 1992)—have served as a blueprint for subsequent studies. The suicide rate of U.S. seniors is 50 percent higher than that for teens or other groups. Osgood has identified a number of factors accounting for this problem. In long-term care facilities she has found that higher staff turnover, lower per-diem costs, and a larger number of clients all correlate with a higher incidence of suicide. Alcoholism and drug abuse are major contributing factors. See her study of 463 long-term care facilities, "Environmental Factors in Suicide in Long-Term Care Facilities," *Suicide and Life Threatening Behavior,* 22 (1992): 98–106.

Osgood's interest in suicide, a problem she views as a national tragedy, has led in a few directions. First, it has led her to call for solutions, including educating caregivers providing specialized geriatric mental health services and restricting the elderly's access to firearms. She has become an important contributor to the cause of suicide prevention, delivering a plenary speech at the 1991 Annual Congress of International Associations of Suicide Prevention (IASP). Putting her solutions into effect, she recently completed a statewide training project for 3,000 older adults, service providers, and family members about alcoholism and drug abuse. Funded by the Administration on Aging, the program yielded a set of training materials and is viewed as a model. Her most recent book, with Helen Wood and Iris Parham, is *Alcoholism and Aging: An Annotated Bibliography* (Westport, Conn.: Greenwood Press, 1995).

Osgood has also contributed two important bibliographic sources. With Ann H. L. Sontz she compiled *The Science and Practice of Gerontology: A Multidisciplinary Guide* (Westport, Conn.: Greenwood Press, 1989); and, with John McIntosh, *Suicide and the Elderly: An Annotated Bibliography and Review* (Westport, Conn.: Greenwood Press, 1986).

Osgood is currently affiliated with the Gerontology and Sociology Departments of Richmond-based Virginia Commonwealth University and the Medical College of Virginia.

JACK OSSOFSKY. Jack Ossofsky was born in 1925 in New York City. He attended City College of New York, where he completed with honors a bachelor's in social science in 1950. He then served as director of retirement and community services for the Wholesale Department Store Union (AFL-CIO) until 1965.

"My career has coincided with America's growing understanding of the needs and capacities of its rapidly increasing older population," Ossofsky once remarked (*Who's Who,* 1986, v. 2, 2124). "In that context I have sought to reaffirm my determination to value all human beings, to nurture each person's potential, to seek fulfillment in all the years, and to cherish each moment of life."

The bulk of that career was spent in service to the National Council on Aging. Ossofsky first served the council as a New York City project director from 1965 until 1967 when he became associate director. In 1969 he moved to Washington, D.C. to become deputy director (1969–1971), then executive director (1971–1986), and finally president until his retirement in 1988.

At the council, Ossofsky helped win passage of Medicare, the Older Americans Act, and amendments to the Age Discrimination in Employment Act. Among the programs he developed to create opportunities for the elderly are the Foster Grandparents Program and the Congregate Meals Program, which extends independent living for the aged. He was a delegate at the 1971 White House Conference on Aging, and a key figure at the 1981 White House Conference on Aging, which outlined aging policy for the decade.

He also convened the United National North American World Assembly on Aging in 1980 and 1981, chaired the Leadership Council of Aging Organizations from 1981–1982, and served as trustee of the Hobart Jackson Fellowship Fund (University of Pennsylvania) from 1979 until 1985. He served as a member of the editorial board of Educational Gerontology, along with several other editorial boards.

For Ossofsky's concerns during this final stage in his career, see "Creating a True Service Continuum: The Challenge to Nursing Home and Community Service Providers," *Journal of the American Health Care Association* (September 1985) 11(5):29–31; and "A Compassionate Man Sums Up," *50 Plus* (April 1988) 28:16+.

Ossofsky was a democratic supporter, serving as vice chairman of senior citizens for Kennedy and Johnson in 1959–1960, and in the same post in 1964 for Johnson and Humphrey.

Ossofsky retired to East Boothbay, Maine, in 1988 where he died of a brain tumor in 1992.

ANDREW OSTROW. Andrew Ostrow has pursued a diverse set of issues relating to the psychological aspects of physical activity in terms of athletics and
aging. His early work pursued the relationship among sports competition, mental
health, and aging.

More recently, Ostrow examined the notion of age-role stereotyping and ageism, as these factors affect participation in physical activity among older adults.
Working with Roger Keener and Susan Perry, Ostrow tested the hypothesis that
children view physical activity as less appropriate among adults of increasing
age. Using a sample ($N = 93$) of preschool children, and photos of individuals
who had been made up to look older, the team found that children do indeed
deem older adults less proficient in physical activity. See "The Age Grading of
Physical Activity among Children," *International Journal of Aging and Human
Development*, 24 (1986–87): 101–11. Working with his graduate students at
Morgantown-based West Virginia University, Ostrow has followed up with similar studies on college students and adults. Among these groups, age role
expectations were far more potent than sex role expectations in terms of assumptions about the appropriateness of physical activity participation.

His latest work has involved older drivers. Ostrow co-directed a two-year
research grant sponsored by the American Automobile Association's Foundation
for Traffic Safety, "Physical Fitness and the Older Driver." The aim of the
study was to test the impact of modifying the functional capacity of the older
driver on his or her driving skills. Most solutions advanced to address the problems of older drivers have centered on vehicle design and driver education.
Ostrow and his colleagues produced some of the first empirical investigations
examining the role of physical fitness in sustaining the driving skills of older
adults.

One such study was reported in his "The Effects of a Joint Range of Motion
Physical Fitness Training Program on Automobile Driving Skills of Older Drivers," *Journal of Safety Research*, 23 (1992): 207–19. The researchers found that
improved shoulder and hip range of motion resulted in improved observation
skills of older drivers.

Despite this important research, Ostrow is proudest of his work as an author,
editor, and publisher of textbooks that promote the importance of sustaining
physical activity through the life course. His 1984 text, *Physical Activity and
the Older Adult: Psychological Perspectives* (Princeton, N.J.: Princeton Book
Co.), summarized the scientific literature on the psychological aspects of aging
in relation to physical activity participation. In 1989, Ostrow followed up by
editing *Aging and Motor Behavior* (Indianapolis: Benchmark Press), which
brought together leading experts in the field.

JOSEPH G. OUSLANDER. Joseph G. Ouslander was born in 1951. He graduated Phi Beta Kappa from Johns Hopkins University in 1973 with a bachelor
of arts degree in natural sciences. He earned a medical degree from Case Western Reserve in 1977, where he worked with W. Leigh Thompson. There, he

became interested in clinical pharmacology and therapeutics. A growing call for geriatric specialists led Ouslander to the field, and he became a fellow in geriatric medicine at the Sepulveda Veterans Affairs Medical Center in 1979. The Sepulveda, California-based hospital is affiliated with the University of California at Los Angeles, and led Ouslander to a post as assistant professor in medicine at the UCLA School of Medicine in 1982.

He has served as the medical director for several nursing facilities, including the Baltimore-based Mason F. Lord Chronic Hospital and Nursing Facility (1986–1987), the Sepulveda VA Medical Center (1984–1986), and Eisenberg Village (1987–1993), operated by the Jewish Homes for the Aging of Greater Los Angeles. He now serves as vice president for medical affairs at the Jewish Home and as associate director of the Borun Center for Gerontological Research at the University of California, Los Angeles. He became an associate professor for the UCLA Multicampus Division of Geriatric Medicine and Gerontology in 1987 and has been a senior natural scientist with the RAND Corporation since 1990.

Ouslander has described the importance of urinary incontinence as a major health problem in geriatrics. See, for example, Joseph G. Ouslander, Robert L. Kane,* and Itamar B. Abrass,* "Urinary Incontinence in Elderly Nursing Home Patients," *Journal of the American Medical Association,* 248 (1982): 1194–98. He has also developed a diagnostic strategy for geriatric urinary incontinence, described in J. G. Ouslander, D. S. Staskin, S. Orzeck, and J. Blaustein, "Diagnostic Tests for Geriatric Incontinence," *World Journal of Urology,* 4 (1986): 16–21.

Working with Daniel Osterweil and J. Morley, Ouslander wrote the textbook, *Medical Care in the Nursing Home* (New York: McGraw-Hill, 1991). He collaborated with Robert L. Kane and Itamar B. Abrass on the textbook, *Essentials of Clinical Geriatrics* (New York: McGraw-Hill, 1984), now in its second printing.

MARTHA N. OZAWA. While pursuing a doctoral degree in social welfare at the University of Wisconsin, Martha N. Ozawa took a course with economics Professor Robert J. Lampman. His important scholarship on income distribution led Ozawa to the field of aging, and Ozawa counts Lampman as her most significant teacher, mentor, and role model.

After earning her doctorate in 1969, Ozawa began to focus on the problem of financing Social Security, and in particular, pursuing an equitable system. In her oft-cited article, "Individual Equity Versus Social Adequacy in Old-Age Insurance," *Social Service Review,* 48 (March 1974): 24–38, Ozawa compared Social Security contributions with subsequent benefits for different classes of wage earners. She was one of the first to explore the balance between individual equity and social adequacy in quantitative terms. In her subsequent work she showed the extent to which the maximum earner, average earner, and minimum earner receive subsidies through Social Security—that is, benefits not accounted for by contributions and interest accrued. She argued, more clearly than had been done previously, that subsidies should be measured in absolute terms. In "Who Receives Subsidies through Social Security, and How Much?" *Social Work,* 27 (March 1982): 128–34, she demonstrated that the subsidy amount differs if the worker is male or female, single, or part of a couple.

By the mid-1980s, Ozawa began to explore issues of intergenerational equity. See, for example, "The 1983 Amendments to the Social Security Act: The Issue of Intergenerational Equity," *Social Work,* 29 (March–April 1984): 131–37. She was one of a group of academics calling for a public debate of such issues as the obligation of the working population to fund subsidies to the elderly. In particular, she linked the development of human capital among the young, and especially among black children, and the financing of Social Security. Her publications on this issue include: "Peace Between the Young and the Old," Guest Editorial Comment, *NASW News,* 9 (February 1984); "Nonwhites and the Demographic Imperative in Social Welfare Spending," *Social Work,* 31 (November–December 1986): 440–47; "The Nation's Children: Key to a Secure Retirement," *New England Journal of Human Services,* 6 (1986): 12–19.

Ozawa observes that the U.S. income security policy was founded on two pillars: social insurance and public assistance. Because of the nation's choice of these two pillars, the United States has paid a high price of not being able to deal with income support for children directly. Thus, in her forthcoming article "Income Security: Overview" in the nineteenth issue of *Encyclopedia of Social Work* (scheduled to come out in print in the spring of 1995), Ozawa recommends that the United States establish a third piller—termed "the investment pillar"— in the income security policy, so that the nation can begin to deal with the issue of income security for children in its own right. "One generation cannot demand public resources to the detriment of the other," Ozawa argues, and this stance has been the keynote of her career. She has sought to put Social Security on the table with other social welfare programs, because the viability of the young as future wage earners is critical to the continued financing of social welfare for the aged.

In recent years, Ozawa's intellectual interest in investigating living conditions of children has accelerated. Thus, she became a co-principal investigator in a federally funded research project on AIDS prevention for children at risk (1989– 1992). Several articles emerged from that project: "Problems in Financing the Care of AIDS Patients," *Social Work,* 38:4 (1993): 369–80 (with V. Slonim-Nevo and W. Auslander); and "Knowledge, Attitude and Behavior Related to AIDS among Youth in Residential Centers: Results from an Exploratory Study," *Journal of Adolescence,* 14 (1991): 17–33 (with V. Slonim-Nevo and W. Aus-lander).

Ozawa is currently affiliated with the George Warren Brown School of Social Work at Washington University in St. Louis.

P

ERDMAN PALMORE. Erdman Palmore was born in Tokuyama, Japan, in 1930. A Phi Beta Kappa graduate of Duke University (1952), he received his M.A. two years later from the University of Chicago. Palmore earned his Ph.D. in sociology in 1959 at Columbia University, where he worked with two giants, Robert Merton and Paul Lazersfeld. During his candidacy, he worked as a research assistant in Columbia's Bureau of Applied Social Research and as a lecturer in sociology at Finch College. He continued his teaching career at Yale.

Palmore's interest in aging began when he was appointed chief of the Social Security Administration's Disability and Family Surveys Branch in the Office of Research and Statistics. One of his early articles, "Retirement Patterns of Aged Men," *Social Security Bulletin,* 27 (1964): 3–10, remains a benchmark for historical studies of retirement. Another publication, *Widows with Children under Social Security* (Research Report No. 16, 1963), was one of the first to delineate the financial situation and living arrangements of this segment of the population. In 1967, Palmore returned to Duke to become a professor of sociology and a professor of medical sociology in Duke's Department of Psychiatry. This arrangement ensured a very close working arrangement with George Maddox,* who was to become his mentor and role model.

Palmore's research interests have fallen into four broad categories. Arguably, his most distinctive contributions have been in delineating *Ageism: Negative and Positive,* to cite the title of a Springer publication (1990). His first contribution on ageism, however, was published nearly two decades earlier: "Attitudes toward Aging as Shown by Humor" in *The Gerontologist,* 11 (1971): 181–86. Six years later, he published his first "Facts on Aging: A Short Quiz," in *The Gerontologist,* 17 (1977): 351–20. The twenty-five-question test covered basic physical, mental, and social aspects of growing older. Palmore phrased issues in such a way as to gauge the extent of misperceptions and biases among different groups of respondents. Results of over 90 studies using this quiz were published in *The Facts on Aging Quiz: A Handbook of Uses and Results* (New York: Springer Publishing, 1988). Prejudice and/or discrimination against an age group may have negative consequences (such as discrimination against older workers) or positive ramifications (such as discrimination in favor of the aged in tax laws). Agreeing with Robert Butler,* Palmore contends that ageism is the third great "ism" in U.S. society and culture, after racism and sexism.

Palmore has also been closely identified with his contributions as an editor and author on the three *Normal Aging* volumes (1970, 1974, 1985) published by Duke University Press. These volumes stressed the advantages of longitudinal and interdisciplinary studies of aging, and discussed patterns of declining health and physical functioning, exceptions to physical decline (as measured by skin conditions, vitamin levels, and sexual activity, among other things), absence of decline in social and psychological functioning, and the wide variations in aging. Shortly after the project disbanded, Palmore encapsulated much of his own insights in *Social Patterns in Normal Aging: Findings from the Duke Longitudinal Study* (Durham, N.C.: Duke University Press, 1981). In addition to offering ways to untangle period, cohort, and age effects in longitudinal analyses (and predictions about human longevity), Palmore stressed an optimistic assessment of people's capacity to adapt to widowhood, illness, and retirement.

Cross-national surveys have been a third major thrust of Palmore's work. His work on Japan—see the first and "revisited" analyses of *The Honorable Elders* (Durham, N.C.: Duke University Press, 1975, 1985)—has been cited by political scientists and cultural anthropologists. His *International Handbook on Aging* (Westport, Conn.: Greenwood, 1980) was selected as an outstanding academic book by *Choice;* he updated the volume with *Developments and Research on Aging* (Westport, Conn.: Greenwood, 1993), which explored problems, programs, and trends in twenty-five countries, including Australia, Brazil, Egypt, and Ireland. This concern for ethnic and cultural variations is also evident in the way Palmore arranged his *Handbook on the Aged in the United States* (Westport, Conn.: Greenwood, 1984) according to demographic, religious, and ethnic groups as well as those (such as addicts and alcoholics, and suicides) presenting special concerns.

Finally, Palmore has maintained an interest in studying institutional aspects of aging, a concern evidenced at the beginning of his career as a researcher on aging. With Springer he published *Retirement: Causes and Consequences* (1985). He also has been studying nursing home outcomes, as well as trends in functional aging and physical well-being.

Palmore has received many professional awards over his career. A president of the Southern Gerontological Society (1984–1985), he was named its Distinguished Academic Gerontologist in 1989. He has also been a fellow and officer of the American Sociological Association, the Gerontological Society, and the Association for Gerontology in Higher Education. He has served on seven editorial boards. Duke University has saluted his accomplishments, and he is held in great respect by such well-known collaborators as Maddox, Linda K. George,* Gerda Fillenbaum, and Ewald W. Busse.* The widespread influence of his prolific publications is illustrated by the fact that he is the second most frequently cited author in the *Encyclopedia of Aging* (New York: Springer, 1987).

HERBERT S. PARNES. Herbert S. Parnes, born in 1919, was educated in the Pittsburgh public school system. He earned his B.A. (1939) and M.A. (1941) from the University of Pittsburgh, and received his Ph.D. in economics from Ohio State University in 1950. Parnes spent the next thirty years in Columbus, rising through the academic ranks; from 1964 to 1980, he was principal investigator of the National Longitudinal Surveys (NLS) of Labor Market Experience, which was funded by the U.S. Department of Labor. Although Parnes's interest in aging-related research issues arose from his involvement in this project, his contribution to gerontological literature did not begin until the 1980s.

The National Longitudinal Surveys originally involved representative national samples selected by the U.S. Bureau of Census of four age-sex subsets of civilian non-institutional population: men forty-five to fifty-nine years of age, women aged thirty to forty-four, and male and female youths between the ages of fourteen and twenty-four. Parnes and his colleagues at the Center for Human Resource Research (CHRR) prepared a series of reports on each of these cohorts that were published by the U.S. Department of Labor. The data tapes were also made available to the entire research community. Originally intended as a five-year study of factors associated with variations in their labor market experience, the study was successively extended: Twelve interviews were conducted between 1966 and 1983, providing a seventeen-year ''motion picture'' of the cohort as a large majority moved from work roles into retirement.

The resulting data bank served as the basis for more than 500 books, articles, monographs, and dissertations. Parnes is probably best known for the analysis he and his colleagues did in *Work and Retirement: A Longitudinal Study of Men* (Cambridge, Mass.: MIT Press, 1981) and in *Retirement among American Men* (Lexington, Mass.: Heath/Lexington Books, 1985). As the titles of these volumes suggest, the extent and nature of the labor market activity of the men changed as increasing numbers moved from the labor force into retirement: The proportion neither working nor seeking employment rose from 5 percent in 1966 to 61 percent fifteen years later. However, for those who did not retire during that period, real average hourly earnings not only were maintained, but actually increased. The wholesale withdrawals from the marketplace, of course, caused family incomes to decrease. However, because of the concomitant decrease in the number of dependents, average per capita family income (adjusted for the increasing price level) rose by about 7 percent.

Summarizing the NLS evidence on men's retirement as of 1981, Parnes suggest that retirement is generally entered into completely voluntarily, found to be pleasant, and not regretted even after many years. He hastens to add, however, that reactions to retirement vary, and that the economic and psychological adjustment to it varies depending on the circumstances under which it occurs. Men forced into retirement by poor health are generally less well off economically and less happy than men who retire voluntarily. Moreover, retirement is not everyone's cup of tea. As of 1981 one out of every seven men age sixty-two to seventy-four had never retired and remained at work full time.

Parnes claims that he "became a gerontologist by growing old" along with the national sample of his age cohort. In late 1988, he was awarded a grant from the National Institute on Aging to resurvey surviving members of the original sample of males and the widows (or other next-of-kin) of decedents. The 1990 data, which were linked to the longitudinal data bank covering the 1966–1983 period, permit a variety of gerontological inquiry in the fields of economics, psychology, public health, and sociology. Illustrative areas of research include the progression of disability from middle age to old age, male mortality in pre- and post-retirement years, patterns of economic adjustment to widowhood in late life, the adequacy of post-retirement medical care benefits, work abilities and proclivities of aged males in the market place, and economic well-being and the quality of life during retirement.

In "Shunning Retirement," *Journal of Gerontology,* 49 (1994): S117–S124, Parnes and his colleague David Sommers report that in the 1990 re-survey, one in six of the men—then sixty-nine to eighty-four years of age—had been employed during the preceding year and that as many as one-third of the employed group had worked full time. The likelihood of continued employment into old age is positively related to good health, level of education, and attitudes suggesting a strong work ethic (measured as long as a decade or two earlier); it is negatively related to level of income in the absence of work and to age. In exploring the implications of their findings for public policy, the authors argue that ethical and economic considerations dictate the importance of maximizing employment opportunities for the elderly. As a long-range means of accomplishing this objective, they allude to measures for improving the health of individuals through the entire lifespan.

BARBARA PITTARD PAYNE. Barbara Pittard Payne, born in 1919, received her M.A. from Emory University in 1955 and her Ph.D. from Emory eight years later. The topic of her dissertation was "The Meaning and Measurement of Commitment to the Church." Payne's interest in pursuing religion and aging arose from four relationships: Virginia Stafford, a staff person in adult education in the United Methodist Church; Clark Tibbitts,* whom she first met at a seminar sponsored by the United Methodist Church on adult education, but with whom she worked closely thereafter; Earl D.C. Brewer, her teacher and mentor at Emory; and her late husband, Raymond Payne. (In 1992, she married a state legislator.)

Payne has devoted much of her life to studying the meaning of religion, psychologically and sociologically, in the aging process. Most experts and observers, she felt, identified and measured "religion" in simplistic terms, by church attendance, number of times a person prayed in a certain time interval, interest in reading devotional literature, and so on. Thus, in her thesis and subsequent work, Payne tried to develop a new theoretical basis for measuring religious commitment. In her view, "commitment" was an analytic complex composed of three levels of clusters of theological, psychological, and sociological categories. As Payne acknowledged, her construct closely paralleled the three independent foci (personality, social systems, and cultures) set forth in Talcott Parsons's theory of the system of actions.

In the 1970s, Payne played a role in establishing the National Interfaith Coalition on Aging. Toward the end of the decade, however, she chafed at the exclusion of religion as part of the aging process. See her "Religious Life of the Elderly: Myth or Reality," in *Spiritual Well-Being of the Elderly,* eds. James A. Thorson and Thomas C. Cook (Springfield, Ill.: C. C. Thomas, 1980). Meanwhile, her own studies were undergoing a paradigm shift. As is clear in "The Older Volunteer: Social Role Continuity and Development," *The Gerontologist,* 17 (1977): 355–61, Payne was moving from structural functionalism to theories of symbolic interactionism.

In addition, Payne came to rely more on secondary data. An analysis of measures of religiosity convinced her that there was a limited number of reliable and valid measures of religious behavior and aging. Even the valid ones, she noted, lacked specificity and an adequate theoretical foundation. See her "Religiosity," in *Social Roles and Social Participation,* eds. David J. Mangum and Warren A. Peterson (Minneapolis: University of Minnesota Press, 1982), 343–82; and "Protestants," in the *Handbook on the Aged in the United States,* ed. Erdman Palmore* (Westport, Conn.: Greenwood Press, 1984), 181–200.

Recently, Payne has focused on spirituality. See, for instance, her "Research and Theoretical Approaches to Spirituality and Aging," *Generations* (Fall 1990): 11–14. Symbolic interactionism has guided her analysis of the ways older adults attain "spiritual maturity and meaning-filled relationships," the title of an essay in *Spiritual Maturity in Later Years,* ed. James Seeber (New York: Haworth Press, 1990), 25–39. See also her use of James Fowler's developmental theory in "Faith Development in Older Men" in *Older Men's Lives,* ed. David Thompson (Thousand Oaks, Calif.: Sage, 1995).

Payne has also actively promoted religion in gerontological education. With Earl Brewer, she published a two-volume report, *Gerontology in Theological Education* (1988) and *Gerontology in Theological Education: Local Church Programming* (Haworth, Long Island, 1989) with Haworth Press. She also offered an interdisciplinary perspective on the study of religion, written with Susan McFadden, "From Loneliness to Solitude: Religious and Spiritual Journeys in

Late Life'' for a *Handbook on Religion and Aging* (1995) edited by Mel Kimble and Susan McFadden for Minneapolis-based Fortress Press.

Thanks to her writings and organizational savvy, Payne has been an institution builder. She was founding director of the gerontology center at Georgia State University (1972–1990). Payne was a founder of the Southern Gerontological Society, serving as its first president (1976–1979). She has served on the Governor's Council on Aging since 1973. In addition, she was a president of the Association for Gerontology in Higher Education (1986). She has also worked closely with the Reverend Elbert Cole in developing the concept of the Shepherd's Center in Kansas City, and then extending it into the Shepherd's Center of America.

JANE PORCINO. Jane Porcino returned to school at the age of fifty, having raised seven children. Because of her "own personal need for information" as she approached menopause, Porcino pursued a master's degree in social work at the State University of New York at Stony Brook, which she earned in 1976, and a doctoral degree in gerontology from the Union Institute, completed in 1980. Attending a Gerontological Society of America meeting in San Francisco in the late 1970s, Porcino organized an ad hoc meeting to discuss issues surrounding midlife and older women. She took the overwhelming response as evidence of the need to confront not only ageism, but sexism as well.

Porcino now directs the National Action Forum for Midlife and Older Women, which grew out of this first meeting. The group, supported by membership dues and volunteers, includes a board of gerontologists and geratricians. It has produced the quarterly newsletter, "Hot Flash," for over ten years, and distributes the publication to all fifty states and fifteen other countries.

She has also created a handbook about and for midlife and older women. *Growing Older, Getting Better: A Handbook for Women in the Second Half of Life* (New York: Crossroad, 1991), an eight-year project, is in its fifth printing. Her second book, *Living Longer, Living Better: Adventures in Community Housing for People in the Second Half of Life* (New York: Crossroad, 1991) is based on interviews with men and women who have chosen alternatives to the traditional retirement and life-care villages.

But elderly women have been Porcino's primary interest. She recalls that studying older women was once a lonely task, noting that most early gerontological research was done with male subjects. She has worked with the White House Conference on Aging and the U.S. House of Representatives Select Committee on Aging. She has taught at the State University of New York at Stony Brook, and currently teaches at New York University while working internationally as a lecturer and consultant.

LAWRENCE ALFRED POWELL. Lawrence Alfred Powell earned a Ph.D. in political science in 1987 from the Massachusetts Institute of Technology, where he worked with Lucian W. Pye, Walter Dean Burnham, and Ithiel de Sola Pool, among others. Since then he has worked most extensively with John B. Williamson, Linda Evans, and Steven P. Wallace. He became interested in what has come to be known as "political gerontology" (the scientific study of power as it relates to the aged) through the work of Robert Hudson, Robert H. Binstock,* Neal R. Cutler,* and Anne Foner.* He credits W. Andrew Achenbaum, David H. Fischer, and Henry J. Pratt* with sparking his interest in the history of aging policy.

Powell's most important contribution to the field has been his co-authorship with John Williamson of *The Politics of Aging: Power and Policy* (Springfield, Ill.: Charles C. Thomas, 1982). *The Politics of Aging* has been received as an important addition to this burgeoning field. It traces political gerontology from preindustrial societies to the present day and argues that "coalition formation" explains the dynamics of gray power, pointing out that the passage of Social Security and legislation enacted during the 1960s and 1970s was linked to concurrent gains made by labor, minorities, and the poor.

Powell's more recent contributions include a history of the evolution of "senior power" in the United States, *The Senior Rights Movement: Framing the Policy Debate in America* (New York: MacMillan-Twayne, 1995). In it, Powell assumes a social constructivist position to argue that senior rights struggles have revolved around the framing of public debates between progressives and conservatives over appropriate social definitions of what constitutes equity or justice in old age. Using political rhetoric and cartoons from the turn of the century to the present, the study highlights the importance of political symbolism in shaping the terms of public debates over old-age policies.

HENRY J. PRATT. Henry J. Pratt attended Dartmouth College, where he was drawn to political science by his teacher, Abraham Holtzman, author of the Townsend Movement. Pratt went on to earn his Ph.D. in the field from Columbia University in 1962 under the direction of David B. Truman, a professor of public law and government. In 1971, while Pratt was serving on the then joint Wayne State University/University of Michigan Institute of Gerontology, Dale Vinyard, a Wayne State colleague, urged him to consider social gerontology. Pratt has continued to teach about public policy and the aged to Wayne State students, though his scholarship has been more directly concerned with the workings of the political process than with particular substance and content.

His most important work remains his application of interest group theory to the understanding of age-group mobilization and seniors' organizations. The fullest statement of his views can be found in his book, *The Gray Lobby* (Chicago: University of Chicago, 1976). His 1983 essay, "National Interest Groups Among the Elderly: Consolidation and Constraint," in *Aging and Public Policy: The Politics of Growing Old in America,* eds. William P. Browne and Laura Katz Olson (Westport, Conn.: Greenwood Press), is a more recent source. Although others have looked at organizations such as the American Association of Retired Persons and the National Council on Aging using the political in-

280   HENRY J. PRATT

terest group framework, Pratt has refined the concept and applied it in great depth. He has also emphasized the elderly in the United States as a leading illustration of the concept of "collective behavior." In this he draws extensively on the work of twentieth-century sociologists and such collective behavior theorists as Neil Smelser, Carl A. Dawson, and Warren Gettys.

Pratt's current work applies his theories in a cross-national context. See his *Gray Agendas: Interest Groups and State Pensions in Canada, Britain and the United States* (Ann Arbor, Mich.: University of Michigan, 1993). He continues to serve as a faculty associate of the Wayne State Institute of Gerontology, which he has done for more than twenty years.

Q _____

JILL QUADAGNO. Jill Quadagno earned her B.A. with distinction and won a Phi Beta Kappa key from Pennsylvania State University in 1964. A National Institute of Mental Health Predoctoral Fellow in 1965, she took her M.A. in sociology from Berkeley in 1966. As a Midwest Council for Social Research in Aging Predoctoral Fellow, Quadagno then earned her Ph.D. in sociology from the University of Kansas in 1976.

For the next decade Quadagno rose through the ranks at the University of Kansas. Initially, she wrote on the Italian-American family and labeling theory. An early article, "Occupational Sex-Typing and Internal Labor Market Distributions: An Assessment of Medical Specialities," *Social Problems,* 23 (1976): 443–53, was widely cited and reprinted. Her first gerontological essay was "Career Continuity and Retirement Plans of Men and Women Physicians: The Meaning of Disorderly Careers," which appeared in *Sociology of Work and Occupations,* 5 (1978): 55–74. Quadagno's subsequent research on aging was supported by a National Science Foundation National Needs postdoctoral fellowship, which enabled her to serve as a visiting scholar at the Cambridge (England) Group for the History of Population and Social Structure in 1979.

Quadagno's next wave of publications established her reputation as one of the nation's foremost gerontologists and historical sociologists of aging. After editing the widely adopted *Aging, The Individual and Society* (New York: St. Martin's Press, 1980), Quadagno issued *Aging in Early Industrial Society: Work, Family and the Social Policy in Nineteenth Century England* (New York: Academic Press, 1982). Not only did this book offer a masterful assessment of trends in Britain, but it also offered a valuable comparison of trends in the

United States and France, which had been set forth by scholars such as Peter Laslett,* Daniel Scott Smith, Peter Stearns, David Hackett Fischer, and W. Andrew Achenbaum, among others. A parallel essay, "From Poor Laws to Pensions: The Evolution of Economic Support for the Aged in England and America," which appeared in the *Milbank Memorial Fund Quarterly,* 62 (1984): 417–46, signaled Quadagno's interest in the evolution of policy issues affecting the aged.

Although Quadagno incorporated a variety of theoretical perspectives in her earlier analyses of historical trends, over time she increasingly articulated a model of her own. In *The Transformation of Old Age Security: Class and Politics in the American Welfare State* (Chicago: University of Chicago Press, 1988), for instance, Quadagno showed a sensitivity to regional variations and differences in labor responses to old-age pension proposals set forth in the private sector and by federal lawmakers. Sensitive to current trends at the national level, she wrote "Generational Equity and the Politics of the Welfare State" for *Politics and Society,* 17 (1989): 353–76, which was reprinted in the *International Journal of Health Sciences* and in *Growing Old in America,* eds. Beth Hess* and Elizabeth Markson* (New Brunswick, N.J.: Transaction Press, 1990). Her differences with structuralists such as Theda Skocpol and with Marxists became evident in *States, Labor Markets and the Future of Old Age Policy* (Philadelphia: Temple University Press, 1991), which she edited with John Myles.*

Quadagno has published general readers and articles on the sociology of aging. See, for instance, her *Social Bonds in Later Life: Aging and Interdependence* (Beverly Hills, Calif.: Sage Publications, 1985), which she edited with Warren Peterson. She also has written broadly on public policy issues. See, for instance, her "Race, Class, and Gender in the U.S. Welfare State: Nixon's Failed Family Assistance Program," *American Sociological Review,* 55 (1990): 11–28, and *The Color of Welfare: How Racism Undermined the War on Poverty* (New York: Oxford University Press, 1994).

Since 1987, Quadagno has served as Mildred and Claude Pepper Eminent Scholar in Social Gerontology and professor of sociology at Florida State University. She taught at Harvard during its fall 1988 term. Quadagno has served as an associate editor of the *Journal of Aging Studies* since 1986, of *Sociological Quarterly* (1986–1989), *The Gerontologist* (1987–1991), *American Sociological Review* (1989–1991), and *Contemporary Sociology* (1992–1995). Quadagno was elected vice president of the American Sociological Association in 1993 and serves as chairwoman of the Section on Aging until 1997. While holding a Congressional Fellowship from the American Sociological Association, a John Simon Guggenheim Memorial Fellowship, and an American Council for Learned Studies Fellowship (1994–1995), Quadagno served as senior policy analyst for the President's Bi-Partisan Commission on Entitlement and Tax Reform (1994).

R

OLLIE ANNETTE RANDALL. Ollie Annette Randall was born in Rawlins Country, Kansas, in 1890. She received her B.A. from Brown University in 1912. After doing library work at Brown and serving as a tutor in a private school in Bryn Mawr, Pennsylvania, Randall moved to New York City, where she served as a statistical assistant to the Russell Sage Foundation. She then held several administrative posts with various civic organizations before she became assistant director for Special Services at the Community Service Society.

Randall's career in aging began in the 1940s, when she served as a welfare consultant to the New York State Joint Legislative Committee on Interstate Cooperation on the Care of the Aged and the Infirm. In 1949, she prepared for the National Social Welfare Assembly a paper titled "A Twentieth Century Philosophy for Homes of the Aged," which proved to be a prescient document. While acknowledging that the fundamental purpose of these homes had remained constant over the centuries, Randall contended that new images of aging and the aged were bound to modify the "rules of conduct" for providing services. She recommended taking advantage of older people's "personal strength and dynamic energy," and providing professional services for those who were capable of maintaining independent living at home. For those who did need to turn to nursing homes in their later years, Randall stressed the advantage of providing good nutrition, rehabilitative surgery, and physical medicine. "Rehabilitation," in her view, was "often achieved by the simple routine of giving to the patient enough personal attention, good nursing care, and by applying what we know *as of now.*" Her emphasis on privacy and respect of individual dignity in retrospect seems to be a clarion call.

As a consultant to the Ford Foundation, Ollie Randall was instrumental in establishing the National Council on the Aging (NCOA) after the 1961 White House Conference on Aging. She served as a major figure in that organization as it moved from New York to Washington, D.C., to serve as an advocate for older Americans. NCOA's highest award is now named in her memory.

ELOISE RATHBONE-McCUAN. Eloise "Lee" Rathbone-McCuan earned her master's degree in social work in 1969 and completed a Ph.D. in research and program evaluation four years later. Both of her advanced degrees were obtained from the School of Social Work at the University of Pittsburgh. She began a limited study of gerontology while earning her master's degree and then entered a self-designed aging research specialization as part of doctoral training. Her academic knowledge was applied to social work practice when she took a position at Baltimore's Levidale Hebrew Geriatric Center and Hospital.

Levidale was the site of one of the first nursing home-based geriatric day care centers in the United States. Seeking to combine social theory, research, and social work practice, Rathbone-McCuan decided to compare the socialization benefits of day care and institutional care as a dissertation. Subsequently, she received a research and demonstration grant from the Administration on Aging as part of the first federal funding wave intended to test day care as a cost-effective alternative to institutional care. That work was informed by Arnold Rose's theoretical formulation of the aging subculture and the then heated debate about the applicability of disengagement theory as relevant to understanding social processes of aging.

Rathbone-McCuan research has contributed to the social work service and family support benefits of day care for impaired elderly. It also established a base for geriatric day care as an alternative to nursing home care and documented the cost-effectiveness of the care model. The results, recounted in Philip G. Welter and Eloise Rathbone-McCuan, *Adult Daycare: Community Work with the Elderly* (New York: Springer, 1978), was named Book of the Year in 1978 by the American Journal of Nursing (AJN). Within the day care population was an elder who suffered from caregiver neglect and isolation as a result of her aging daughter's alcohol abuse. Obtaining funding from the NIAAA, her research group surveyed alcohol abuse patterns among the elderly in different residential and community settings.

Rathbone-McCuan won the same AJN book award again in 1982 for her *Isolated Elders* (Rockville, Md.: Aspen Systems, 1982), co-written with Joan Hashimi. Her interest in isolation grew out of her work in aging and mental health for the Missouri Mental Health Association while continuing her interest in gerontological social work and while on the faculty of Washington University in St. Louis.

She expanded her social research interests into cross-national social policy while at the University of Vermont as coordinator of the social work program. Noting the lack of comparisons between the United States and Canada, she joined with other researchers in the Canadian Studies Program at University of Vermont. With funding from the Canadian Embassy, Rathbone-McCuan collaborated on a comprehensive social policy text for comparative gerontology. The result, co-edited with Betty J. Havens,* is *North American Elders: U.S. and Canadian Perspectives* (Westport, Conn.: Greenwood, 1988).

Her latest book, co-edited with Dorothy Fabian, is *Self-Neglect in the Elderly: Clinical Dilemma* (New York: Auburn House, 1992). It is the result of Rathbone-McCuan's effort to help craft elder abuse legislation for the state of Vermont and to provide training for the Adult Protective Services Division of the Tennessee Department of Human Services.

Her interest in geriatric practice, policy, and research continues in her present position as a research social worker at the Colmery O'Neil VA Medical Center in Burlington, Vermont. There she conducts research on veteran caregivers, strengths-based long-term case management, and practitioner intervention effectiveness.

THOMAS A. RICH. Tom Rich was born in 1928. He became interested in gerontology while working as a research assistant for Robert W. Kleemeier* at the Moosehaven Research Laboratory in Orange Park, Florida, in 1955. While participating in a range of research projects in aging, he also took a course on the sociology of aging with Irving L. Webber* of the University of Florida. Rich recalls that it was a lonely time for gerontology: Webber was the only sociologist at the University of Florida interested in aging, and Rich was the only student in his course.

He went on to earn a doctorate in clinical psychology from Florida University under the direction of Henry Wunderlich, who encouraged him to apply psychological theory to issues of aging. Completing his Ph.D. in 1957, Rich found no job openings in the field for someone with his credentials. He then turned to community mental heath and directed a small community health center. During this time he earned his S.M.Hyg. in community mental health at the Harvard School of Public Health in 1960.

Upon taking a position at the Tampa-based University of South Florida, Rich found the field needed better education about the aging process. Along with medical doctor Alfred Lawton,* he developed the first master's degree programs in social gerontology. This effort was supported with funding through the Older Americans Act with support from Clark Tibbitts.* In addition to the master's degree, the institute, and now the department of gerontology, also grants a bachelor's degree in gerontology and a bachelor's of science in nursing home administration.

Rich's primary effort over nearly four decades in the field has been the conceptualization and development of educational programs in gerontology. He has promoted the teaching of gerontology as a multidisciplinary venture. His early efforts in this area include his collaboration with Alden Gilmore, in *Basic Concepts in Aging: A Program Manual,* published by the U.S. Department of Health, Education and Welfare in 1969. His more recent efforts include editing the

Standards and Guidelines for Gerontology with J. Richard Connelly and Elizabeth B. Douglass for the Association for Gerontology in Higher Education (Washington, 1990), and co-editing, with D. W. Rich and L. C. Mullins, *Old and Homeless—Double Jeopardy: An Overview of Policy and Service Needs* (Westport, Conn.: Greenwood Press, 1995).

Rich is currently professor of gerontology and sociology and director of the gerontology program at West Georgia College in Carrolton, Georgia, where his major role is the development of the recently initiated master's degree program in gerontology.

KLAUS F. RIEGEL. Klaus F. Riegel was born in Germany in 1925. He earned his Vordiplom at the University of Hamburg in 1953. After receiving an M.A. from the University of Minnesota in 1955, he returned to Germany. From 1957 to 1959, Riegel served as an assistant professor in the Psychologisches Institut at the University of Hamburg, where he earned his Ph.D. in 1958.

James E. Birren* invited Riegel to serve as a visiting scientist in the Section on Aging at the National Institute of Mental Health the following year. In 1959, Riegel joined the faculty of the University of Michigan, where he remained until his untimely death. During his tenure, he chaired Michigan's program in developmental psychology (1964–1965) and its program in psycholinguistics (1973–1975). Riegel also held visiting appointments at Bowling Green State University, the Educational Testing Service, and the University of British Columbia's Psychology Department. He retained his German citizenship although he became a permanent U.S. resident.

Riegel's primary research interests fell into two domains. Early on, he was interested in language and cognitive development, with an emphasis on methodology and theories. He was interested in bilingualism, particularly in the ways people learn second languages. Much of his work in this area was underwritten by the U.S. Public Health Services and the Ford Foundation. Riegel's mature thinking in this area can be found in his essay, "Semantic Basis of Language: Language as Labor," in *Structure and Transformation: Developmental and Historical Aspects* (New York: John Wiley, 1975), 167–92.

Riegel's interest in linguistics soon attracted him to the elderly. One of his first publications in English was "A Study on Verbal Achievements of Older Persons," *Journal of Gerontology,* 14 (1959): 453–56. That same year, he also published "Personality Theory and Aging" in *Aging and the Individual,* ed. James E. Birren (Chicago: University of Chicago Press, 1959), 797–851. This essay offered a brilliant survey of major theories about the unconscious, genetics, the self, inner personal structures, social roles, learning, and the environment as they relate to the aged, processes of aging, and to personality. Noting that "no theory exists which takes full account of the aging personality," Riegel hoped "that one day all these different aspects may become integrated into a single system."

For the rest of his career, Riegel engaged in precisely the sort of theory-building that he found lacking in research on aging. He published several articles with James Birren and with his wife, Ruth Riegel, on age differences in response speed in speech patterns, in associative behavior, and in intelligence tests. See, for instance, Riegel and Birren's "Age Differences in Associative Behavior," *Journal of Gerontology*, 20 (1965): 125–30; and their "Age Differences in Verbal Associations," *Journal of Genetic Psychology*, 108 (1966): 153–70.

Riegel continued to write essays that tried to integrate theoretical approaches in gero-psychology. For instance, "On the History of Psychological Gerontology," in *The Psychology of Adult Development and Aging*, eds. Carl Eisdorfer and M. Powell Lawton* (Washington, D.C.: American Psychological Association, 1973), offered a quantitative analysis of works in this area as they relate to findings in other areas of developmental psychology. Riegel raised questions concerning research and theory in communication, education, and the development of humans and society.

In 1969, with the publication of "History as a Nomothetic Science: Some Generalizations from Theories and Research in Developmental Psychology," *Journal of Social Issues*, 25 (1969): 99–127, Riegel began to expand his theoretical purview to take greater account of social structures and dialectical historical processes that affect human behavior over the life course. Sometimes this exploration took Riegel into the realm of macro-analysis. See, for instance, his "Developmental Psychology and Society: Some Historical and Ethical Considerations," in *Life-Span Developmental Psychology: Methodological Issues*, eds. John R. Nesselroade and Haynes W. Reese (New York: Academic Press, 1973), 1–23; and "Toward a Dialectical Theory of Development," in *Human Development*, 18 (1975): 50–64. At other times, however, his sensitivity to "noise" in the background alerted him to phenomena that others missed. For instance, in "The Prediction of Death and Longevity in Longitudinal Research," in *Prediction of Life-Span*, eds. Erdman Palmore* and F. C. Jeffers (Lexington, Mass.: Heath Lexington Books, 1971), 139–52, Riegel suggested ways that repeated testing of elderly subjects might predict, for example, through certain patterns of memory loss, their likelihood of dying sooner.

In 1975, Riegel was awarded the Gerontological Society's Kleemeier Award.

MATILDA WHITE RILEY and JOHN W. RILEY, JR. In terms of chronological age and stature, Matilda and Jack Riley are probably gerontology's "first couple," though both did not begin their research in the field of social aging until relatively late in their careers. Each surely warrants a separate biographical entry, yet (like "the Kanes") most specialists in the field think of "the Rileys" as if they were one. Not only has theirs been an exemplary marriage of individuals who epitomize "the new old," but they have proved to be wonderfully compatible intellectual soulmates for more than six decades. Their first major joint publication, "The Use of Various Methods of Contraception," appeared in the *American Sociological Review*, 5 (December 1940): 890–903. Accordingly, this entry will combine their separate biographies to show how their contributions to research on aging have been intimately entwined.

Jack graduated from Bowdoin College in 1930; the college also gave him an honorary degree in 1972. He received his Ph.D. in 1936 from Harvard University, where he studied with Talcott Parsons and Pitirim Sorokin. He spent most of his career building the Sociology Department at Rutgers University into one of the major departments in the nation. His career had the usual hallmarks of a successful academic career: He won five merit and research awards, and was a visiting scholar at the Center for Advanced Study in the Behavioral Sciences in Stanford, California. He served as president of the Sociological Research Association and of the American Association for Public Opinion Research, and as secretary of the American Sociological Association. In World War II and the Korean War, he served in the Psychological Warfare Division.

In 1960, Jack Riley joined The Equitable, a large insurance company based in New York. Riley had no job description; he was expected to be the "resident intellectual," and he was accorded resources to research and to support research. In this capacity, he organized two programs of retirement planning. Thus, Jack might be considered the first partner to do aging-related research. He tried to serve as an advocate for other age-related corporate programs, such as training for older workers and family-related leaves. His peers in the American Sociological Association saluted the importance of Riley's "applied" work by awarding him the Distinguished Career Award for the Practice of Sociology in 1987.

However, Riley's intellectual focus at The Equitable was on death, not aging. His studies challenged the taboo on death as a topic for serious sociological research. Riley's work demonstrated the validity of two important propositions. First, people will talk about death in formal social surveys. Second, most people are more concerned about the consequences of their own death for others than they are personally afraid of death. See, for instance, his entries in the *International Encyclopedia of the Social Sciences* (1968), *The Annual Review of Sociology* (1983), and *The Encyclopedia of Sociology* (1991) as well as his monograph, *The Dying Patient* (1970). His first work in social gerontology came at the behest of his wife, who had been his collaborator since their marriage in 1931.

Born in Boston in 1911, Matilda White Riley was a Phi Beta Kappa graduate of Radcliffe College (B.A., 1931). After serving as a research assistant at Harvard, she studied at the University of Vienna and earned her A.M. from Radcliffe in 1937. From 1938 to 1949, Matilda was vice president and research director of the Market Research Company of America. During World War II she served as chief consulting economist for the War Production Board. From 1949 to 1960, as executive officer of the American Sociological Association, Matilda helped to guide a fairly small central agency as it became a large organization. From 1950 to 1973, she was affiliated with Rutgers University.

In the mid-1960s, when the Ford Foundation was phasing out its funding of social-science research on the middle and later ages (a program on which Ollie

Randall had served as an adviser), unexpended funds were turned over to the Russell Sage Foundation. Orville G. Brim, who headed Russell Sage, persuaded Matilda to undertake a summary of the research findings in gerontology to date in return for support of her work at Rutgers on intergenerational relations. Riley accepted the challenge, though it interrupted her research at Rutgers. Indeed, it took five associates (in addition to her husband) seven years to sift through the record. A tough-nosed methodologist and rigorous theorist (like Jack, Matilda had studied with Sorokin and Parsons, and she had worked closely with Robert Merton), Matilda found most studies too flawed to be useful. Nonetheless, she laid out the state of the field in three path-breaking volumes: *Aging and Society, Vol. 1: An Inventory of Research Findings,* with Anne Foner,* Mary E. Moore, Beth Hess,* and Barbara Roth (New York: Russell Sage Foundation, 1968); *Aging and Society, Vol. 2: Aging and the Professions,* with John W. Riley, Jr., and Marilyn Johnson (New York: Russell Sage Foundation, 1969); and *Aging and Society, Vol. 3: Sociology of Age Stratification,* with Marilyn Johnson and Anne Foner (New York: Russell Sage Foundation, 1972). In the last volume, Matilda began to set forth a paradigm for thinking about age stratification and the universal dynamics of aging that would greatly influence the profession.

Perhaps Matilda Riley's most important conceptual contributions have been the indentification and specification of aging and cohort flow as universal processes. Biopsychological aging from aging to death, the continual entry into society of new cohorts (and, analogously, generations—though the Rileys do not use the terms interchangeably; they tend to reserve the latter for parent-child bonds), as well as their ultimate exit from it, are the dynamic components of an age stratification system. Although Leonard Cain had anticipated some of these ideas in his contribution to the 1964 edition of the *Handbook of Sociology,* Matilda Riley deserves (and has received) enormous credit for refining, elaborating, and popularizing these concepts.

Riley's model revolutionized earlier gerontological notions of aging as an individual, or species-specific, biologically driven process, and of age as simply an ingredient of populations and social structures. Her model takes on additional power because of its methodological rigor. Riley has demonstrated that the process of aging is not primarily biological in nature; neither is it characterized by inevitable declines in physiological and cognitive functioning. Rather, it is a biological and psychosocial process that is open to interventions and change.

To trace the evolution of her age-stratification model since the publication of the three Russell Sage Foundation volumes, see her "Aging and Cohort Succession: Interpretations and Misinterpretations," *The Public Opinion Quarterly,* 37 (1973): 35–49; "Age and Aging: From Theory Generation to Theory Testing," in *Sociological Theory and Research,* ed. Hubert Blalock, Jr. (New York: The Free Press, 1981), 339–48; and, with her long-time associates Anne Foner and Joan Waring, "Sociology of Age" in *Handbook of Sociology,* ed. Neil Smelser (Newbury Park, Calif.: Sage, 1988).

Having written widely on the proposition that aging is a life-long process from birth to death, Riley strongly opposed in 1973 the separation of the adult development and aging components from the National Institute of Child Health and Human Development. She lost; the National Institute on Aging was approved in 1974. Although Matilda was mentioned as a candidate to become the first director, she was not interested, having recently moved with Jack to Maine, where she concurrently headed the Sociology Department at Bowdoin College in Maine (1973–1979) and served as a staff sociologist at Russell Sage and a senior research associate at Columbia University's Center for the Social Sciences. In 1979, however, Matilda agreed to become associate director of Behavioral and Social Research at NIA, a position she would hold until the age of eighty.

Starting with a small backlog of grants from the National Institute of Child Health and Human Development and the National Institute of Mental Health, Riley ably set a rigorous "scientific" agenda. Under her direction, the program initially tried to spark interest in four areas: the dynamic character of aging, the interrelatedness of old age, cultural variability, and the multiple facets of aging. All of these issues, she felt, would contribute to a multidisciplinary, theoretical construct of aging and yield practical payoffs. Riley's list proved durable. During its first decade of operation, the Behavioral and Social Research Division collaborated with eighteen governmental agencies, thirty-five public or private associations or foundations, and nine international organizations. For her assessments of the record, see National Institute on Aging, *The Behavioral and Social Research Program at the National Institute on Aging* (1990–91).

While constantly fighting for a greater share of NIA's research budget, Matilda Riley found time to edit or contribute to important collections. See, for instance, her interdisciplinary collections, *Aging from Birth to Death* (Vol. 1, 1979; Vol. 2, with Ronald Abeles and Michael Teitelbaum, 1982), and her increasing focus on gender, with NIA colleague Marcia Ory. Much of her work since 1983 has been co-written with Jack Riley. In 1986, for instance, the couple contributed "Longevity and Social Structure: The Added Years" to *Our Aging Society,* eds. Alan Pifer and Lydia Bronte (New York: W.W. Norton, 1986). The "problematics of the individual life course in an aging society require deeper scientific understanding and wider public recognition so that they may form the basis for improved public policy and professional practice," they declared, combining individual and collective sociological interest. "Fortunately, a knowledge base is developing that can guide such decisions toward correcting the structural lag and enriching the prolonged life course. Fortunately too, as members of an aging society we have been given not only added years, but also the privilege—too often taken for granted—of thinking about such problems and participating in attempts to solve them."

At a time when many gerontologists retire, the Rileys seem as vital and intellectually curious as they were, say, a half-century ago. Jack and Matilda have traveled around the world, considering the global implications of societal aging. (Of the two, Jack has had probably the stronger interest in cross-national research. He was senior consultant to the International Federation on Ageing and did studies for the World Health Organization. He was an early member of the American Association for International Aging, and senior editor of the *International Glossary of Social Gerontology*.) And the couple has launched, with NIA support, a new project to study "structural lags." They are engaged in multilevel, micro-macro studies that call attention to the mismatch between increasing numbers of capable and motivated older people and decreasing role opportunities for them in the social structure.

Matilda White Riley received an honorary D.Sc. (with Jack) from Bowdoin College in Maine in 1972. Rutgers awarded her an L.H.D. in 1983. *Ladies Home Journal* named her one of "American's 100 Most Important Women" in 1988. The Gerontological Society cited her Distinguished Creative Contribution to Gerontology (1990) and gave her the Kent Award two years later. As president of the American Sociological Association in 1986, Matilda edited a two-volume series, *Social Change and the Life Course* (Beverly Hills, Calif.: Sage, 1988). The second volume, *Sociological Lives,* offers her voice.

Both Jack and Matilda Riley are listed in *Who's Who in America* and *Who's Who in the World.* Matilda was elected to the National Academy of Sciences in 1994.

MORRIS ROCKSTEIN. Morris Rockstein was born in Toronto in 1916. After earning his A.B. and Phi Beta Kappa key from Brooklyn College in zoology and mathematics (1938), Rockstein earned his M.A. in science from Columbia University in 1942. During World War II he was a weather forecaster in the Army Air Forces. He received his Ph.D. nine years later from the University of Minnesota, where he was greatly influenced by A. Glenn Richards. His doctoral thesis examined aspects of the aging of the brain. Nathan W. Shock,* who was advancing bio-medical research in gerontology in Baltimore, encouraged Rockstein to continue his inquiry. For much of his career, Rockstein was a professor of physiology and biophysics at the University of Miami Medical School. There he was active in its Institute for the Study of Aging.

Rockstein's fundamental contribution, which remains of critical importance, was to show that only certain systems of the body really age in terms of age-related diminution in structure (that is, in terms of numbers of cells and fibers) and in functions. The deterioration of the skin, for instance, is more cosmetic than life-threatening. Yet the brain and nervous system show an age-related, irreversible loss of neurons and other cells with senescence. Similarly, muscles—particularly skeletal and heart—have fibers that diminish in mass with age. As they become demonstrably, irreversibly weaker in their decline, their diminished functional capacity leads to ever greater inability to support major bodily functions and to meet environmental assaults and insults. See, for instance, M. Rockstein and K. Brandt, "Changes in Phosphorus Metabolism in the Gastrocnemius Muscle in Aging White Rats," *Proceedings of the Society for Experimental Biological Medicine,* 107 (1961): 377–80; and Rockstein and

K. Brandt, "Muscle Enzyme Activity and Weight Changes in Aging White Rats," *Nature*, 196 (1962): 142–43; M. Rockstein and D. Gutfreund, "Age Chances in Adenine Nucleotides in Flight Muscle of Male House Fly," *Science*, 133 (1961): 1476–77; and two articles with J. Hrachovec, "Biochemical Criteria for Senescence in Mammalian Structures," *Gerontologica*, 6 (1962): 237–48; and "Age Changes in the Chemical Composition of the Rat Liver and Muscle," *Gerontologica*, 7 (1963): 30–43.

For a later work along these lines, see his study, with three associates, "Age Related Changes in Actomyosin ATPase and Arginine Phosphokinase in *Drosophila melanogaster Meig*. Male Flies," *Gerontology*, 27 (1981): 301–305. Like Shock, Rockstein attacked aging problems throughout his career by quantitative evaluation of important organic systems. Enzyme systems, he held, were responsible for normal functioning of the brain, skeletal muscle and heart. Without these systems functioning, the body's resistance weakened. This theme became central in a textbook he published with Marvin Sussman,* *Biology of Aging* (Belmont, Calif.: Wadsworth Publishing, 1979). More representative of his scientific style, however, was his article with H. Klefenz, "Fructose-1, 6-Biphosphatase from Young and Adult Rats," *Journal of Gerontology*, 31 (1976): 409–12.

In the middle of his career, Rockstein was fascinated with the genetic basis for longevity. Although his thesis can be reduced to a bumper-sticker expression—"You are as old as your genes allow"—here, too, his research was meticulous. See his "The Role of Molecular Genetic Mechanisms in the Aging Process," in *Molecular Genetic Mechanisms in Development and Aging*, eds. M. Rockstein and George T. Baker III* (New York: Academic Press, 1972); and his introduction, "The Genetic Basis for Longevity," in *Theoretical Aspects of Aging*, ed. M. Rockstein (New York: Academic Press, 1974): "It is apparent, both from life insurance statistics, intraspecies records, evidence from sex differences favoring the females in most animal species, as well as that from longevity data for identical versus non-identical twins, that the primary basis for longevity of an individual, strain, or a species is the genetic material which is incorporated in the fertilized egg at the climactic moment when the spermatozoan meets the unfertilized egg."

Toward the end of his career, Rockstein considered ways to prevent or at least decelerate senescence. He contended that exercise begun at an early age markedly diminished age-related declines in muscle mass and energy-related enzymes in skeletal and heart muscle in white rats. See his work, with J.A. Chesky and T. Lopez, "The Effect of Exercise on Biochemical Aging of the Mammalian Heart," *Journal of Gerontology*, 36 (1981): 297–305; and "Effects of Exercise on the Biochemical Aging of Mammalian Myocardium," *Mechanisms of Ageing and Development*, 6 (1981): 379–83.

In addition to his research, Rockstein was very active in the Gerontological Society. He headed its publications committee and served as president in 1966. An active member and past chairman of the Biological Sciences Section, Rockstein promoted multidisciplinary perspectives on aging. In addition to working with Shock on the International Association of Gerontology, Rockstein trained several scholars from such countries as India, France, Canada, Turkey, and West Germany.

Several of Rockstein's students have attained prominence in gerontological circles: George T. Baker III, who has been affiliated with the University of Maryland's Center on Aging and the National Institute on Aging, and Jeffrey Chesky, now the head of the Gerontology Program at Sangamon State University in Illinois. Rockstein also reached scores of biomedical students through his training seminars in aging and geriatrics, the proceedings of which were published by Academic Press. See his *Development and Aging in the Nervous System* (1973); *The Physiology and Pathology of Human Aging,* eds. R. Goldman and M. Rockstein (1975); and *Nutrition, Longevity and Aging,* eds. M. Sussman and M. Rockstein (1976).

A professor emeritus since 1983, Rockstein is listed in *Who's Who* and *Who's Who in the World.* He also is a Knight Commander of Merit, Sovereign Order of St. John Knights of Malta.

CAROLYN J. ROSENTHAL. Carolyn J. Rosenthal received her Ph.D. in 1981 from McMaster University. She first became attracted to the field of aging in 1976, when she began delving into the literature on aging and intergenerational relations. She was particularly interested in the paradigms set forth by Vern L. Bengtson,* and, as she progressed, by the theories of aging analyzed by Victor W. Marshall.* Rosenthal's own intellectual development was to be greatly shaped by Marshall, who has been one of her significant teachers, mentors, and primary collaborators. (Very conscious of the importance of gender in career development, she counts Lillian E. Troll,* Anne Martin Matthews, Ingrid Connidis, and Sarah Matthews as her chief role models.) She recently returned to McMaster after twelve years at the University of Toronto. She is a member of the Department of Sociology at McMaster University and director of its Office of Gerontological Studies.

Rosenthal is particularly pleased with contributing two concepts to the research literature on aging. She introduced the concept of ''the familial division of labor'' to refer to roles such as family kinkeeper, comforter, as well as head of the family, which are taken on by people in the extended family, thereby contributing to family solidarity. See, for instance, her ''Kinkeeping in the Familial Division of Labor,'' *Journal of Marriage and the Family,* 47 (1985): 965–74. There, she limned the status of a person in the wider extended family, who, more than others, takes responsibility for keeping family members in touch with one another. See also her article, ''The Comforter: Providing Personal Advice and Emotional Support to Generations in the Family,'' *Canadian Journal of Aging,* 6 (1987): 228–40.

Rosenthal came to appreciate the significance of this concept as she grappled with issues of family relationships across ethnic lines. In ''Aging, Ethnicity, and the Family: Beyond the Modernization Thesis," *Canadian Ethnic Studies,* 15 (1983): 1–16, she related assumptions about high family support in non-mainstream ethnic groups to the modernization theory of aging. See also her papers with Victor Marshall, "The Head of the Family: Social Meaning and Structural Variability," in *Canadian Journal of Sociology,* 11 (1986): 183–98, and "Generational Transmission of Family Ritual," *American Behavioral Scientist,* 31 (1988): 669–84.

Rosenthal also has coined the term "quasi-widowhood" to refer to the transition that occurs when a spouse enters a long-term care institution. See, for instance, her study, "Wives of Institutionalized Men: The Transition to Quasi-Widowhood," *Journal of Aging and Health,* 3 (1991): 315–34. This line of research has brought her back to larger questions of the variability in family relations and issues of intergenerational succession. See, for instance, her summary of the literature (with Vern L. Bengtson and Lynda C. Burton), "Families and Aging: Diversity and Heterogeneity," in the third edition of the *Handbook of Aging and the Social Sciences,* eds. Robert H. Binstock* and Linda George* (New York: Academic Press, 1990).

With Victor Marshall, Anne Martin Matthews, and others, Rosenthal is a major participant in a research initiative that has linked researchers in major Canadian universities with partners in the corporate sector. Her current work focuses on ways that employed persons, especially women, balance their job responsibilities with family responsibilities related to older relatives. See, for example, a review of the issues (with Anne Martin Matthews), "Balancing Work and Family in An Aging Society: The Canadian Experience" in *Annual Review of Gerontology and Geriatrics,* eds. G. Maddox* and P. Lawton* (New York: Springer, 1993), 96–119. She also has been active in regional and national professional associations for gerontologists in Canada and has been the social sciences editor for the *Canadian Journal on Aging.*

IRVING ROSOW. Irving Rosow was born in Cleveland, Ohio, in 1921. He earned his B.A. in 1943, majoring in economics and political science. He spent six months in Germany as an interviewer and coder with the Morale Division of the U.S. Strategic Bombing Survey. While working as a technical aid for the Detroit City Planning Commission, he published his first article, "Home Ownership Motives," *American Sociological Review,* 13 (1948): 751–56. Rosow earned his M.A. in 1948 from Wayne State. He then went to Harvard University, where he worked with Ale Inkeles and Raymond Bauer at the Russian Research Center. He collaborated with them in publishing *The Soviet Citizen* (Cambridge, Mass.: Harvard University Press, 1959). Rosow earned his Ph.D. in sociology in 1955.

From 1954 to 1957, Rosow served as senior sociologist for Nuffield Research at Belmont Hospital, Sutton, Surrey, England. After spending a year at Purdue, he joined the faculty at Case Western Reserve University. There, he directed the Ford Foundation Aging Study (1958–1965), and held appointments in the

Sociology Department and the School of Applied Social Sciences. His first gerontologic essays built on his earlier interests in the social effects of the physical environment. They dealt with issues of "retirement housing and social integration." An article by that title first appeared in *The Gerontologist,* 1 (1961): 85–91; it was reprinted in *Social and Psychological Aspects of Aging,* eds. Clark Tibbits* and Wilma Donahue* (New York: Columbia University Press, 1962), and *Gerontology: A Book of Readings,* ed. Clyde Vedder (Springfield, Ill.: Charles C. Thomas, 1963).

In 1969, Rosow became professor of medical sociology in the Department of Psychiatry at the Langley Porter Institute at the University of California at San Francisco (UCSF). From 1984 to 1988, he directed the Human Development and Aging Program at UCSF.

Rosow retired in 1989.

Rosow is probably best known for his theories on role changes through the lifespan and his views on criteria of adult socialization. He presented his ideas in such important works as *Social Integration of the Aged* (New York: Free Press, 1967) and *Socialization to Old Age* (Berkeley: University of California Press, 1974), which was translated into Japanese in 1983. Rosow emphasized that because role losses exclude the aged from meaningful social participation, many older people found themselves judged invidiously. The sense of devaluation and consequent loss of self-esteem differ from that which occurs at earlier stages of life, since the resulting feelings do not affect just victims of race, class, gender, and economic discrimination; they represent the "systematic status loss for an entire cohort." Adults, Rosow contended, are not socialized to anticipate this major discontinuity in later years. Their sense of isolation is heightened, moreover, because society itself provides no norms or guidance. Hence, old age is a time of "crisis." For more on this, see his "Status and Role Change through the Life Cycle," in *Handbook of Aging and the Social Sciences,* 2nd edn., eds. Robert H. Binstock* and Ethel Shanas* (New York: Van Nostrand Reinhold, 1985), 62–93.

Rosow has also been very interested in sharpening the conceptual tools that he and other gerontologists use. See, for instance, his 1977 address for Division 20 of the American Psychological Association, "What is a Cohort and Why?" which appeared in *Human Development,* 21 (1978): 65–75; "Seven of My Research Instruments," in *Research Instruments in Social Gerontology,* vols. 1–2, eds. David Mangen and Warren Peterson (Minneapolis: University of Minnesota Press, 1981 and 1983); and "Morale: Concept and Measurement," in *Measuring Morale: A Guide to Effective Assessment,* ed. Corrine Nydegger (Washington, D.C. Gerontological Society, 1977), 39–45.

For his contributions, Rosow received the 1975 Prochovnik International Award from the Israel Gerontology Society and prizes from the Section on Aging of the American Sociological Association (1986), of which he was a founding member. He was also a founding member of the International Sociological Association's research committee on the sociology of aging. The Behavioral and Social Sciences Section of the Gerontological Society honored Rosow a year later for his achievements on more than a dozen committees between 1973 and 1982. Rosow received the 1993 Kleemeier Award, giving a lecture on "Lessons from the Museum: Claude Monet and the Social Roles," *The Gerontologist,* 34 (1994): 292–98.

GEORGE S. ROTH. George S. Roth received his Ph.D. from Temple University School of Medicine in 1971. There, he was taught by Lolita Daves-Moore and Gerald D. Schockman. Roth worked very closely with Richard C. Adelman,* who first introduced him to research on aging. The pair worked on altered enzyme adaptation during aging.

Roth's primary work has been to elucidate the mechanisms of altered hormones and neurotransmitters' actions during aging. He was the first to demonstrate the loss of receptors as a cause of reduced responsiveness during aging. Roth was also the first to compare and contrast "receptor" and "post-receptor" mechanisms in altered signal transduction during aging. In "Changes in the Mechanisms of Hormones and Neuro-Transmitter Action during Aging: Current Status of the Role of Receptor and Post-Receptor Alterations: A Review," in *Mechanisms of Ageing and Development,* 20 (1982): 175–94, Roth and Gerald D. Hess assessed the disagreement among their peers concerning the extent and importance of receptor alterations. Based on a review of 179 reports, they confirmed that receptors did appear to change with age in many, but not all, systems; they acknowledged that at that time only a few scientists had been able to localize particular post-receptor alterations responsible for changes in response. Nonetheless, they wrote, "localization of changes at both the receptor and post-receptor levels during aging continues to be an essential approach toward elucidating age-related impairments in the mechanisms of hormone and neurotransmitter actions." Roth and Hess felt that future progress would depend on standardizing experimental systems and effecting methodological advances in analyzing subcellular components and events that mediate such processes.

During the 1980s, working at the National Institute on Aging's Gerontology Research Center with Reuben Andres,* Richard Cutler, Donald Ingram, and James Joseph, Roth refined his hypotheses. The impaired ability of old animals to regulate physiological functions and overall homeostasis, Roth asserted, may be due to altered hormone and neurotransmitter signal transduction components and events at both the receptor and post-receptor levels. More recently, his hypothesis has been confirmed by a number of laboratories, particularly with respect to loss of dopamine receptors and impaired coupling/uncoupling of certain G-protein linked receptors. See Roth's assessment in the *Annual Review of Gerontology and Geriatrics,* 10 (1990): 132ff.

JOHN W. ROWE. John W. Rowe was born in Jersey City, New Jersey, in 1944. He graduated from Canisius College in Buffalo, New York, in 1966 and earned his M.D. at the University of Rochester four years later. He went on to Harvard

Medical School and Beth Israel Hospital for residency training in internal medicine. From 1972 to 1974, Rowe completed his service obligation by working in Nathan W. Shock's Gerontology Research Center. The next two years were spent completing his residency training as a clinical fellow in nephrology at Massachusetts General Hospital and Harvard Medical School.

From 1976 to 1988, Rowe was of critical importance in building a geriatrics and gerontology program at Harvard. He rose through the academic ranks to become a professor of medicine. He directed the Division of Aging at Harvard Medical School. Concurrently, Rowe was senior physician at Brigham & Women's Hospital and Beth Israel Hospital. He also directed the Geriatric Research, Education and Clinical Center at Boston's Veterans Administration medical center. Since 1988, Rowe has been president of the Mount Sinai Medical Center at the Mount Sinai Hospital and School of Medicine as well as professor of geriatrics and adult development.

Rowe has held many important positions, including the presidency of the Gerontological Society and membership in the National Academy of Sciences. He has consulted with several foundations and federal blue-ribbon panels. Among his several publications, three are worth noting in some detail.

With Robert Kahn, Rowe published "Human Aging: Usual and Successful" in *Science,* 237 (July 1987): 143–49. In the absence of identifiable pathological manifestations, the authors argued, gerontologists and geriatricians have tended to attribute age-associated cognitive and physiological deficits to advancing age. This overstates the role of senescence as a sufficient explanatory variable in accounting for changes in a heterogeneous population. Stressing such factors as carbohydrate metabolism. osteoporosis, extrinsic psycho-behavioral factors, lifestyles, and diet, Rowe and Kahn stressed the importance of extrinsic factors. They encouraged investigators to distinguish between usual and successful aging, taking into account a full range of functional variables, including the capacities for autonomy and self-support. Such inquiries might generate the discovery of interventions that might prevent disease.

In the "Interface of Geriatric Medicine and Geriatric Psychiatry" in the *Journal of Geriatric Psychiatry,* 20 (1987): 3–9, Rowe reflected on his years of combining geriatric research and training. He doubted the likelihood that geriatrics would ever become a single specialty. Rather, he predicted, two subspecialities, likely based in internal medicine and psychiatry, would be merged in most clinical programs.

Finally, in the third edition of the *Handbook of the Biology of Aging* (New York: Academic Press, 1990), which he edited with Edward L. Schneider,* Rowe (with San Y. Wang and Dariush Elahi) outlined the "Design, Conduct, and Analysis of Human Aging Research." A comparison of this essay with an earlier paper, "Clinical Research on Aging: Strategies and Directions," *New England Journal of Medicine,* 297, (1977): 1332–36, suggests how far Rowe's thinking had progressed beyond that earlier analysis of *in vitro* studies of human tissues. In this recent piece, Rowe shows considerable sophistication in discussing issues of selective mortality and drawbacks in longitudinal studies (as evidenced from work in the Framingham Study). But his forte remains his ability to show how clinical findings must be interpreted with common sense and an appreciation of the multiplicity of extrinsic and intrinsic factors that might distort results:

> Ideally, in studying an aging change in humans, one would like to precisely quantitate a change, study the detailed mechanisms of the change, pinpoint effector agents causing the change, and show that one can produce the change by appropriate manipulation of the mechanism or effector agents. . . . The exciting and accelerating developments in the study of the neurobiology of aging show the potential of these approaches for the future.

Such advances, however, depend upon advances in medical research as a whole.

LAURENCE Z. RUBENSTEIN. Laurence Z. Rubenstein earned his B.A. *cum laude* in anthropology from the University of California at Santa Cruz in 1970 and his medical degree four years later from Albert Einstein College of Medicine in New York. He began work in geriatrics in 1978 while pursuing a master's degree in public health from the University of California at Los Angeles School of Public Health (1979). His mentors included Itamar B. Abrass,* Robert L. Kane,* John Beck, and Victor Sidel; his teachers included Robert Brook, Sheldon Greenfield, and Lester Breslow.

Rubenstein did his residencies in internal and preventative medicine. His most important contributions to the field of gerontology have been in the area of geriatric health services research, specifically in the systematic study of the effectiveness of clinical interventions in geriatric health services across a variety of settings. His primary collaborators in this area have been Darryl Wieland, Karen Josephson, and Robert Kane. It was Kane's research that first attracted him to gerontology.

Rubenstein was one of the developers of the concept of comprehensive geriatric assessment in the United States. He directed the first randomized clinical trial of a hospital-based geriatric evaluation and management unit. See his "Effectiveness of a Geriatric Evaluation Unit: A Randomized Clinical Trial," *New England Journal of Medicine,* 311 (1984): 1664–70. This study and subsequent follow-up studies have contributed to the creation of such units internationally. He has also tested other geriatric evaluation management approaches, including out-patient, home visit, and in-patient consultation through randomized trials and formal meta-analysis.

The incidence of falling among the elderly has been another important subject for Rubenstein. He has identified important predictors for falls and has directed a randomized clinical trial to test the efficacy of post-fall assessment interventions with frail nursing home patients. His team, which included Alan S. Robbins and Josephson, was able to document a significant reduction in subsequent hospitalization; see their "The Value of Assessing Falls in an Elderly Population: A Randomized Clinical Trial," *Annals of Internal Medicine* 113 (1990): 308–16. He has also documented the systematic biases in self-rated functional status measures, identified determinants of hospital outcomes for elderly patients, measured the value of routine diagnostic testing and screening for elderly populations, and documented the benefits of academic nursing homes.

Rubenstein is currently affiliated with the Veterans Affairs Medical Center in Sepulveda, California, and is a professor of geriatric medicine at UCLA School of Medicine. He has been a section editor of the *Journal of the American Geriatrics Society* and a member of the electoral boards of the *Journal of Gerontology* (1983–1988), and the *Annals of Internal Medicine* (1989–1992). Rubenstein has won awards from the VA and the American Geriatrics Society.

ISAAC MAX RUBINOW. Isaac Max Rubinow was born in Grodno, Russia, in 1875; he migrated to the United States at the age of eighteen. A cosmopolitan kin network facilitated his entry into American life. Rubinow enrolled in Columbia University, earning a B.A. in 1895 and a medical degree three years later.

In the course of caring for New York City's poor between 1898 and 1903, Rubinow discovered that the illnesses and disabilities he treated were as much a socioeconomic problem as they were physiological or pathological maladies. Eager to corroborate this hypothesis, he abandoned his medical practice and began to conduct the sort of investigative studies of the urban working class being done at the time by Charles Booth in England. Rubinow's penchant for gathering and interpreting social statistics was hardly amateurish. He took graduate courses in mathematics while working for a Ph.D. in political science at Columbia. Under the direction of E.R.A. Seligman, Rubinow investigated trends in workers' wages and purchasing power. He completed his second doctorate in 1914.

Rubinow's graduate studies prepared him for a sequence of positions that advanced his career as a social investigator, teacher, and reformer. He was an examiner for the U.S. Civil Service Commission (1903–1904). He then served as a researcher and statistician for the U.S. Department of Agriculture (1904–1907) and the U.S. Department of Commerce and Labor (1907–1908). For the next three years, Rubinow worked on the Commissioner of Labor Statistics's report on *Workmen's Insurance and Compensation Systems in Europe.* As a government employee, Rubinow published his first series of articles, including "The New Russian Workingmen's Compensation Act," which appeared in the *U.S. Labor Bulletin,* 58 (May 1905): 955–59.

From 1911 to 1916, Rubinow worked as chief statistician for the Ocean Accident & Guarantee Corporation. During this period, he also served as president of the Casualty Actuarial Society. In addition, Rubinow lectured on social insurance at the New York School of Philanthropy; he proudly declared that he offered the first course exclusively devoted to the topic at any American university.

In 1913, Henry Holt and Company published Rubinow's *Social Insurance,* arguably the most impressive statistical and theoretical rationale for adopting new forms of protection for the aged and the poor issued in the United States to that date. Rubinow hoped that the 525-page text would stimulate nascent scholarly and public interest in accident pensions, widows' pensions, retirement annuities, and state-financed life insurance. Social insurance, in Rubinow's opinion, went far beyond relief. He wrote: "The ideal purpose of social insurance, the purpose to which the best insurance systems tend (and the others slowly follow), is to prevent and finally eradicate poverty, and the subsequent need of relief, by meeting the problem at the origin, rather than waiting until the effects of destitution have begun to be felt" (p. 481). Few of Rubinow's contemporaries were yet prepared to accept his thesis, but *Social Insurance* became a classic.

For the rest of his life, Rubinow worked for better workmen's compensation laws, unemployment insurance, old-age pensions, and national health insurance programs. Along with a growing number of experts, Rubinow felt that these provisions should be financed through general public reserves, taxes on employees' wages, and employers' contributions. Not all reformers shared Rubinow's opinions. Leaders of the American Association for Labor Legislation (AALL), for instance, were greatly influenced between 1916 and 1920 by Rubinow's views on health insurance and mothers' pensions. Thereafter, however, AALL placed greater emphasis on the "preventive" than on the "redistributionist" features of social insurance. AALL laid less stress than Rubinow on class differences and the inevitability of federal action.

In 1916, Rubinow became executive secretary of the American Medical Association's Social Insurance Commission. A year later, he was appointed director of the Bureau of Social Statistics of New York City's Department of Public Charities. In the meantime, he continued to lecture on social insurance at the New York School of Philanthropy and became a contributing editor of *Survey.*

After World War I, Rubinow became increasingly involved in the second major cause of his distinguished career: He organized and promoted social services in the Jewish community. From 1918 to 1922, Rubinow headed the Hadassah medical unit in Palestine, supervising the modernization of hospitals and clinics in the country. He was director of the Jewish Welfare Society in Philadelphia for the next five years. In addition, he worked as editor of the *Jewish Social Service Quarterly* between 1925 and 1929. Rubinow served as secretary of the B'nai B'rith in Cincinnati from 1929 until his death. In this latter capacity, he was instrumental in launching an antidefamation movement and took steps to aid Jews who wished to flee Nazi Germany.

In 1934, Henry Holt published Rubinow's second major book, *The Quest for Security.* Rubinow saw no need to replicate recent works such as Barbara Nachtrieb Armstrong's *Insuring the Essentials* (Berkeley, Calif.: University of California Press, 1932) or Abraham Epstein's *The Challenge of the Aged* (New

York: Vanguard, 1928). Confident that he would be recognized as the authority he was, Rubinow discarded tables, figures, quotations, and citations in setting forth his argument. He pitched the book to "the average intelligent and educated but not specialized adult mind," to people who might be persuaded to make an "effort toward a more desirable social order" (p. vi). Eschewing images of a utopian or Arcadian society, he appealed to New Dealers to do what was possible: "Social insurance must therefore become—if it is not already—an essential aspect of the New Deal."

Rubinow's message was heard. FDR wrote him to express "great interest" in his suggestions about the president's probable role in enacting social security legislation. But Rubinow did not play a central role in drafting the 1935 Social Security Act, though he was a member of Ohio Commission on Unemployment Insurance (1932) and chaired the Cincinnati Board on Old Age Pensions (1934–1935). Some historians have suggested that he was too pugnacious and "ethnic" to gain the confidence of those who had to accommodate diverse interests to get Social Security enacted. Rubinow died in New York City on September 1, 1936, at the age of sixty-one.

The best biographical details on Rubinow's life appear in *Who Was Who in America,* vol. 1 (1943), 1064, and in his obituary in the *New York Times,* September 3, 1936, 21. Additional details can be gleaned from Rubinow's two major works, *Social Insurance* (1913) and *The Quest for Security* (1934). The significance of Rubinow's ideas and efforts to promote social insurance are discussed in Roy Lubove, *The Struggle for Social Security* (Cambridge, Mass.: Harvard University Press, 1968); Daniel J. Boorstin, *The Americans: The Democratic Experience* (New York: Vintage Press, 1974); and W. Andrew Achenbaum, *Old Age in the New Land* (Baltimore: Johns Hopkins University Press, 1978) and *Social Security* (New York: Cambridge University Press, 1986).

ROBERT L. RUBINSTEIN. Robert L. Rubinstein earned a master's degree from Bryn Mawr College in 1974 and completed his Ph.D in anthropology there four years later, under the direction of Jane Goodale. Like a surprisingly large number of gerontologists, Rubinstein came to the field by happenstance. In 1981, he was hired by M. Powell Lawton* of the Philadelphia Geriatric Center, which needed an anthropologist for a one-year position. Rubinstein counts Lawton and Miriam Moss of the Philadelphia Geriatric Center, along with Jennie Keith* of Swarthmore College, as his mentors in the field.

His major contribution has been in the examination and explication of the role of personal meaning and interpretation in the lives of older people. The concept of "personal meaning" bridges the gap between the sociocultural and the personal aspects of life by representing the ways in which older people interpret and give meaning to their lives according to community and personal values. This construct has been used in qualitative studies of the environments of older people, the lives of older men, and the lives of childless older men and women, among other topics.

As an anthropologist, Rubinstein's emphasis has been on cross-cultural, ethnographic research, but his methods have been more recently applied to single-culture, ethnographically based research in the United States. His references include "Narratives of Elder Parental Death," *Medical Anthropology Quarterly,* 1995; and *Elders Living Alone: Frailty and the Perception of Choice* (New York: Aldine de Gruyter, 1992).

In addition to his research, Rubinstein has worked with the Association for Anthropology and Gerontology and the Qualitative Interest Group of the Gerontological Society of America. He is director of research at the Polishen Research Institute at the Philadelphia Geriatric Center.

CAROL D. RYFF. Carol D. Ryff received her B.A. in 1973 from Colorado Women's College. She then earned her M.A. (1975) and Ph.D. (1978) from the Pennsylvania State University. The writings of Erik Erikson and Carl Jung first attracted her to research on aging. Paul B. Baltes* has been a key teacher, mentor, and role model. With Baltes, Ryff wrote one of her early, important papers, "Values Transitions and Adult Development in Women: The Instrumentality-Terminality Sequence Hypothesis," which appeared in *Developmental Psychology,* 12 (1976): 557–68. As a member of the MacArthur Research Network on Successful Mid-Life Development, she has also been greatly influenced by Orville G. (Bert) Brim, with whom she had collaborated earlier. See Brim and Ryff, "On the Properties of Life Events," in *Life-Span Development and Behavior,* eds. Paul Baltes and Orville Brim (New York: Academic Press, 1980), vol. 3: 368–88.

Ryff has focused thus far on developing a theoretical and empirical model for assessing positive psychological functioning in adulthood and aging. See, for instance, her essay, "Happiness Is Everything, or Is It? Explorations on the Meaning of Psychological Well-Being," in the *Journal of Personality and Social Psychology,* 57 (1989): 1069–81, as well as an essay with one of her collaborators, Marilyn Essex, "Psychological Well-Being in Middle and Later Adulthood: Descriptive Markers and Explanatory Processes," in *Annual Review of Gerontology and Geriatrics,* eds. K. Warner Schaie* and M. Powell Lawton* (New York: Springer Publishing, 1991), vol. 11: 144–71. Much of this work elaborated Ryff's greatest contribution thus far: the explication of the meaning of "successful aging" in the psychological sense. For an early attempt in this area, see her "Successful Aging: A Developmental Approach," *The Gerontologist,* 22 (1982): 209–14. There, she reformulated earlier conceptions of "successful aging" (a term that she traced back to the Kansas City Studies of Adult Life) to make them more responsive to a theory-guided developmental perspective, especially those proposed by Erik Erikson and Charlotte Buhler's optimization theory of personality development. Ryff dealt with issues of operational definitions, selective sampling, and stage theory: "Whereas the present perspective relied largely on developmental theories, it is possible that insight will be gained from the clinical literature."

After serving two years as a consultant for the Foundation for Child Development (1976–1978), Ryff was affiliated with Fordham University's Department of Psychology (1978–1985). She has been at the University of Wisconsin at Madison since then, becoming the associate director of its Institute of Aging and Adult Life in 1989 and a professor of psychology two years later. Ryff has served as a consulting editor of *Psychology and Aging*. In addition to support from the MacArthur Foundation, Ryff has received major grants from the National Institute on Aging.

S

GEORGE A. SACHER, JR. George Alban Sacher, Jr. was born in Newark, New Jersey, in 1917. After spending a year at Rutgers University College of Pharmacy, he earned his B.S. in 1939 from the University of Chicago. From 1939 to 1942, he did graduate work in psychology at Chicago. Sacher also worked on the Manhattan Project, and after the war he conducted studies in cell physiology. He worked in the metallurgical laboratory at the University of Chicago from 1942 to 1946, before joining the Argonne National Laboratories in Argonne, Illinois. In 1959, Sacher became a senior biologist in the Division of Biological and Medical Research at the Laboratories, a position he held until his death in 1981.

In addition to his research at Argonne, Sacher held many concurrent positions. He began to lecture in 1969 on biological aspects of human development at the University of Chicago. In 1980, he became a research associate with professional rank in the university's Department of Biology and Committee on Human Development. For most of his career, he was on the advisory committee of the radiation registry of physicians for the National Academy of Science/National Research Council. From 1960 to 1963, Sacher was a member of a National Institutes of Health advisory committee for computation for research; from 1965 to 1975, he served on various U.S. Public Health Service committees dealing with aspects of radiation in research. For the National Academy of Sciences, Sacher served on a committee on the use of ionizing radiation treatment in benign diseases (1975–1977), and on animal models in research on aging (1978–1981). In 1976, he joined the U.S. Department of Commerce's committee on electromagnetic radiation management.

Sacher's research focused on mammalian environmental pathophysiology, the biology of aging, and evolutionary biology. He tried to develop a mathematical theory of aging and mortality. He also was interested in diet cycles of energy metabolism and thermoregulation. With Austin M. Brues, he published a collection of essays from an interdisciplinary conference underwritten by the American Institute of Biological Sciences and the National Heart Institute on *Aging and Levels of Biological Organization* (Chicago: University of Chicago Press, 1965). Participants focused on metazoan aging at all levels of organization, ranging from cells to ecosystems, stressing relationships between genetics and the environment, and changes in the structure and performance of cells with age. That same year, he also edited a volume on *Radiation Effects on Natural Populations* for the Argonne National Laboratory. In 1974, Sacher contributed the article on "Aging: Biological" for the fifteenth edition of the *Encyclopaedia Brittannica*. He published roughly another hundred articles and book chapters.

Sacher's breadth of vision is perhaps most evident in his 1977 Kleemeier Award Lecture, published as "Longevity, Aging, and Death: An Evolutionary Perspective" in *The Gerontologist,* 16 (April 1978): 112–19. From an evolutionary perspective, Sacher claimed, biogerontology became primarily the biology of longevity, not the biology of aging and death, as most gerontologists would have it. With mathematical formulae and comparative data, he argued that mammalian lifespan was primarily related to two quantitative measures: the cephalization coefficient and an index of lifetime metabolic activity that has the physical dimensions of action. The bold hypothesis presented in the Kleemeier lecture, as an alternative to more widely accepted theories of senescence, was that natural selection acts to maintain and extend mammalian longevity by modifying a set of longevity assurance mechanisms that all mammals have in common. Hence, with a conviction reminiscent of Metchnikoff,* Sacher believed that gerontology "points to the possibility of an evolutionarily and humanistically meaningful transcendence of that finitude as a result of future biological research."

Sacher served as president of the Gerontological Society in 1979.

ANDREA SANKAR. Anthropologist Andrea Sankar earned a B.A. in Far Eastern languages and literature from the University of Michigan in 1970 and a Ph.D. in anthropology from Michigan in 1987. She is associate professor of anthropology and director of the Medical Anthropology Program at Wayne State University in Detroit. Her current work focuses on adapting and testing theories and findings developed in gerontology to community-based care for minorities with AIDS. In this project she is adapting quality-of-life measures developed for white gay male populations to African American men who have sex with men and to African American women.

In her dissertation work on culture and aging, Sankar conducted fieldwork in Hong Kong with aging single Chinese women and documented the role of non-kin relationships in providing care in old age. She found that when these associations, known as sisterhoods, were supplemented by a religious structure that was provided if the sisterhood joined or formed a Buddhist or Taoist nunnery, the association was able to provide care for aging members. Sisterhoods that remained secular became dysfunctional as the members aged and no new recruits appeared.

Sankar also examined the different uses of old age as a diagnosis in Chinese and Western medical systems and found that the Chinese tend to treat "old age" with a range of remedies but do not treat terminal illness. In contrast, Western medicine believes nothing can be done for "old age" but aggressively treats a terminal illness. See "It's Just Old Age: Diagnosis in Chinese and Western Medicine" in *Age and Anthropological Theory*, eds. David Kertzer and Jennie Keith* (1984). She has continued this interest and recently published a comprehensive work on gerontological research in China. See her "Gerontological Research in China: The Role of Anthropological Inquiry," *Journal of Cross-Cultural Gerontology,* 4 (1989): 199–224; as well as "Cultural Alternatives to the Vulnerable Elderly: The Case of China Past and Present," *Studies in Third World Societies*, 23 (1983): 21–51.

Since her postdoctoral work at UCSF, Sankar's research has focused around the deinstitutionalization of health care and the impact this is having on the community system of care and on the "speed up" of domestic life. In a study of medical decision-making in the home, she described the integration of non-biomedical data into the medical decision-making process. See "Out of the Clinic into the Home: Control and Communication in the Patient-Physician Relationship," *Social Science and Medicine,* 22 (1986): 973–82. In line with this focus on home care, with Jaber F. Gubrium* she co-edited *The Home Care Experience* (New York: Sage, 1990).

In a study of real-time, naturalistic problem-solving between caregivers and the family member they cared for, Sankar developed a observational instrument to document these interactions. This instrument allowed her to identify patterns of conflict and styles of decision-making. She found that caregivers who maintained a private space in their home where the practices and compromises of caregiving were not apparent, for example, keeping a glass bell collection intact, experienced less stress and solved caregiving problems with less conflict than those caregivers who turned their entire home into a caregiving context. "Home Observation: A Qualitative and Quantitative Approach" was delivered at the American Anthropological Association annual meeting in 1987.

A study of caregivers of the dying, reported in her book *Dying at Home* (Baltimore: Johns Hopkins University Press, 1991), found that social support for the caregiver, not the dying person, was related to caregiver outcomes with caregivers who received instrumental support during the caregiving process coping better with bereavement than the caregivers who did not. Most caregivers in a home death saw themselves as "in control," which allowed them to bracket the reality of the impending death; this was not possible in the hospital. See

Sankar's "Culture and Practice in the Care of People Dying at Home," *Medical Anthropological Quarterly,* (June 1995).

In a research project on high-tech home care for AIDS patients, Sankar found that most of the care was provided by mothers and that many had to quit their jobs to monitor the infusion therapy. Many caregivers reported being extremely anxious about giving this therapy to demented patients.

Sankar also has a long-term interest in social science theory and methodology. She recently co-edited with Jaber Gubrium, *Qualitative Methods in Aging Research* (New York: Sage, 1994).

K. WARNER SCHAIE. K. Warner Schaie was born in 1928 in the town of Stettin, in what was then Germany but is now Poland. Escaping the Nazis by going east, he settled in China before entering the United States. He became a U.S. citizen in 1953, two years after receiving an A.A. degree in the social sciences from the City College of San Francisco and a year after earning his B.A. in psychology from Berkeley, where Read T. Tuddenham introduced him to the literature on psychometric intelligence. Schaie did his graduate work in psychology at the University of Washington (M.A., 1953; Ph.D., 1956). In addition to working on his degrees, Schaie served as a research assistant, extension instructor, project coordinator, and executive secretary for the university's Committee on Gerontology (1953–1956), which deepened his interest in aging. After training at Western State Hospital in Fort Steilacoom, Washington, Schaie became a Diplomate in clinical psychology; he also is a psychologist licensed to practice in California and Pennsylvania.

Schaie took a postdoctoral fellowship in medical psychology at Washington University's School of Medicine. After seven years in the Psychology Department at the University of Nebraska (with summer appointments in the universities of Saar, Germany, and Washington), Schaie moved to West Virginia University (1964–1973), where he chaired the Psychology Department, gaining for it national attention in the area of lifespan and developmental psychology, and directed its Human Resources Research Institute. From 1973 to 1982, Schaie was on the faculty of the University of Southern California, directing the Gerontology Research Institute at its Andrus Gerontology Center. Since 1981, he has held an appointment at the Pennsylvania State University. He became director of Penn State's Gerontology Center in 1985, and the Evan Pugh Professor of Human Development and Psychology a year later. Since 1992, Schaie has also been an affiliate professor of psychiatry and behavioral science at the University of Washington.

Schaie has been the co-author or co-editor of more than two dozen books; eight monographs, manuals and technical reports; and several hundred peer-reviewed journals and book chapters. His first publication (with Fred Rosenthal and Robert Perlman), "Differential Mental Deterioration of Factorially 'Pure' Functions in Later Maturity," *Journal of Gerontology,* 8 (1953): 191–96, was based on his presentation at the Second International Gerontological Congress two years earlier in St. Louis. The article presented the results of a pilot study using the Thurstone Primary Mental Abilities test battery on sixty-one subjects between the ages of fifty-three and seventy-eight. Schaie and his associates found that spatial and reasoning abilities declined faster than number, verbal-meaning, and word-fluency when the time limit (which others, such as Alan Traviss Welford,* were confirming, was a handicap) was removed. He then noted the value of using this instrument, even though it had been designed for younger subjects. Thus the article not only shows Schaie's early concern for methodological rigor, but it also presages his fascination with studying conti-nuities and changes in adult intelligence over the lifespan.

Schaie's major intellectual contributions to gerontology fall into three do-mains: (1) his efforts to promote the lifespan development movement; (2) his methodological and conceptual refinements of a general developmental model of aging, which differentiates among the dimensions of age, time-of-measure-ment, and cohort; and (3) his creation of the Seattle Longitudinal Study of Adult Intellectual Development. One way to trace his intellectual odyssey is to read several of his seminal essays. Schaie himself is particularly pleased with ''A General Model for the Study of Developmental Programs,'' which appeared in *Psychological Bulletin,* 64 (1965): 92–107. Then go to his ''Quasi-Experimental Designs in the Psychology of Aging,'' in the first edition of the *Handbook of the Psychology of Aging,* eds. James E. Birren* and Schaie (New York: Van Nostrand Reinhold, 1977). Schaie's *Longitudinal Studies of Adult Psychological Development* (New York: Guilford Press, 1983) offers a good primer on the design and findings of the Seattle studies, as does his 1988 Kleemeier Lecture, published as ''The Hazards of Cognitive Aging'' in *The Gerontologist,* 29 (1989): 484–93. In the latter article, Schaie discusses the application of event-history analysis to data involving changes of states in individual behavior that is related to senescence. The dependent variable is the calendar or functional age in which the event occurs. A more comprehensive account of the Seattle Longitudinal Study, ''Intellectual Involvement in Adulthood: The Seattle Lon-gitudinal Study,'' has been published (New York: Cambridge University Press, 1995).

Schaie's ''Intellectual Development in Adulthood,'' his contribution to the third edition of the *Handbook of the Psychology of Aging,* eds. Birren and Schaie (New York: Academic Press, 1990), offers a representative sample of Schaie's interest in substantive and methodological issues, though he also briefly dis-cusses meta-theoretical concerns. He acknowledges his continuing adaptation of L. L. Thurstone's factorial analyses of children's mental abilities, but then quickly adds that the field of adult intelligence has been reconfigured by meth-odological disputes over ways to design studies and assess results. He notes internal validity threats (due to the use of cross-sectional data or the effects of history), and disputes over the appropriateness of various instruments for meas-uring levels of cognitive processes and products. Schaie then turns to patterns of intellectual aging, using his Seattle Longitudinal Study as a baseline, in addition to offering profiles of individual aging and the role of cohort effects.

Schaie then considers factors that affect intellectual aging, such as "normal" versus "pathological" aging, speed of performance, as well as the effects of social structures and personality correlates on intellectual aging. Reflecting his years of collaboration with Paul Baltes, Schaie offers definitions of "practical intelligence," which move beyond psychometric criteria, being based instead on judges' ratings, performance of everyday tasks, and quasi-ethnographic studies of situational competencies. Building on work he has done with his wife, Sherry Willis,* he then discusses the efficacy of interventions in adult intellectual development. Schaie notes that "much of the cohort-related aspect of older person's intellectual disadvantage when compared with those at midlife may well be amenable to compensation by suitable educational interventions."

Throughout this review essay and other works, Schaie unfailingly cites the work of his primary role model (James Birren) and principal collaborators (Paul Baltes, Christopher Hertzog, Gisela Labouvie-Vief, John Nesselroade, Iris Parham, and Sherry Willis). Nonetheless, the orientation to gerontological issues is unmistakably his own. Schaie is eager to decompose aggregate data so as to elucidate precise influences on individual behavior and, ideally, to predict individual risks of intellectual decline as well as ways to maintain performance. Empirical work, he believes, shows that intellectual decline is not necessarily irreversible. Longitudinal analyses, moreover, should permit the identification of individuals who may (shortly) be at the threshold of cognitive impairment. Ever the methodologist, he is convinced that scholars should develop new techniques that might in turn promote the emergence of comprehensive theoretical formulations of adult intellectual development.

Schaie has been often honored over the course of his distinguished career. Division 20 of the American Psychological Association gave him the Distinguished Contribution Award in 1982; a decade later, APA offered him its Distinguished Scientific Contribution Award. In addition to receiving the Kleemeier Award, Schaie has served as chairman of the Gerontological Society's research and awards committees. He earned a MERIT Award (Method to Extend Research in Time) from the National Institute on Aging in 1989. He has served on innumerable editorial boards, and was an editor of the *Journal of Gerontology: Psychological Sciences* from 1988 to 1992.

EDWARD L. SCHNEIDER. Edward L. Schneider earned his B.S. from Rensselaer Polytechnic Institute (RPI) in Troy, New York, in 1961 and his M.D. *cum laude* from Boston University in 1966. (RPI gave him its Distinguished Alumnus Award in 1990.) Alex Comfort* first attracted Schneider to work in aging at a meeting in 1972. His primary role models were Robert N. Butler* and T. Franklin Williams, with whom he worked at the National Institute on Aging.

Schneider has been an able researcher and institution builder. In the research

310   EDWARD L. SCHNEIDER

domain, he is best known for his work with cell cultures from young and old
human subjects. Demonstrating how the impairment of cellular replicative capacities with aging affects human lymphocytes, Schneider has shown that there
was an altered response to DNA damage in human cells *in vitro* and animal
cells *in vitro* with aging, by sister chromatid exchange induction.

This research also motivated Schneider's interest in ways to affect human
longevity. He acknowledged various environmental, chemical, hormonal, and
pharmacological interventions, and affirmed that caloric reduction is as important in humans as in rats. But unlike those who opt for a *global* approach, which
takes the maximum lifespan as the end point, Schneider has been interested in
possible strategies for life extension at various points within the life course. "If
there are multiple etiologies for aging processes," Schneider pointed out with
National Institute on Aging colleague John Reed (in "Modulations of Aging
Processes," *Handbook of the Biology of Aging,* 2nd edn., eds. Caleb E. Finch*
and Edward L. Schneider (New York: Van Nostrand Reinhold, 1985), 45–76,
"future emphasis should be on 'segmental interventions.' These segmental interventions can best be assessed through the measurements of specific biomarkers of aging." For his early work on biomarkers, see his collection (with M.
E. Reff), *Biological Markers of Aging* (Washington, D.C.: U.S. Department of
Health and Human Services, 1982). Much of Schneider's work was made possible by establishing a cell bank for cultures that were derived from participants
of the Baltimore Longitudinal Study of Aging.

As an associate director and then deputy director of NIA, Schneider oversaw
the institute's Extramural Biomedical Programs. He was also chief of the Laboratory of Molecular Genetics at NIA's Gerontology Research Center. With
Evan Hadley, Schneider developed the Teaching Nursing Home program at
NIA.

Upon James E. Birren's* retirement, Schneider became the second executive
director of the Andrus Gerontology Center and dean of the Leonard Davis
School of Gerontology at the University of Southern California. There, with
some mentoring from his colleagues Warren Bennis and Robert Biller, Schneider
managed during his first five years to make a first-rate center even more impressive. During his tenure, pledges to the endowment rose from $6 million to
more than $25 million and helped to establish named chairs and professorships
for eight faculty members. Tuition income doubled, and research grants substantially increased from $2.4 million to $8 million.

Schneider has become a major advocate for the need for more aging research
to combat rising health care costs. With his former colleague at NIA, Jacob
Brody, he examined actuarial data and found, contrary to the compression-of-
mortality thesis set forth by James Fries, that the maximum life expectancy at
birth has been increasing, and that these increases were unlikely to stop at the
eighty-five-year limit. See Schneider and Brody, "Aging, Natural Death, and
the Compression of Morbidity: Another View," *New England Journal of Medicine,* 309 (1983): 854–56. In "Cutting the Costs of Aging," *Issues in Science*

and Technology, 7 (1991): 47–49, Schneider stressed the need for greater uses of molecular genetic approaches, which could lead to drugs that restore the replicative capacities of aged immune cells, thereby protecting people from bacterial and viral diseases. He also urges more longitudinal studies, such as the Baltimore Longitudinal Study of Aging, and work in social, behavioral, and epidemiological research. Schneider also stresses the need for preventive and therapeutic methods for the diseases and disorders of aging: "By investing now to conquer [chronic, disabling] diseases, we will provide the dual benefits of reducing health care costs while ensuring for ourselves and future generations long and healthy lives."

In addition to his administrative duties at Andrus and work on more than half a dozen journals, Schneider also serves as scientific director of the Buck Center for Research on Aging in Marin County, California.

DAVID SCHONFIELD. David Schonfield describes himself as an "early propagandist for aging studies, and services for the aged, in Canada." He was a founding member and vice president of the Canadian Association of Gerontology, and of the Alberta Council on Aging. He has served as the psychology editor for the *Canadian Journal on Aging.* But he was educated in England, and it was there that he first became interested in gerontology while training older workers with Sir Frederic Bartlett. He earned his M.A. from the University of Cambridge in 1950, and became licensed to practice psychology in 1951 from the University of London.

Perhaps his most important research has been the study of memory retrieval. In particular, he has examined age-associated increases in the difficulty of retrieving memories that are not the focus of attention. References include his "Memory Changes with Age," *Nature* 208 (1965) 818; "Delineating the Loci of Loss," *Design Conference on Decision Making and Aging,* eds. L. W. Poon and J. L. Fozard* (Boston: Geriatric Research Center, 1976). A more recent project has been the study of the relationship between future commitments and successful aging. With a sample of non-institutionalized elderly women, Schonfield found that levels of well-being and happiness were correlated with the number of specific events individuals have to look forward to. See his "Future Commitments and Successful Aging I: The Random Sample," *Journal of Gerontology* 28 (1973): 189–96.

Schonfield has also turned his investigations toward the study of the elderly themselves. He attempted to demonstrate the presence of age differences. His investigations have been aimed at understanding the special difficulties of memory recall in elderly subjects. He has pursued testing strategies with a sensitivity to age changes in general, and thereby refined standard tests of cognitive abilities. The choice of changes that will "work" requires some "feel" about age changes in general as these apply in specific situations. See "The Coding and Sorting of Digits and Symbols by an Elderly Sample," *Journal of Gerontology* 23 (1968): 318–23.

In a 1982 study he challenged the accepted literature on age bias. "Who Is Stereotyping Whom and Why?" (*The Gerontologist,* 22 (1982): 267–72), argues that evidence does not support the view that a negative attitude toward older people pervades in the United States. Finally, he has encouraged the humorous side of the "aging enterprise" in many papers, including, "Geronting: Reflections on Successful Aging" (*The Gerontologist,* 7 (1967): 270–73. He is currently affiliated with the University of Calgary in Alberta. At Calgary he has help lead the development of graduate and undergraduate studies in gerontology since the early 1960s.

JAMES H. SCHULZ. James H. Schulz received his B.A. at Miami University in Oxford, Ohio. While there, he was greatly influenced by Delbert Snider and Fred Cottrell, the latter a sociologist who was interested in aging, among other things. In 1966, he earned his Ph.D. in economics at Yale University, where he studied with Charles E. Lindblom, who was renowned for his global interpretations of politics and economics. Schulz's interest in research on aging was sparked early in his career by his father-in-law, Clark Tibbitts,* who was a moving force at the U.S. Administration on Aging.

Schulz was one of the first economists, along with Juanita Kreps, to specialize in aging topics. Thus he rightly deserves credit for blazing the subfield of the economics of aging. Schulz was, for instance, the first academic economist to study the policy issues related to employer-sponsored pensions and to draw attention to their inadequacies in supplementing Social Security. See his monograph, *Private Pension Benefits in the 1970s: A Study of Retirement and Survivor Levels in 1974 and 1979* (Bryn Mawr, Pa.: McCahan Foundation, 1982).

Schulz also introduced simulation modeling into policy analysis in gerontology. Specifically, his work involved evaluating the impact of public and private pensions on the aged's income status. See his "Problems of American Pensions: Microsimulation Policy Analyses," in *Zeitschrift fur die gesamte Staatswissenschaft,* 138 (1982): 527–45. He also collaborated with researchers at the Employee Benefit Research Institute, one of the nation's premier independent organizations concerned with broad issues in human resources management and worker compensation. See his work with a frequent co-author, Thomas Leavitt, *Pension Integration: Concepts, Issues, and Proposals* (Washington, D.C.: Employee Benefit Research Institute, 1983).

Schulz is probably best known for his textbook, *The Economics of Aging.* First published by California-based Wadsworth Publishing in 1976, it appeared in its sixth edition nineteen years later through Auburn House in New York. "Policy makers and the elderly themselves generally agree that economic security in old age is one of the most important problems needing a solution," Schulz noted in the third edition of the text. "This book attempts to present a wide range of existing knowledge, which permits a more sophisticated view of the many issues and which, in some cases, challenges the conventional wisdom."

Schulz's chapter titles for his most recent edition suggest the scope: (1) "The Economic Status of the Aged"; (2) To Work or Not to Work"; (3) "Retirement Income Planning"; (4) Social Security Old Age and Survivor Benefits"; (5) Social Security Financing: Who Pays? Who Should Pay?"; (6) "Health, Disability, and Ssi Benefits"; (7) "What Role for Employer-Sponsored Pensions?"; and (8) "Population Aging: Generational Conflict."

The fact that half of *The Economics of Aging* is devoted to public and private pensions underscores their importance in Schulz's mind. He stressed their impact on younger workers as much as he focused on the needs of retirees. Risking complaints from his fellow economists, Schulz eschewed heavily quantitative analyses in order to elucidate the economics of aging to a broad spectrum of non-economists; he wrote, "I have tried to cover technical topics in a relatively nontechnical and concise manner." Well-written and judicious in tone, Schulz's text is accessible to those with no formal training in economics.

While *The Economics of Aging* is his best-known work, Schulz has also made important theoretical contributions to the scholarly literature. He has challenged the widespread use of the notion of a "dependency ratio," which measures the proportion of those too young and too old to work compared with the numbers of men and women who are gainfully employed. See, for instance, his discussion in *The Economics of Population Aging* (New York: Auburn House, 1991). In the early 1970s, Schulz introduced the concept of "pension replacement rates" into U.S. discussions of the economics of aging. Although widely used in postwar Europe, the concept was not extensively used in the United States prior to his *Providing Adequate Retirement Income* (Hanover, N.H.: University of New England Press, 1974).

In recent years, Schulz has contributed to the growing body of research into the nature and causes of wide-scale poverty among older women; (see *The Economic Status of Divorced Older Women* (Waltham, Mass.: Brandeis University, 1993).

This early interest in cross-cultural patterns has become manifest in Schulz's writings since the late 1980s. With Deborah Davis-Friedmann he edited *Aging China: Family, Economics, and Government Policies in Transition* for the Gerontological Society of America (Washington, D.C.: *The Gerontological Society*, 1987). In his *The Economics of Population Aging*, he published research on the economics of aging in Japan; and with two Japanese collaborators, he looked at Japan's older-worker employment policies in *When "Lifetime Employment" Ends* (Waltham, Mass.: Brandeis University, 1989).

With John Myles,* he prepared "Old Age Pensions: A Comparative Perspective" for the third edition of the *Handbook of Aging and the Social Sciences,* eds. Robert H. Binstock* and Linda K. George* (New York: Academic Press, 1990). The chapter offers a pellucid summary of various theoretical perspectives on the evolution of the so-called welfare state and growth of employer-sponsored pensions during the past century in industrializing nations. In the last few years, Schulz has undertaken major international projects with the United

Nations, the International Social Security Association, and the World Bank. See, for example, *The World Aging Situation* (New York: United Nations, 1991).

Schulz has held positions in the U.S. Office of Budget and Management and at the University of New Hampshire, but he spent most of his academic career at Brandeis University. A former director of its Policy Center on Aging, he is currently professor of welfare economics and Kirstein Professor of Aging. Schulz has been active in the Gerontological Society, serving as its president in 1982.

FRANCES G. SCOTT. Frances G. Scott did her undergraduate and master's degree work in sociology with Ivan C. Belknap at the University of Texas. He continued his mentoring role when Scott moved to the University of California at Los Angeles, where she completed her Ph.D. in 1960. She also counts Talcott Parsons of Harvard University as an influential teacher. Although she never had a class with Parsons, her doctoral dissertation was based on his theoretical constructs.

Scott's most important legacy is the University of Oregon Center for Gerontology, among the first gerontology training programs established by the Administration on Aging. As the center's first director, Scott oversaw planning beginning in 1968 and presided over the first baccalaureate degrees, granted in 1978. The training program was marked by a multidisciplinary approach and a concentration on the field placement of students. Among the center's innovative work was training in pre-retirement education programs.

In addition, Scott developed a curriculum in death education for the center. The highlight was a 1970 seminar on "Confrontations of Death." It was developed with the expectation that preparing students to work with dying clients required preparing them to cope with their own eventual deaths. Seminar students were led through a simulated death experience. "In the death-denying U.S., one's own death is a scare idea, pushed away as rapidly as it arises," Scott says. She has produced a number of films and videotapes on the subject, including, "Sallie: 1893–1974" (distributed by Continuing Education Film Library, Portland, Oregon).

Scott's primary intellectual collaborations have been with her husband, Saul Toobert. As a clinical psychologist, Toobert served for several years as a paid consultant to the University of Oregon center.

Since retiring from the field in 1981, Scott has pursued a career as a novelist and travel writer.

MILDRED M. SELTZER. Mildred M. Seltzer was born in 1921. She received her B.A. in sociology and psychology from Miami University in 1942. She then earned her M.A. from the University of Chicago School of Social Service Administration in 1949 and her Ph.D. in experimental social psychology from Miami University in 1969. Fred Cottrell, an eminent sociologist and the third director of the Scripps Foundation in Population Research (established in 1922), introduced Seltzer to gerontology. He showed her the Kansas City study and other work being done by the University of Chicago's Committee on Human Development. Because Seltzer had known some of these individuals during her Chicago days, she was quickly attracted to the study of aging by Cottrell's own work, especially his two chapters in the Clark Tibbitts's* *Handbook of Social Gerontology* (Chicago: University of Chicago Press, 1961). Seltzer's decision to earn a doctorate and continue in the field of aging was also stimulated by another Cottrell protégé, Robert C. Atchley,* and by her husband.

Together, Atchley and Seltzer were to build at Miami University arguably the best master's-level program in gerontology in the nation. (A doctoral program in gerontology is now in the works.) Of the two, Seltzer is probably the better known as a spokesperson for academic gerontology.

In 1978, with frequent collaborators Tom Hickey* and Harvey Sterns, Seltzer issued *Gerontology in Higher Education: Perspectives and Issues* (Belmont, Calif.: Wadsworth Publishing, 1978), which contained papers from the 1977 meeting of the Association for Gerontology in Higher Education. This work stimulated a series of editorials, articles, and discussions, which gave greater visibility and direction to pedagogical, curricular, and organizational issues in academic gerontology.

Seltzer's other distinctive contribution to the field has been her infusion of humor into what could be dry sessions. She introduced the "Speculative Excursions" series to the annual GSA meetings—humorous commentaries on the foibles and failings of gerontology. The first of these spoof sessions, the brainchild of Martin Loeb, Vivian Wood, and Seltzer, took place in 1975. Seltzer felt that these sessions "have been important in providing us with opportunities to look at ourselves and our pomposity; to remind us that professional life is not always real and earnest and that a sense of humor provides us with some perspective and enables us to see ourselves as sometimes others see us."

Seltzer has pursued other research interests. She has written and spoken about "time" and "timing" as significant variables in the study of aging, and related this to humor. See, for example, her "Timing: the Significant Common Variable in Both Humor and Aging" in *Humor and Aging* (New York: Academic Press, 1986); and with Jon Hendricks,* "Explorations in Time: Introduction to the Fourth Dimension in Gerontology," *American Behavioral Scientist* (1986): 653–61.

Seltzer was among the first researchers to stress the importance of gender-specific issues in the processes of becoming an old woman; she has explored various aspects of retirement and fictive kin. With her friend and collaborator, Lillian E. Troll,* she explored Bortner's concept of the "Expected Life History" in an article by that name that appeared in *American Behavioral Scientist,* 29 (1986): 1446–64. Yet in all of these domains, Seltzer's chief accomplishment probably has been to suggest ideas and to raise questions that could be developed and expanded by others. Hence Seltzer characterized herself as an "eclectic gerontologist"—one who moves from topic to topic without becoming identified with any specific area.

Seltzer has served as secretary of the Gerontological Society, and has chaired and served on a variety of its committees. During her tenure as president of the Association for Gerontology in Higher Education, some of the early explorations of cooperative arrangements with GSA were held. Seltzer was also a founding member and a president of the Ohio Network of Education Consultants in the Field of Aging. This organization of academicians who work closely with practitioners in Ohio's aging network has become a model for other states.

The winner of numerous awards, Seltzer was the 1994 co-winner of the GSA Donald Kent Award. Until her death in November 1994, she was a Senior Fellow of the Scripps Gerontology Center and Professor Emerita of the Department of Sociology and Anthropology of Miami University.

WILLIAM J. SEROW. William J. Serow was born in 1946 in New York City. He began his study of economics and demographics at Boston College and went on to graduate work at Duke University, earning a Ph.D. in 1972. His dissertation, supervised by Joseph J. Spengler, is a study of the economic and demographic implications of a stationary population in the United States.

Following a brief period with the U.S. Army Finance Corps, Serow took his first major position in 1972 as research director of the Tayloe Murphy Institute's population study center in Charlottesville, Virginia. He also held the title of associate professor at the University of Virginia from 1975 until 1981. Serow began his current affiliation with Tallahassee-based Florida State University in 1978, and became a full professor of economics in 1982 and director of the Center for the Study of Population in 1990.

His study of gerontology began with an interest in studies done during the 1920s and 1930s on the economic impact of population decline and the economic consequences of aging. See, for example, "Population and Other Policy Responses to an Era of Sustained Low Fertility," *Social Science Quarterly,* 62 (1981): 323–32. He has explored migration in older populations, including his recent article, in collaboration with William H. Haas III, "Measuring the Economic Impact of Retirement Migration: The Case of Western North Carolina," *Journal of Applied Gerontology* (June 1992). Cross-national comparative studies are Serow's latest interest. See his study, "Trends in the Characteristics of the Oldest Old: 1940 to 2020," *Journal of Aging Studies,* 2 (1988): 145–56.

Serow's most significant contribution has been made in collaboration with sociologist Charles F. Longino, Jr.* Together they have identified and measured a rather surprising phenomenon: elderly people returning from popular retirement destinations to the places where they spent most of their lives. See, "Regional Differences in the Characteristics of Elderly Return Migrants," *Journal of Gerontology,* 47 (1992): S38–S43.

ETHEL SHANAS. Ethel Shanas began her long career in gerontology at the University of Chicago in January 1947. It was at the moment that she had a choice. On the one hand there was Philip M. Hauser offering a chance to help develop a program in demography and community research; on the other hand, Ernest W. Burgess* and Robert J. Havighurst* offered Shanas the opportunity to join in a new research program. She opted for the new research, aging, and completed her Ph.D. in 1949.

Since then she has been a steady contributor to the field. Her most important contributions have come in the study of the health care and health needs of the elderly, studies of the family life of older persons, and comparative cross-national research.

In 1957, she directed a national study of the health needs of older people. The survey sampled persons aged sixty-five and over, their "responsible relative," usually a son or daughter, and a cross-section of the American public for their attitudes toward the elderly. The public believed that old age and illness were synonymous. In contrast, most older persons considered themselves well, not sick. Further, the conventional wisdom notwithstanding, older people in general were not isolated from their families either physically or socially. In fact, the great majority of the elderly were functioning well in the community. More than anything else, these findings emphasized the heterogeneity of the elderly. The survey stimulated academic and government research, as well as community programs for the elderly. See her *The Health of Older People: A Social Survey* (Cambridge, Mass.: Harvard University Press, 1962).

In 1962, with colleagues in Denmark and Britain, Shanas conducted a major comparative study of the social integration of the elderly in the United States, Denmark, and Britain. The research combined national samples, comparative interview schedules, and similar analytical techniques. Again, in each country most older people were found to be "securely knitted into the social structure." Yet some of the elderly in each country experienced poverty, isolation, and inadequate health care.

The rigor and careful comparative framework of this study have helped it stand the test of time well. See Ethel Shanas, Peter Townsend, Dorothy Wedderburn, Henning Friis, Poul Milhoj and Jan Stehouwer, *Old People in Three Industrial Societies* (New York: Atherton and Routledge and Kegan Paul, 1968). In 1975, Shanas, together with Danish colleagues, repeated national surveys of the elderly.

Shanas reiterated the results of her findings in a 1979 article for *The Gerontologist*, "Social Myth as Hypothesis: The Case of the Family Relations of Older People," 19(1). Old people in industrial societies are neither alienated from their families nor rejected by their children, Shanas says. She has demonstrated that the family is the first resource for older persons in need of emotional and social support.

For more on Ethel Shanas, see Gordon F. Streib's* entry in *Women in Sociology,* ed. Mary Jo Deegan (Westport, Conn.: Greenwood Press, 1991).

DENA SHENK. Dena Shenk studied under anthropologist Sylvia Forman at the University of Massachusetts, completing her Ph.D. in 1979. She became intrigued by the conception of aging as a cultural experience and has devoted her career to exploring the diversity in the aging experience based on gender, cultural, and environmental contexts.

Shenk is particularly well known for her application of anthropological gerontology to the study of populations in the United States, especially ethnic groups, and most recently, the social networks of rural older women. Her most important work examines the formal and informal support systems of rural older women, focusing on a group of thirty older women in central Minnesota. Through an in-depth study, Shenk examined ways that older women manipulate the social support system to provide for themselves and others. She found a strong desire for independence and a correlated sense of autonomy. Her findings are recorded in "Someone to Lend a Helping Hand: Older Rural Women as Recipients and Providers of Care," *Journal of Aging Studies,* 4 (Winter 1991): 347–58. See also her work supported and published by the Central Minnesota Council on Aging, *Someone to Lend a Helping Hand: The Lives of Rural Older Women in Central Minnesota* (1987).

Shenk recently completed a comparative study of thirty older women in rural Denmark. Her publications based on this research include "The Dynamic System of Care for the Aged in Denmark" (published simultaneously in the *Journal of Aging and Social Policy,* 5 (1993): 169–86 and in *International Perspectives on State and Family Support for the Elderly,* eds. Scott A. Bass* and Robert Morris* (New York: Haworth Press, 1993), 169–86.

She has also helped to develop higher education in gerontology. Shenk outlined her approach to the study of ethics in "Using a Case Study Approach to Teach Ethics in Gerontology," *Educational Gerontology,* 16 (May–June 1990), 79–88. Her keen interest in the use of images for teaching has found an outlet in two ways. For higher education, Shenk has promoted the use of visual aids in "An Evolving Visual Methodology for Aging Research," Gerontology Society of America 1991 (with Bob Schmid and Eleanor Stokes); and "Visual Images of Aging Women," with Bob Schmid in *Generations* (Spring/Summer 1993): 71–74, also published in *Changing Perceptions of Aging and the Aged,* eds. Dena Shenk and W. Andrew Achenbaum (New York: Springer Publishers, 1994), 71–74.

For the general public, she has collaborated with Bob Schmid of St. Cloud State University, Minnesota to create photographic exhibits to bring the aging experience to a larger population. These have been shown in public buildings, including libraries, banks, senior centers, and nursing homes. She has developed and directs a continuing education program for those working with older adults in the community and has published "Meeting the Educational Needs of Service

Providers: The Effects of a Continuing Education Program on Self-Reported Knowledge and Attitudes About Aging," in *Educational Gerontology* (in press) based on this project.

Shenk is currently coordinator of the interdisciplinary program in gerontology at the University of North Carolina in Charlotte. She is also a professor of anthropology in the Department of Sociology, Anthropology, and Social Work.

SUSAN R. SHERMAN. Susan R. Sherman completed her doctoral work with M. Brewster Smith at the University of California at Berkeley in 1964. With a newly minted Ph.D. in hand she was hired by Daniel Wilner at the University of California at Los Angeles to work on an NIMH-funded study of retirement housing. Since 1974, she has been at the School of Social Welfare of the University of Albany, and she served as director of the Institute of Gerontology from 1975 to 1980. She has served as president of the Association for Gerontology in Higher Education and the New York State Association of Gerontological Educators.

Sherman found a congenial match between the "person-in-environment" approach of social psychology and the study of the elderly. Sherman sees social psychology as a methodological beacon for social welfare theorists and social planners in search of a balance between the individual and the environment. The social ecology of aging has been Sherman's primary area of interest. Her major studies for the past three decades have been concerned with environments for the elderly, including foster family homes, retirement villages and hotels, life-care communities, domiciliary care facilities, and age-integrated community housing. In addition to the physical variations of these settings, Sherman has examined the interpersonal and normative aspects of the environment. The subjects in these studies have ranged from well elderly to frail dependent elderly, including mentally ill and mentally retarded older persons. Sherman recently summarized her work in "Housing," a chapter for the *Handbook of Gerontological Services,* 2nd edn., edited by A. Monk (New York: Columbia University, 1990). See also Sherman's article, "A Social Psychological Perspective on the Continuum of Housing for the Elderly," *Journal of Aging Studies,* 2 (1988): 229–41.

Sherman's research themes have integrated theory and application. In the 1960s, the controversy over the effects of age segregation was a critical consideration in planning environments for the elderly. The 1970s brought the challenge of caring for the recently deinstitutionalized and finding alternatives to institutions. In the 1980s and 1990s, interests turned to developing and extending theory, and exploring long dormant options. It was in that context that Sherman extended theories pertaining to age homogeneity along a continuum from highly age-segregated to age-integrated environments, as well as employing a theoretical approach to understanding questions of family and community integration for frail individuals in non-institutional environments. Her references include S. R. Sherman and E. S. Newman, *Foster Families for Adults: A Community Al-*

ternative in Long-Term Care (New York: Columbia University Press, 1988); and R. A. Ward,* M. LaGory, and S. R. Sherman, *The Environment for Aging: Interpersonal, Social and Spatial Contexts* (Tuscaloosa, Ala. University of Alabama Press, 1988). Sherman's other areas of interest and scholarship include images of middle-aged and older women, intergenerational relations, and social psychology of age identity. See S. R. Sherman, "Changes in Age Identity: Self Perceptions in Middle and Late Life," *Journal of Aging Studies,* 8 (1994): 397–412.

A professor of social welfare of public health at the University of Albany of the State University of New York, Sherman has received research grants from NIMH, AARP Andrus Foundation, New York State Health Research Council, and SUNY Research Foundation. She is a Fellow of the Gerontological Society of America, and has received the Walter M. Beattie, Jr. Award for Distinguished Service in Gerontology, State Society on Aging of New York.

SYLVIA SHERWOOD. Sylvia Sherwood earned her B.A. in sociology from Hunter College in 1945. Her first peer-reviewed article, with D. Robinson, on "A Public Opinion Study of Anti-Semitism in New York City," was published in the *American Sociological Review,* 10 (1945): 511–16, a few months later. After serving as an instructor in the Statistics Laboratory at New York University, Sherwood took her graduate degrees in sociology from the school (M.A., 1950; Ph.D., 1955). While in graduate school she served as an instructor at Brooklyn College. For the next decade, Sherwood held teaching posts at Adelphi, Hofstra, and C. W. Post colleges. She also did work with the Long Island Business Research Associates.

In 1965, Sherwood became director of the Department of Social Gerontological Research at the Hebrew Rehabilitation Center for the Aged in Boston. Her first project studied converging community services on a home for aged waiting list. Sherwood then received support from the U.S. Department of Housing and Urban Development and the Administration on Aging, as well as agencies of the Commonwealth of Massachusetts, to study sheltered housing, medically oriented specialized housing, and alternatives to institutionalization for the elderly and chronically ill. Sherwood increasingly became identified with efforts to develop assessments of needs for domiciliary care and ways to create effective informal support systems.

Much of Sherwood's early ideas about alternatives to institutionalization were captured in three books that she edited: *Research Planning and Action for the Elderly,* edited with Donald P. Kent* and Robert Kastenbaum* (New York: Behavioral Publications, 1972); *Long-Term Care: A Handbook for Researchers, Planners, and Providers* (New York: Spectrum Publications, 1975); and *An Alternative in Long-Term Care: The Highland Heights Experiment* (Cambridge, Mass.: Ballinger Publication Company, 1981), which Sherwood edited with D. S. Greer, J. N. Morris, and Vincent Mor,* and associates.

In the 1980s, Sherwood focused specifically on high-risk elders and care for

NATHAN W. SHOCK 321

frail older persons. See, for instance, her essay with J. Morris on the "Quality of Life of Cancer Patients at Different Stages in the Disease Trajectory," *Journal of Chronic Diseases,* 40 (1987). Lately, Sherwood has been writing about aging in place. See, for example, her two essays, "CCRCs: An Option for Aging in Place," and "Aging in Place: A Longitudinal Example," in *Aging in Place,* eds. David Tilson and Charles E. Fahey* (Glenview, Ill.: Scott, Foresman and Company, 1989).

Sherwood has been on the editorial board of the *International Journal of Aging and Human Development* since 1969 and was an associate editor of *The Gerontologist* from 1967 to 1970. She has served on numerous task forces in the Commonwealth of Massachusetts and for the federal government. In 1983, she received the American Association of Homes for the Aging Distinguished Service Award for Research in recognition of her efforts to improve long-term care. In 1991, Sherwood received both the Northeastern Gerontological Society's Ollie Randall* Award and the Association of Massachusetts Homes for the Aging's Public Service Award.

NATHAN W. SHOCK. Nathan Wetherwell Shock was born in Lafayette, Indiana, on Christmas Day, 1906. He received his undergraduate degree in chemical engineering (1926) and master's degree in organic chemistry (1927) from Purdue University. Although he often claimed that he had intended to pursue a doctorate in engineering at the University of Chicago, he was initially put off by the long lines at registration and moved instead to the shorter queue for psychology. The switch was fateful.

By 1930, he had earned his Ph.D. in physiological psychology under the tutelage of A. Baird Hastings,* one of the preeminent biological chemists of this century, and L. L. Thurstone, who made his reputation by demonstrating the value of factor analysis in the social sciences. Shock's dissertation on "Studies of Acid-Base Balance of the Blood" showed early on some of his intellectual and practical strengths. Shock's concern for measurement issues was evident; he designed a pipette that could measure several components on the same small sample of blood. "Never did I have a better, more successful student," Hastings recalled in a letter published in *Experimental Gerontology,* 21 (1986), on the occasion of Shock's eightieth birthday. "When I would suggest duplicate analyses, they would usually appear in triplicate. That describes Nathan Shock and his search for accuracy in Gerontology."

Shock then spent nine years at Berkeley, collaborating on a major longitudinal study of adolescent growth. There, he met Lawrence K. Frank,* a foundation officer keenly interested in issues of development and aging, and received additional training from such eminent developmental psychologists as Harold and Mary Cover Jones and Jean MacFarlane. He made semi-annual physiological and psychological measurements on fifty girls and fifty boys as they matured from ages ten to eighteen. Ultimately, Shock published thirty-four chapters and articles for a variety of scholarly journals.

Some of Shock's studies begun in Berkeley were completed in Baltimore, where he had moved, on Baird Hasting's recommendation, to head the U.S. Public Health Services Unit on Gerontology. Shock found that he had to rely on the Baltimore City Hospitals for laboratory space and access to patients in the Old People's Home, since the National Institutes of Health in Bethesda had no hospital or facilities for clinical research. As he recalled forty years later, "Our first laboratory was a kind of closet, about twelve by fifteen feet. It had a sink in it and that was about all. We didn't have a budget for equipment, so we scrounged what we could." World War II delayed Shock's immersion into gerontology, though he did recruit his first two physicians—James O. Davis and Dean Davies—to begin an extensive series of measurements of the effects of age on a variety of physiological systems.

After the war ended, Shock's primary task was to promote research and training in aging at the federal level. No government scientist did more in this regard than he. With additional staff and resources, Shock launched an ambitious research program, much of which was devoted to describing in quantitative terms age differences in the specific organ systems as well as integrated responses by normal human adults between the ages of twenty and one hundred to physiological stresses. The first studies on aging focused on the kidney. See Nathan W. Shock, "Insulin, Diodrast and Urea Clearance Studies on Aged Human Subjects," *Federal Proceedings, Baltimore*, 4 (1945): 65; "Age Changes in Kidney Function of Human Subjects," *Federal Proceedings, Baltimore*, 5 (1946): 94–95; and "Kidney Function Tests in Aged Males," *Geriatrics*, 1 (1947): 232–39.

Shock directed what was to become NIH's intramural Gerontology Research Center in Baltimore from 1941 until his mandatory retirement in 1976; he served as a Scientist Emeritus until his death in 1989. The program expanded within the National Heart Institute (1949–1965) and then was transferred to the National Institute of Child Health and Human Development (1965–1975) before becoming part of the newly established National Institute on Aging. A rat colony was established in 1954; senescent rats were raised to study decrements in various systems over time. As programs developed, increasing emphasis was placed on isolated tissues to learn more about cellular and molecular aspects of aging.

In addition to supervising basic laboratory studies of his own, Shock tried to encourage other scientists to do research on aging. With support from the Forest Park Foundation, he compiled a *Classified Bibliography of Gerontology and Geriatrics* (Stanford, Calif.: Stanford University Press, 1951), which featured 16,036 entries. References to the biology of aging (items No. 116 to No. 3,164) and organ systems (items No. 3,165 to No. 11,784) dominate the volume. Another 2,170 entries dealt with geriatric medicine. The remaining 4,080 citations mixed social and economic aspects of aging with historical features, psychological processes, and other items. Supplements to the bibliography were published as bound volumes in 1957 and 1963. Additional entries appeared regularly in the *Journal of Gerontology* until the 1980s.

As part of his effort to lay the foundations for a research program at Stanford University, a venture that never got off the ground, Shock began to think systematically about how work in gerontology had been emerging over the past several decades and how it should be organized to take advantage of tremendous advances in science. "In the broadest sense, problems of growth, development and maturation are as much a part of gerontology as are those of atrophy, degeneration, and decline," Shock wrote in "Gerontology (Later Maturity)," in *Annual Review of Psychology,* 11 (1951), but he stressed mainly "changes that occur in later maturity and senescence." From this thinking came two editions of *Trends in Gerontology* (Stanford, Calif.: Stanford University Press, 1951, 1957). In the second edition he stressed that gerontology institutes should focus on four major areas: (1) the general biology of aging; (2) the physiological and psychological aspects of aging in humans; (3) the clinical problems of aging persons; and (4) the socioeconomic problems of an aging population. "The goal of research in gerontology is not to extend the life span, but to minimize disabilities and handicaps of old age," Shock wrote. "The ultimate goal of action programs in the field of aging is to minimize the individual and social handicaps of old age as they now exist."

By 1960 Shock had organized the Gerontology Research Center's program into three categories. The section on basic biology of aging focused on molecular biology, biophysics, cellular and comparative physiology, intermediary metabolism, nutritional biochemistry, and morphology. Researchers in human physiology assessed age differences in cardiovascular and renal systems, endocrinology and metabolism, and pulmonary physiology and exercise. Those who engaged in behavioral analyses dealt with physiological issues (such as the role of the nervous system and deficits in the senses and motor skills) and did experimental research on changes in learning and memory as well as alterations in personality characteristics.

Many scientists under Shock's supervision worked on the Baltimore Longitudinal Study on Aging (BLSA). This study began in 1958 with assistance from W. W. Peter, a retired medical officer in the U.S. Public Health Service. For more on this, see Joseph T. Freeman's account, "Bits of Fossils," *Experimental Gerontology,* 21 (1986): 219–28. Initially, every two years the researchers measured physiological and psychological aspects of 650 male subjects between the ages of twenty and ninety-six; women were added to the sample in 1978. The first comprehensive report from the BLSA analysis, *Normal Human Aging* (Bethesda: National Institute of Health, 1984) presented results test by test, differentiating longitudinal and cross-sectional analyses of performance scores. Shock contributed two chapters to the collection: "Energy Metabolism, Caloric Intake, and Physical Activity of the Aging" (Bethesda: National Institute of Health, first published in 1972); and (with Reuben Andres,* Jordan Tobin, and A. H. Norris) "Patterns of Longitudinal Changes in Renal Function" (Bethesda: National Institute of Health, first published in 1979), which demonstrated that some individuals maintained their renal function. Relying on Shock's "functionalist" approach to measuring age-related changes, other scholars have used these findings to integrate their understanding of physiological mechanisms over the lifespan.

Shock (co)wrote more than 350 publications dealing mainly with biochemical, behavioral, and physiological aspects of human aging. He trained more than 200 postdoctoral fellows, including three future presidents of the Gerontological Society—Reuben Andres,* James E. Birren,* and John W. Rowe.* In part to accommodate the growing needs of investigators associated with the BLSA survey and burgeoning specialized studies, plans were made to construct a separate building for the Gerontology Research Center (GRC) on the grounds of the Baltimore City Hospitals. In June 1968, a four-story building with 200,000 square feet of laboratory and office space was dedicated for studies of the molecular biology of aging, comparative physiology of aging, clinical psychology, and behavioral sciences. At the time, friends affectionately called it "The House that Nathan Built." In 1989, the GRC was formally renamed the Nathan W. Shock Aging Research Laboratories.

Although Shock's skills as a research manager grew over time, his views about how scientific gerontological inquiries should be conducted changed little. Compare, for instance, his "Current Concepts in the Aging Process," *Journal of the American Medical Association,* 176 (February 25, 1961): 656, with "Theoretical Concepts Governing Gerontological Research" (with George T. Baker III*) in *Potential for Nutritional Modulation of Aging Processes,* ed. D. K. Ingram et al. (Trumball, Conn.: Food and Nutritional Press, 1990). Toward the end of his life, Shock talked at length with George T. Baker III about six tenets that should animate all research on aging:

1. Give a testable hypothesis. It is worth a thousand theories.

2. Formulate questions to address basic mechanisms of aging and design scientifically rigorous protocols to examine those questions.

3. Focus research on the processes of aging over the entire lifespan. Studies on older individuals may tell one about diseases in later life but are not likely to yield information about the basic mechanisms of aging.

4. Aging and disease are not synonymous. There are processes of aging and etiologies of disease. The relationships between the two are important but not inevitable.

5. Aging is a dynamic equilibrium. The rates of aging differ for various systems in any given organism, however. It is the whole organism that ages and dies.

6. Well-documented observations and good scientific data are timeless. Also, don't overlook studies in other scientific fields. Much of our knowledge of gerontology today is a byproduct of non-aging research.

Because he believed that biological aging was a universal phenomenon, Shock closely followed research developments in evolutionary and comparative biology. In addition to his rat colony, he kept species of *Drosophila,* rotifers, and other animals at the GRC. His breadth of interest in turn spurred him to build other institutions intended to promote research on aging in a variety of disciplines.

For instance, Shock was very active in the Gerontological Society, which was incorporated in 1945. He served as president in 1960–1961, then became editor-in-chief of the *Journal of Gerontology* (1963–1968), and chaired the Publications Committee (1966–1974). While he welcomed well-trained investigators to do research on aging, he was keenly aware that professional standards had to be set high. He repeatedly warned, for instance, that biologists would only join a multidisciplinary group that was as rigorous scientifically as any constituent group in the American Institute of Biological Sciences. He held equally strong opinions about quality control in the journals. In 1959, when members of the Gerontological Society's Section on Social Welfare considered forming a *Journal of Applied Gerontology,* Shock said that "if the Social Welfare people have research results that will meet the standards on research, they would go in the *Journal of Gerontology* [JG]. If someone makes a general talk about the implications of biological research for medicine and social science, this kind of what I call hot-air artistry would go in the bulletin. If someone has a specific study with some numbers and some data it would then go into the *JG*" (from the transcript of the November 11, 1959, meeting of the GSA council). As funds fell short for annual meetings and publications, Shock occasionally provided costs that the society could not meet out of his own pocket, or he allowed work to be done at the GRC. In addition, Shock held leadership positions in the American Psychological Association, the Society for Experimental Biology and Medicine, and the American Heart Association.

Shock was also very active in establishing the International Association of Gerontology. He knew that European scholars had been doing solid research and convening scientific symposia on aging long before U.S. investigators met in 1937 at Woods Hole, Massachusetts—the event that probably marks the birth of gerontology in this country. As late as the 1950s, Britain, not the United States, set the pace for researchers on aging in the international community. A British Society for Research on Ageing had been founded in 1939; no U.S. aging-related research facility enjoyed the prestige, resources, and reputation of the Oxford Gerontological Research Unit, which was started in 1945 under the direction of the Russian-born experimental pathologist V. Korenchevsky.

Shock was an official representative at the First International Congress in Liege, Belgium, held in July 1950. He was active in all of the next twelve congresses and served as president of the Eighth International Congress, which met in Washington in 1969. With the assistance of George T. Baker III,* Shock wrote his memories in *The International Association of Gerontology: A Chronicle—1950 to 1986* (New York: Springer Publishing, 1987). Because of the increasing involvement by North American gerontologists and influence of U.S. scientific institutions, the volume serves in part as a way to gauge Shock's own sense of the development of the field. Also to be consulted is his "Historical Perspectives on Aging," in *Environmental Physiology: Aging, Heat, and Altitude,* ed. Yousef Horvath (New York: Elsevier North Holland, 1980).

Shock's contributions to the science of gerontology were amply rewarded. He received the first Brookdale Award from the Gerontological Society of America as well as the first award of the American Federation for Aging Research. He delivered a Kleemeier Lecture for the Gerontological Society and won the American Geriatrics Society's Willard O. Thompson Award. Both the American Heart Association and the American Aging Association honored his research. Besides honorary degrees from Purdue and Johns Hopkins University, he won the Chancellor's Award from Syracuse University. The National Council on the Aging gave him the Ollie Randall Award. The federal government honored Shock by bestowing the Department of Health, Education, and Welfare Superior Service and Distinguished Service awards.

In "Obituary: Nathan's Last Words," delivered *in absentia* by George Baker at the 1989 Gerontological Society's annual meetings and reprinted in *Experimental Gerontology,* 25 (1990): 205–209, Shock summed up his life's career:

> To my many good friends and cherished colleagues. I have appreciated the opportunity to know and work with many of you. I have had a good life and have no regrets. For those of you here and others in the field of gerontology, I would remind you that we were formed and nurtured in the firm belief that the biological phenomenon we call 'aging' was worthy of scientific pursuit. We have achieved some degree of success. I would caution, however, that our future will be determined only, and only, by the quality of scientific research on understanding the basic mechanisms of the aging process.

On his death in 1989, much of his estate went to the Nathan W. and Margaret T. Shock Aging Research Foundation.

HERBERT SHORE. Herbert Shore earned his master's degree in social work from Columbia University in 1952. He completed his doctorate in education from the University of North Texas in Denton, Texas, in 1969. His long career in gerontology began with the encouragement of Graenum Berger, head worker of the Bronx House Community Center. As a licensed institutional administrator, social worker, and educator, Shore has worked as a gerontologist-practitioner for over forty years. He became a fellow of the Gerontological Society in 1982.

He was one of the founders and is a past president of the American Association of Homes for Aging. Shore created the organization to help refocus the care of the institutionalized aged away from a heavy emphasis on the medical model. He balanced the existing emphasis on medical aspects and physical care and treatment with the social components of care. By devoting an annual meeting to the topic of social components, out of which came a publication, Shore was able to help create recognition of the psychosocial needs of the elderly.

As a practitioner and educator, Shore has long been concerned with sensitizing "hands on" employees to the aging process. With Marvin Ernst in 1975, he developed a training model and co-wrote *Sensitizing People to the Processes of Aging*. The volume is now in its second edition (Denton, Texas: Center for Studies in Aging, Texas State University, 1988), and has been widely used.

Shore also worked to further therapeutic interventions and treatment modalities. In particular, he has sought alternatives to institutionalization and explored the relationship between institutional and non-institutional services. He has advanced the campus concept for elder care, "parallel service" provision, and a continuum of care.

An interest in how perceptions of the elderly are communicated led Shore to create a stamp album with the late Joseph T. Freeman* of older people on stamps, or "Gerontophilately."

In addition to teachers such as Gertrude Landau, Shore counts such familiar names as Clark Tibbits* and Wilma Donahue* among his mentors. (Shore taught a class on retirement housing management with Donahue from 1967 to 1970). He is currently affiliated with the North American Association of Jewish Homes and Housing for the Aging, and teaches at the Center for Studies in Aging at the University of North Texas. He has served as chairman of the Senior Affairs Commission of the City of Dallas, president of Senior Citizens of Greater Dallas, and on the board of the Texas (State) Department of Health. Shore was a delegate to the 1961, 1971, and 1981 White House Conferences on Aging.

JACOB S. SIEGEL. Jacob S. Siegel earned his B.A. and M.A. at the University of Pennsylvania. His aging-related work began in 1972, after he had made his mark as a demographer with the federal government. In that year, Arthur Campbell, deputy director of the Center for Population Research in the National Institute of Child Health and Human Development (NICHHD), invited Siegel to contribute a document on the demography of aging to the NIH's First Conference on the Epidemiology of Aging. Siegel attended the NICHHD meeting. His paper was published as "Some Demographic Aspects of Aging in the United States," in *Epidemiology of Aging,* eds. Adrian M. Ostfeld and Don C. Gibson (Baltimore, Md.: National Institutes of Health, 1972). He then became increasingly interested in developing the field. He contributed an updated version of this paper to the Second Conference on the Epidemiology of Aging in 1977. With the support of the National Institute on Aging, he elaborated these papers into a series of Census Bureau publications, culminating in the publication in 1984 of *The Demographic and Socioeconomic Aspects of Aging in the United States* in the Census Bureau's Current Population Reports series.

Siegel justifiably considers himself one of the "fathers" of a subfield that lies at the intersection of gerontology and demography. Taking advantage of his role as a major figure in demography, Siegel gave attention to aging issues in a sort of second career. He introduced the term "gerontic" (to replace "geriatric") into the technical vocabulary that gerontologists and demographers use to describe the elderly population. Through International Population Union and with the International Glossary of Social Gerontology of the International Federation on Aging, he has contributed to standardizing and refining the terminology at the intersection of demography and gerontology. Siegel made aging the subject of his presidential address before the Population Association of America; see "On the Demography of Aging," *Demography,* 17 (1980): 345–64. "Gerontic" themes were featured prominently in *The Methods and Materials of Demography,* which he published with Henry S. Shryock (a colleague both in the U.S. Bureau of the Census and the Department of Demography, Georgetown University), and associates. The two-volume text was first published by the U.S. Bureau of the Census in 1971 and reprinted three times (last printing in 1980); with Edward Stockwell, Siegel issued a "condensed" version (New York: Academic Press, 1976).

Siegel claims that his primary role has been that of synthesizer, data producer, and interpreter rather than that of original researcher. See, for instance, the paper he produced originally for the 1982 World Assembly on Aging in Vienna, with Sally L. Hoover, "Demographic Aspects of the Health of the Elderly in the Year 2000 and Beyond," *World Health Statistics Quarterly,* 35 (1982): 133–202. Yet at other times he was prepared to speculate, though rarely straying far from his data. See the essay, "Demographic Dimensions of an Aging Population," which Siegel wrote with Cynthia M. Taeuber for *Our Aging Society,* eds. Alan Flier and Lydia Bronte (New York: W. W. Norton, 1986), 79–110). There, he spelled out the consequences of low-middle fertility, extremely low mortality, and middle immigration: He envisaged the possibility of a "gerontic dependency" ratio three and a half times that at present. Under these assumptions, major technological innovations and institutional adjustments would be necessary by the middle of the next century.

More recently, Siegel published a major work on aging—one of the volumes in the latest census monograph series, *The Population of the United States in the 1980s,* titled *A Generation of Change: A Profile of America's Older Population* (New York: Russell Sage Foundation, 1993).

In the last decade, Siegel has been a sort of roving lecturer on the demography and sociology of aging, presiding over graduate courses at the University of Maryland, the University of California at Berkeley, Cornell University, and George Mason University. His recent research has concerned the measurement of trends in retirement age (with Murray Gendell), historical shifts in the share of elderly women with adult children, developing a typology of measures of population aging, and designing cohort and period generalized patterns of age-cycle changes in various socioeconomic characteristics.

Siegel's major mentors are former senior Census Bureau officials and professors of demography at Georgetown, Henry Shryock and Conrad Taeuber. Two of his major role models—Nathan Keyfitz and Ansley Coale, professors emeriti of demography at Harvard and Princeton, respectively—have written extensively on population aging. Yet of all of his "seniors," it is John W. Riley* whose career pattern most closely resembles Siegel's. Neither man would wish to be considered primarily a researcher on aging, yet each, through his efforts in collaboration with others, has enriched the field through insights cultivated outside the field of gerontology.

ALEXANDER SIMON. Alexander Simon was born in New York in 1906. He was educated at Columbia University, where he received his B.A. (1926) and M.D. (1930). After an internship at St. Joseph's Hospital in Paterson, New Jersey (1930–1931), Simon did a residency in psychiatry at St. Elizabeth's Hospital in Washington, D.C. (1931–1934). From 1935 to 1943, he was an associate in neurology at the George Washington University Medical School.

From 1945 to 1974, Simon was a professor of psychiatry at the School of Medicine in the University of California at San Francisco. He chaired the department from 1956 to 1974. From 1943 to 1956, Simon was assistant medical superintendent of the Langley Porter Neuropsychiatric Institute; he was medical director from 1956 to 1974. Concurrently, Simon was a consultant to the Letterman Army Hospital in San Francisco; from 1949 to 1958, the Palo Alto Veterans Administration Hospital; and several Air Force units from 1953 to 1963.

Toward the end of his career, Simon published "Physical and Socio-Psychologic Stress in the Geriatric Mentally Ill," *Comprehensive Gerontology,* 11 (May 1970): 242–47. There, he argued that patients rarely required just one type of treatment or service; the deprivations suffered in late life tended to be multiple. He stated that geriatricians should try to provide services conducive "to a comfortable, safe, and satisfying life within the limitations of their physical and mental capacities." Simon was also one of the first to study the demographic characteristics of psychiatric patients suffering from alcoholism. In "Alcoholism in the Geriatric Mentally Ill" (with Leon Epstein and Lynn Reynolds) in *Geriatrics,* 23 (October 1968): 125–31, the authors noted that more than a quarter of those men and women over age sixty admitted to an institution had a serious drinking problem; 38 percent had evidence of alcoholic chronic brain syndrome, and another 20 percent had arteriosclerotic chronic brain syndrome.

Simon served on many local, state, and national commissions dealing with the problems of the elderly. He was a delegate to the 1961 and 1971 White House Conferences on Aging, a trustee of the San-Francisco-based Pacific Institute for Living (1964–1970), and commissioner of the California Commission on Aging (1976–1979). Simon was a member of the (federal) Government Interdepartmental Committee on the Problems of the Aging (1960–1966). From 1956 to 1965, he served on several review panels for the National Institute of Mental Health. In the 1960s, he was on several advisory committees for the Federal Housing Administration.

In 1967, the U.S. Army gave him its Outstanding Civilian Service Medal. The Western Gerontological Society honored him in 1977, and he received the Gerontological Society's Kent Award five years later.

LESTER SMITH. Biologist Lester Smith earned his Ph.D. from the University of California in San Francisco in 1969. There he worked with the late Richard Fineberg. He was initially attracted to the field of gerontology by Lester Packer, by doing research on the aging of mitochondria, at the University of California at Berkeley.

His significant contributions to the field have been primarily related to the organization and implementation of programs for the National Institute on Aging, in particular, the first national program on the biology of aging. In 1980, he was responsible for grant and contract activity in excess of $26 million, covering 175 academic institutions. He created the Biology of Aging Summer Institute for postdoctoral students in aging research. The program lasted four years and served some 150 participants. Most of these students remain active researchers and teachers in gerontology and geriatrics.

As director of the Immunology Program at the NIA, Smith oversaw the program's funding of more than thirty laboratories. It focused on the fundamental and clinical aspects of the immunological basis of aging. The nature of the program is reflected in *Immunological Aspects of Aging,* eds. by Lester Smith and Diego Segre (New York: M. Dekker, 1981). As chairman of the minority task force of the Biological Sciences Section of the Gerontological Society of America in 1989, Smith, along with onetime GSA President Richard C. Adelman,* emphasized the relevance of biological studies to resolving the problems of the non-white minority elderly. In a witty editorial, "Message to Biologists from the GSA Taskforce on Minority Issues in Gerontology" (January 1989, 44:B1-3), the authors discussed "ethnically" distinct rat populations that could be used to study variations in the aging process. As a result, they argued, "it may be possible to design animal model experiments that address the appropriateness of current social policies that are applied to elderly people."

Smith also served as the first director of the Multidisciplinary Center for the Study of Aging at the State University of New York, in Buffalo. His current project is developing a geriatric program for the medical students and residents of Howard University's College of Medicine.

JOAN SMITH-SONNEBORN. Joan Smith-Sonneborn completed her doctoral work in zoology at the University of Indiana in 1962. There, she became fascinated by the resistance of single-celled organisms to radiation.

Her most important contribution to the study of aging came in the late 1970s and was sparked by this fascination. Studying a single-celled protozoan, she discovered that ultraviolet (UV) radiation could extend lifespan. High doses of UV radiation had been known to cause DNA damage and to shorten lifespan. However, Smith-Sonneborn found that the lower doses stimulated a stress response, which in turn lengthened lifespan. She advanced the theory that the induced damage could be stimulating repair and subsequent resistance to higher doses. See "DNA Repair and Longevity Assurance in Paramecium Aurelia," *Science,* 203: 1115–17. She has subsequently advanced the more general theory that toxic agents at certain doses could stimulate beneficial responses, including increased longevity.

In addition, she has contributed the idea that there are suites of genes that are essential for health and long life. Imperfection in any of the suites will shorten lifespan. Aging, therefore, is not caused by a single gene, but by a relatively small number of suites. For example, one suite is related to DNA repair, while another affects cholesterol metabolism. The combination of suites shapes the aging process for individuals. We do not all age in the same fashion, but in a "family" way according to a combination of suites. See Smith-Sonneborn's chapter, "How We Age," in *The Promise of Productive Aging,* edited by R. Butler,* M. Oberlink, and M. Schechter (New York: Springer, 1990).

Smith-Sonneborn cautions that she has not finished her research. "The best is yet to come," she says. She is currently affiliated with the Program in Aging and Human Development and the Department of Zoology and Physiology at the University of Wyoming.

MICHAEL A. SMYER. Michael A. Smyer graduated with a B.A. from Yale University in 1972 and earned his Ph.D. in psychology from Duke University in 1977. The work of Margaret Gatz* and Ilene Siegler attracted him to the study of the elderly. Their work on evaluating the effects of alternative services for older adults in state mental hospitals led Smyer to an interest in variability between individuals and within individuals across the lifespan.

Smyer has applied psychological theory and practice to the problems of impaired older adults, especially those in long-term care settings. Much of his work has incorporated the concept of plasticity, or adaptability, in later life. Some of his studies have explored the consequences of non-normative events, such as mid-life divorce. In other studies his team has focused on the behavioral functioning of impaired residents in long-term care settings. He most recently directed the Penn State Nursing Home Intervention project, which assessed interventions designed to affect the performance of nursing assistance through training and job redesign. The study found that while knowledge could be increased significantly, performance was not improved. See Michael A. Smyer, Diane Brannon, and Margaret D. Cohn, "Improving Nursing Home Care Through Training and Job Redesign," *Gerontologist,* 32 (1992): 327–33.

Smyer is currently affiliated with Boston College.

JAY SOKOLOVSKY. Jay Sokolovsky was born in 1947 in Brooklyn, New York. He majored in anthropology at Brooklyn College, earning a B.A. in 1969. He did graduate work at Pennsylvania State University (M.A. 1971, Ph.D. 1974). His dissertation included ethnographic field research in San Jeronimo Amatango,

332   DAVID O. STAATS

Mexico, which sought to understand indigenous forms of ecological adaptation and community organization. In particular, he looked at ways these structures were transformed in response to regional urbanization.

Upon completion of his doctorate, Sokolovsky held positions at four institutions simultaneously between 1974 and 1976. He was a visiting assistant professor at Seton Hall University (South Orange, New Jersey), and an adjunct assistant professor at Fordham University at Lincoln Center, Marymount Manhattan College, and the New York Institute of Technology. He accepted a permanent post at the University of Maryland in Baltimore County in 1976, and he quickly rose through the ranks, becoming a full professor in the Department of Sociology and Anthropology in 1986.

Work in the field of gerontology began in 1975 when the Office of Urban Health Affairs of the New York University Medical Center contracted Sokolovsky to coordinate urban ethnographic research of the social networks of geriatric populations living in mid-Manhattan residential hotels and "Skid Row."

Throughout this urban research, Carl I. Cohen has been an ever-present collaborator. In addition to numerous articles, the pair collaborated on *Old Men of the Bowery: Survival Strategies of the Homeless* (New York: Guilford Press, 1989). The book was a product of an National Institute of Mental Health-funded study of the social networks and health of elderly men in downtown New York.

More recently, Sokolovsky has been interested in aging in the former Yugoslavia. His research has included a study of aging and social support in rural Croatia, done in the mid-1980s with the Zagreb-based Andrija Stampa School of Public Health. Currently, he is working on a study of self-help groups for the aged in Zagreb. See J. Sokolovsky, S. Sosic, and G. Pavlekovic, "Self Help Groups for the Aged in Yugoslavia: How Effective Are They?" *Journal of Cross-Cultural Gerontology,* 6 (1991): 319–30.

Sokolovsky has not turned his back on his original interest in Latin America. He began in 1993 a study of abandonment of the frail elderly in Tepexpan, Mexico. He also has worked on a study of the voluntary relocation of elderly to the planned community of Columbia, Maryland (1982–1983), and a study of board and care homes for the elderly throughout the state (1989–1991).

DAVID O. STAATS. David O. Staats attended the University of Chicago Medical School, completing his M.D. in 1976. He began clinical studies at the Michael Reese Hospital where, he says, "fine physicians showed me the right way to care for sick old persons."

His primary area of interest has been the nursing home. In a chapter for *Geriatric Medicine,* edited by C. K. Cassel and John R. Walsh (New York: Springer-Verlag, 1984), Staats showed that small improvements in one area of a patient's treatment can bring about large functional improvements in another. "Physical Environments" emphasizes the value of searching for treatable conditions afflicting older persons.

Staats has also written on "The Role of the Nursing Home Medical Director,"

Clinics in Geriatric Medicine, 4 (1988): 493–506, from his experience at the West Side Veterans Administration Medical Center of Chicago. He pointed to the interdisciplinary role of the medical director, who must cope with a variety of issues to best serve residents and staff. He outlined an algorithm to describe the way decisions are made in a nursing home; it shows where and how to intervene in nursing homes to upgrade care.

However, it is his role as a teacher that Staats finds most fulfilling. He is currently a professor at the College of Medicine of the University of Illinois at Chicago.

E. PERCIL STANFORD. E. Percil Stanford first became interested in research on aging in 1960. He was attracted to the field by Dr. Earl Moses, a professor of sociology at Morgan State University. Stanford went on to earn his M.A. (1967) and Ph.D. (1968) from Iowa State University. From 1961 to 1972, he worked in Washington, D.C., as a specialist in aging at the U.S. Administration on Aging and as a staff member to Senator Alan Cranston and Representative Shirley Chisholm. Stanford has spent most of his academic career since 1972 at the University Center on Aging at San Diego State University.

Most of Stanford's work has focused on research, training, and practice in the field of minority aging. He is particularly proud of *Elder Black* (San Diego: Campanile Publishing, 1978). The book focused on a segment of the aged population that has generally been underplayed because of the emphasis placed on the needs of older African Americans who live in urban areas, and because of the stereotypical notion that most suburbs are white refuges. Nonetheless, Stanford demonstrated that a small but important segment of blacks in America were in fact growing old in suburbs and exurbs that were themselves aging.

In subsequent writings, Stanford elaborated the notion of "diverse life patterns." Nearly all racial and ethnic groups have life histories that are unique. They cannot be evaluated and analyzed without comparison with a majority group that has a different social, political, and economic history. See, for instance, his "Diverse Black Aged," in *Black Aged: Understanding Diversity and Service Needs,* ed. Zev Harel (Cleveland: Cleveland State University Press, 1990), 33–49. To this end, Stanford has also been engaged in a study of the health and functional dependency of older minorities and whites. This study has provided a unique opportunity to examine cross-sectional similarities and differences among ethnic and racially different older people. Especially notable is the representation of Mexican-Americans in the sample of 2,105 subjects.

The establishment of the National Institutes of Minority Aging, under the auspices of the U.S. Administration on Aging, has probably been Stanford's most significant accomplishment. Begun in 1973, these institutes have served a vital training function, generating data well utilized by scholars, students, and practitioners. Ten books and monographs have been written as a result of these institutes. Perhaps most important has been that the institutes provided the first broad forum for bringing together researchers from multiple ethnic and racial backgrounds to focus on aging.

Stanford has also been involved in developing several model demonstration projects. One, designed to promote advocacy by minority elders, has become a national model for shaping coalitions of minority leaders who can effectively serve as advocates on their own behalf.

Percil Stanford has been very active in professional gerontological organizations. He is a past president of the California Council on Gerontology and Geriatrics and the American Society of Aging. He has frequently served on the Gerontological Society's council. Stanford considers Clark Tibbitts* and Bernice L. Neugarten* to be his primary mentors; Donald P. Kent* and Arthur M. Flemming* are his chief role models.

R. KNIGHT STEEL. The valedictorian of the Class of 1957 at the Trinity School in New York City, Steel graduated with honors in philosophy from Yale University four years later. After earning his M.D. from Columbia University's College of Physicians and Surgeons in 1965, he completed his house officer training under Dr. Louis Welt at the North Carolina Memorial Hospital of the University of North Carolina (UNC) at Chapel Hill. Steel was chief resident of the Department of Medicine and an assistant professor of medicine at UNC between 1970 and 1972. From 1968 to 1970, he served as a lieutenant commander in the U.S. Public Health Service, working in the Heart Disease and Stroke Control Program and at the National Institutes of Health.

From 1972 to 1977, Steel was associate medical director at Monroe Community Hospital, an 800-bed, multiple-level facility affiliated with the University of Rochester School of Medicine. There, he worked closely with T. Franklin Williams, who was later to become the director of the National Institute on Aging (1979–1991).

In 1977, Steel joined the faculty of Boston University School of Medicine, where he remained for fourteen years. While at Boston University he became professor of medicine, professor of socio-medical sciences, director of the Boston University's Gerontology Center, and director of the Home Medical Service, Boston University Medical Center, the largest academic home-care program in the United States, providing approximately 6,000 home visits annually by doctors and fourth-year medical students. As founding chief of the Geriatrics Section, Steel established fellowships for both basic science and health services research, arranged for the granting of an M.P.H. degree to fellows in geriatrics, and implemented an obligatory rotation for house staff in the Department of Medicine.

Steel was supported by, among others, the National Institute on Aging, the Administration on Aging, the Massachusetts Department of Elder Affairs, and many private foundations, including the Henry J. Kaiser Foundation, the Robert Wood Johnson Foundation, the Commonwealth Fund, and the Hartford Foundation. Boston University established the R. Knight Steel Award for Excellence in Geriatric Medicine in 1991 to recognize an outstanding junior assistant resident.

In 1986–1987, Steel chaired the first certifying examination committee in geriatric medicine for the American Board of Internal Medicine, meeting jointly with the American Board of Family Practice. Four thousand two hundred and eighty-two physicians sat the examination in April 1988. He also was the first chairman of the Council of Medical Societies for the American College of Physicians between 1980 and 1983. He oversaw the writing of the first national guidelines for training in geriatric medicine and participated in rewriting the requirements for the training of all house officers in internal medicine while serving on the Residency Review Committee for Internal Medicine of the Accreditation Council for Graduate Medical Education. Steel has served as president and chairman of the board of the American Geriatrics Society and was a founding member of the American Federation for Aging Research. He has been a member of the Council of the Gerontological Society of America, served on multiple committees of the Institute of Medicine and was on the editorial boards or served as a reviewer for twelve journals. He won the Milo D. Leavitt Award from the American Geriatrics Society in 1989.

In 1991, Steel moved to Geneva, Switzerland, where for twenty-one months he served as chief of the Health of the Elderly Programme of the World Health Organization. While there, he developed support for cross-national research efforts in successful aging, osteoporosis, Alzheimer's Disease, the immunological aspects of aging, and home care. In the fall of 1993, Steel returned to the United States to become president of the World Organization for Care in the Home and Hospice (WOCHH), a newly founded, not-for-profit organization in Washington, D.C., dedicated to home care research, education, and policy development.

EDWARD J. STIEGLITZ. Edward Julius Stieglitz was born in Chicago in 1899. A 1918 graduate of the University of Chicago and 1921 graduate of its Rush Medical College, he was a National Research Fellow at Johns Hopkins during the 1922–1923 academic year. Stieglitz then served on the medical school faculty of the University of Chicago from 1923 to 1938. In 1939, he accepted the invitation of Thomas Parran, the surgeon general of the United States, to start a gerontological research unit in the U.S. Public Health Service. Stieglitz arranged through the Baltimore Department of Public Welfare to establish a research laboratory in its City Hospitals, which included an Old People's Home with approximately 1,000 ambulatory patients. He also established a national board, which included Anton J. Carlson,* Lawrence K. Frank,* and A. Baird Hastings.* Building on his own prior research on renal secretion and hisophysiology, Stiegliz launched a study of uric-acid excretion among aged subjects.

Before resigning for personal reasons a year after his appointment, Stieglitz did much to publicize the creation of the federal research center on aging and to underscore the importance of gerontological and geriatric investigations. See, for instance, his article, "Gerontology," in the *Annals of Internal Medicine,* 14

(October 1940): 739; and his plea, "The Social Urgency of Research in Ageing," in the second edition of *Problems of Ageing,* ed. Edmund V. Cowdry* (Baltimore: Williams and Wilkins, 1942): "The more we know about the biologic mechanisms of the aging processes, the more effectively can clinical medicine treat the ageing and the aged."

After World War II, Stieglitz continued to pursue his interests in geriatrics, gerontology, and the psychiatry of later maturity. He became the attending internist and chaired the staff of Suburban Hospital in Bethesda. He was also attending internist in geriatrics for the Chestnut Lodge in Rockville, was affiliated with the Washington Home for the Incurable and the Washington School of Psychiatry, and served as a consultant to the Veterans Administration. Stieglitz served as the first secretary of the Gerontological Society in 1945. Philadelphia's W. B. Saunders Company published two editions of his *Geriatric Medicine.* The subtitle of the first (1943) edition was "Diagnosis and Management of Disease in the Aging and in the Aged," but the 1949 edition was simply "The Care of the Aging and the Aged." Stieglitz divided his subject, "the problems of gerontology," into three parts—the biology of aging, the clinical problems of aging man, and the socioeconomic problems of aging mankind. His crossdisciplinary interests underscored at the outset: "The triad of primary categories is intimately and inseparately related. Though widely differing disciplines and techniques of scientific research must be applied to study of the various fields, the observations and conclusions derived from such investigations will fit into the broad pattern and thus amplify the whole."

ROBYN STONE. Robyn Stone was attracted to gerontology by the work of Robert N. Butler,* and that of Ethel Shanas.* She earned a master's degree in public administration from the University of Pittsburgh's Graduate School in Public and International Affairs in 1978 and became a doctor of public health at the University of California at Berkeley in 1985.

Her most important work has been an assessment of informal care networks for the disabled elderly. Her research confirmed through a national survey what other research had tentatively shown about informal caregivers. Typically, caregivers are female, and often they are themselves over age sixty-five; most are the wives and daughters of the recipients. The 1982 National Long-Term Care Survey found that there are some 2.4 million aged individuals receiving unpaid help with one or more instrumental activities of daily living. Through this work, Stone refined the concept of the competing demands of caregiving and employment, and then looked at the predictors of work accommodation on the ability to provide informal care. The survey, conducted with Gail Lee Cafferata and Judith Sangl, is reported in "Caregivers of the Frail Elderly: A National Profile," *The Gerontologist,* 27 (1987):616–26.

Using this profile of caregivers, Stone then provided policymakers with the first national estimates of spouses and adult children facing long-term care decisions. See Robyn Stone and Peter Kemper, "Spouses and Children of Disabled

Elders: How Large a Constituency for Long-Term Care Reform?'' *Milbank Memorial Quarterly* 67, 3 and 4 (1989):485–506. She differentiated between ''potential'' and ''active'' caregivers to demonstrate the magnitude of the long-term care problem for families facing critical care decisions.

In more theoretical work, Stone examined the causes of ''The Feminization of Poverty among the Elderly,'' for *Women's Studies Quarterly* 17, 1 and 2 (1989):20–34. In addition to outlining the major causes of the relative poverty of elderly women as compared with men, she is sensitive to the impact of racial differences. ''We need to focus more attention on the racial gap in poverty rates among the elderly population and the feminization of poverty among minorities,'' she writes.

As part of her effort to translate her insights into policy, Stone has worked as a senior research analyst for the Pepper Bipartisan Commission on Comprehensive Health Care, and she has created visibility for informal caregiving in the mass media. She worked as a research fellow at the National Center for Health Services Research and Health Care Technology Assessment, and she is currently affiliated with Project HOPE's Center for Health Affairs in Chevy Chase, Maryland.

BERNARD L. STREHLER. Bernard Louis Strehler was born in Johnstown, Pennsylvania, in 1925. After service in the U.S. Naval Reserve, he was educated at the Johns Hopkins University, where he earned his B.A. (1947) and Ph.D. (1950). Strehler served as an assistant professor of biological chemistry before joining Nathan W. Shock* at the Gerontology Branch of the Baltimore City Hospitals.

Strehler's interests in gerontology have been wide-ranging. He has studied firefly luminescence, bioenergetics, bacterial bioluminescence, vitamin metabolism, photosynthesis, and chemiluminescence ATP in photosynthesis. Strehler is probably best known for *Time, Cells, and Aging* (New York: Academic Press, 1962; 2nd edn., 1977). The work was inspired by the efforts of Alexander Comfort* in the *Biology of Senescence* and by symposium volumes issued by the National Science Foundation and the American Academy for the Advancement of Science to try to develop a ''theory'' of aging. While he doubted that *Time, Cells, and Aging* set forth a theoretical framework, his concept of adverse change in a variety of chemical loci that resulted, he claimed, from ''evolutionary inadvertencies'' nonetheless did have an impact on the field. This ''evolutionary dereliction,'' Strehler suspected, could never be altered through interventions. Like his colleague James E. Birren,* who would recruit him in the mid-1960s to the Gerontology Center at the University of Southern California (USC), Strehler was convinced that an understanding of the subjective and objective properties of ''time'' was essential to understanding the processes of aging.

After a few years at USC, Strehler moved to UCLA, where he has continued to do his research.

GORDON F. STREIB. Gordon F. Streib was born in Rochester, New York, in 1918. He received a master's degree from the New School for Social Research and his Ph.D. in sociology from Columbia University in 1954, where he studied with two giants in the field, Robert K. Merton and Paul F. Lazarsfeld. Two years earlier, as a young instructor at Cornell University, he became a member of a research group that was studying occupational retirement. The timing was serendipitous: Streib saw opportunities for his career by engaging in a field that was itself just emerging. Streib had never taken a course in gerontology or the sociology of aging, but he was to become over more than four decades one of gerontology's most incisive, trenchant analysts.

Streib is probably best known for his work on the longitudinal study of retirement that he conducted with his colleagues at Cornell University. The most cited product of this endeavor is a book he published with Clement J. Schneider, *Retirement in American Society* (New York: Cornell University Press, 1971); for an early study, see his "Morale of the Retired," *Social Problems,* 3 (1956): 270–76. Streib's pathbreaking analysis established that retirement is not a major traumatic event in the lives of most retirees. This finding contradicted conventional expert wisdom of that time, for many professionals had considered retirement to be a major stress factor resulting in psychological maladaption. Some claimed that quitting the work force hastened the deaths of retirees.

The Cornell retirement study was methodologically forward-looking in the sense that its team of interviewers revisited participants in the original sample rather than trying to make inferences about attitudes about retirement and retirees' behavior based on cross-sectional data. Streib and his colleagues also included a large number of older women in the project. They found that retirement for women sometimes had somewhat different outcomes (in terms of economic security and health status) than it did for men. *Retirement in American Society* remains the most important study we have of patterns of older workers' experiences with retirement for that era in U.S. history sometimes characterized as "the age of affluence." Subsequent studies with more precise samples and larger numbers of respondents (such as the Panel Studies of Income Dynamics at the University of Michigan's Institute for Social Research) have verified the Cornell study's central tenet that retirement is not universally experienced as a traumatic life event. However, some professionals in the health care field and related domains still claim that retirement is a serious stress factor in the lives of older persons.

From his considerations of the interrelationships among aging, race, ethnicity, gender, and class, Streib developed and refined over the course of his career a social stratification perspective for studies in gerontology. At a conference at the University of Michigan in the 1960s, he reminded his colleagues that a well-rounded study of the older population demanded disciplined attention to the sociology of stratification. See, for instance, Streib's "Are the Aged a Minority Group?" in *Applied Sociology,* eds. A. W. Gouldner and S. M. Miller (New York: Free Press, 1965), 311–28. Since then, other gerontologists, such as Vern

L. Bengtson,* James Dowd, Linda K. George,* and Jill Quadagno,* have enunciated this perspective.

Social stratification, Streib contends, antedates one's standing in relation to age stratification. One's class position is the one persistent factor relating to well-being throughout the life cycle. Accordingly, explicating the dynamics of social stratification and age stratification is one of the most challenging policy issues related to the study of the life course and to the application of research results into policies and programs involving health care and social services. Streib stressed the interconnections of ethnicity/race, aging, and stratification, examining variations not only in regions in the United States but across national boundaries, in "Social Stratification and Aging," in the *Handbook of Aging and the Social Sciences,* eds. Robert H. Binstock* and Ethel Shanas* (New York: Van Nostrand Reinhold, 1976), 160–85. In the second edition of the *Handbook of Aging and the Social Sciences* (1985), which featured a chapter by Jacqueline Johnson Jackson on "Race, National Origin, Ethnicity, and Aging," Streib underscored the importance of age as an observable indicator of stratification: "Researchers on stratification in the latter part of the life cycle must recognize age and aging as the strategic characteristics, linked causally to other stratification indices, and primary reasons for downward mobility."

Streib's efforts to sharpen gerontologists' conceptualizations of social stratification models led, in turn, to his refinement of disengagement theory. Streib suggested a more precise term—differential disengagement—to discuss distinctive aspects of the aged's social stratification, such as socialization to role loss and to downward mobility. He stressed that disengagement occurs at different rates in different amounts for various roles in the complex of role sets. Disengagement from the work role may provide an opportunity for engagement in other roles. See Streib's "Disengagement Theory in Socio-Cultural Perspective," in *International Journal of Psychiatry,* 6 (1968): 69–76 as well as Chapter 13 in *Retirement in American Society: Impact and Process,* eds. Gordon F. Streib and Clement J. Schneider (Ithaca, N.Y.: Cornell University Press, 1971).

Streib recognized that the family is the institution that most conditions individual behavior and adjustment to society. Yet the family, he contended in an essay with Wayne E. Thompson, "The Older Person in a Family Context," in the *Handbook of Social Gerontology,* ed. Clark Tibbitts* (Chicago: University of Chicago Press, 1960), has been "singularly neglected as an area for study of the older aged groups." He stressed the importance of viewing relationships and exchanges from a generational perspective. With Ethel Shanas (whom, along with Bernice L. Neugarten,* Edward Suchman, and Edward Folts, he considers his major intellectual colleagues), Streib underscored the importance of generational relations in the field. See, for instance, *Social Structure and the Family,* eds. Ethel Shanas and Gordon F. Streib (New York: Prentice-Hall, 1965).

It is indicative of Streib's status as a senior social scientist in the field of aging that Robert Binstock invited him to co-write the lead essay, "Aging and the Social Sciences: Changes in the Field," in the third edition of the *Handbook of Aging and the Social Sciences,* eds. Robert Binstock and Linda George (San Diego: Academic Press, 1990). The chapter's major headings underscore Streib's sense of the state of the art: demography and aging, gender-oriented research, political economy of aging, global gerontology, and theoretical and analytical approaches. Binstock and Streib devote the most space to the last topic, especially to techniques of research synthesis, such as meta-analysis and secondary analysis. They asserted that issues of "old age and equity" would loom large in the future. Throughout the essay, one senses Streib's balanced, disciplinary grounded judgments aimed at enriching a field of study that has stimulated him so much.

After teaching at Cornell University for twenty-six years, he joined the Department of Sociology at the University of Florida. Intrigued by the large number of persons who moved to Florida after retirement, Streib initiated a new line of research in the field of environment and housing for the aged. With colleagues he carried out research on small group homes that resulted in the book, *Old Homes—New Families: Shared Living for the Elderly* (New York: Columbia University Press, 1984). With another set of colleagues, he conducted the first comparative study of thirty-six retirement communities in four states, focusing on different levels of community size, age, location, and organizational structure. See G. F. Streib, W. E. Folts, and A. J. La Greca, "Autonomy, Power, and Decision-Making in Thirty-Six Retirement Communities," *The Gerontologist,* 25 (1985): 403–409.

Since retirement in 1990, he has continued his research on retirement communities. See his "The Life Course of Activities and Retirement Communities," in *Activity and Aging,* ed. John R. Kelly (Beverly Hills, Calif.: Sage, 1993), 246–63.

MARVIN B. SUSSMAN. After earning a B.A. in history from New York University in 1941 and a master's degree in group behavior work from George Williams College in 1943, Marvin B. Sussman went on to doctoral work in sociology in 1948 and completed his Ph.D. at Yale University in 1951. His dissertation on help patterns in the middle-class family demonstrated the endurance and viability of kin networks in complex, urbanized, and highly differentiated societies. It also elaborated ongoing exchanges and continuities of family members of different generations, and transfers of knowledge and equities over time. His study of ninety-seven families contradicted the then-current notion that families in American society, indeed in all developed societies, were nuclear in structure and isolated from extended kin networks.

In refuting this impression of the modern family, Sussman undermined assumptions that family life and family structure depend on the economic system. Because the economic system determines where individuals work and live and creates a readiness and expectation of regular relocations, the isolated, fractured family system was taken to be the result. Following Sussman's early work, a number of studies in the 1960s and 1970s sustained the view that family members maintained connections with their children, parents, and kin in a new urban environment. See "The Isolated Nuclear Family: Fact or Fiction," *Social Problems,* 6 (1979): 333–40.

Once the significance of family bonding has been ascertained, it provides explanations of the motives and practices of caregiving and care receiving. Sussman's subsequent work has been to describe the implications of such a realistic view of family structure (as opposed to the myth of the isolated nuclear family) for bureaucratic organizations working with older adults. He has proposed a reciprocal model for the interaction between families and bureaucracies. "Family members functioning on behalf of their kin can influence and modify the normative demands of large-scale systems," Sussman writes. "Thus, a model that is based on the complementarity of organizational and family values has robust explanatory power." For more on this approach, see *The Family, Bureaucracy, and the Elderly,* eds. Marvin Sussman and Ethel Shanas* (Durham, N.C.: Duke University Press, 1977).

He has also explored family inheritance systems with Judith N. Cares and David T. Smith in *The Family and Inheritance* (New York: Russell Sage Foundation, 1970). The study examines what happens in a family at the death of one of its members. The findings represent a random sampling of 659 decedents, which yielded a survivor population of 2,239, of whom 1,234 were interviewed. This study established the power and robustness of family continuity over generational time. Data from this study of intergenerational transfers of property within kinship networks provided clarification of the relationship among such variables as family size, occupation, education, ages of members, sex distribution and patterns of service, exchange, and reciprocal expectations. For Sussman's more recent thoughts in this area, see his article, originally presented as the Burgess Award Lecture, "Law and Legal Systems: the Family Connection," *Journal of Marriage and the Family,* 47 (1983): 9–21.

Sussman also studied connecting children and adolescents with older adults. With grants from the W. T. Grant Foundation and the AARP Andrus Foundation, he developed activity programs and studied their efficaciousness in promoting intergenerational linkages and connections.

Sussman is currently investigating the use of an "inheritance contract" in relation to caregiving. The major question is whether the use of this resource, inheritance, can enhance or negate caregiving practices of family and kin members. Currently the Unidel Professor of Human Behavior (Emeritus) at the University of Delaware, Sussman is also a professor at the Union Institute.

ALVAR SVANBORG. Alvar Svanborg was educated in his native Sweden, completing a medical degree in 1948 and a Ph.D. in 1951 at the Karolinska Institutet in Stockholm. He felt an urgent need for better understanding of the biology of aging and its clinical implications at that time. Most of his important research was done in Gothenburg, Sweden. After retiring, he became affiliated with the University of Illinois Section of Geriatric Medicine in Chicago.

He initiated, planned, and led a broad, detailed longitudinal study of aging, morbidity, health care needs, and sought preventive measures for Gothenburg's elderly. A follow-up study included elderly from seventy to eighty-five years. By dividing an age cohort into two groups, Svanborg and his team were able to determine the effects of a systematic intervention program. Their efforts demonstrate the causative relationship between lifestyle and environment and aging.

The study has produced more than 200 reports internationally. It has contributed to a more comprehensive understanding of morphological, physiological, and psychosocial consequences of aging, as well as a better knowledge of the incidence and prevalence of diseases. It has also shown how to differentiate between aging itself and diseases that might accompany aging. The study continues to bear fruit; see, for example, "A Medical-Social Intervention in a 70-year-old Swedish Population: Is it Possible to Postpone Functional Decline in Aging?" *Journal of Gerontology,* 48 (1993): 84–88.

As important as the research project itself is to Svanborg, he is equally proud of his ability to recruit and lead a team of interdisciplinary researchers. He has been able to create synergy between basic biological, physiological, and clinical research, as well as behavioral science research. Because of his European connections and interests in plasticity and productive aging, he has worked closely in the United States with such giants as Robert N. Butler* and James E. Birren.*

In addition to his research, Svanborg serves as an adviser to the World Health Organization and to governmental and university organizations in France, Germany, Greece, Hungary, Israel, Japan, Poland, and Thailand. He is also the founding president of the Federation of Gerontology of the Nordic Countries, a position he has held for fifteen years. He is scientific adviser to the Swedish National Board of Health and Welfare, and was a onetime adviser to the director of the U.S. National Institute of Aging.

Svanborg's primary collaborators to date include Ove Dehlin, Staffan Edén, Ann-Kathrine Granerus, and Bertil Steen, all of whom now chair university departments in Sweden. Physicians Sten Landahl, Dan Mellstrom, and Ake Rundgren have also collaborated with Svanborg.

JAMES T. SYKES. "I like to think of myself as a humanist," James T. Sykes told the members of the Colorado Gerontological Society in 1989. "I am simply one who attends to the human values of gerontology and one who believes deeply that there is within each human being a sacred self, a soul, a spirit seeking to be all that one can be, through relationships to the awesome and to fellow human beings." As a senior lecturer in preventive medicine at the University of Wisconsin-Madison, and as one who has traveled to nearly fifty countries to examine cultural variations, Sykes has repeated this theme often.

Sykes developed his approach to gerontology while at Kent State University, where he earned a master's degree in English. Later, at the University of Wisconsin, he studied under Carl Rogers, who promoted putting the individual at the center of a caring environment. Sykes has developed his own gerontological analog of "caring with care" in presentations, public service, and teaching.

As chairman of the Dane County, Wisconsin, Board of Public Welfare, and Wisconsin's Board on Aging, Sykes examined the problems of institutionalized older persons. His nursing home visits instilled in him a desire to improve conditions for older persons in the community and in institutions. He applied Kurt Lewin's "force-field" theory to diagram and address the challenge of providing a nurturing environment through community building and public policy. He put his gerontological ideas into practice by developing a model community-based, long-term care system, the Colonial Club of Sun Prairie, Wisconsin. The twenty-acre campus contains a senior center, an adult day care center, and more than 260 units of elderly housing. The result is a continuum of care, a dynamic community, and a neighborhood in which elders are both the recipients and the providers of care, as well as the staff, faculty, owners and residents. The Colonial Club exemplifies how private and public efforts can achieve an attractive, accessible, affordable care community.

Sykes founded the Colonial Club in two basement rooms of the town's museum with major funding for what is now a model caring community from Helen and Garvin Cremer. These two entrepreneurs asked Sykes to identify the needs of rural Dane County and, with corporate and foundation resources, respond to those needs. In the process, Sykes became recognized as an expert in housing for the elderly, its management, design, financing, and services related to residential environments. He chaired the Wisconsin Housing and Economic Development Authority and the Dane County Housing Authority.

In 1994, Sykes served as chairman of the National Council on the Aging and on numerous boards. He is an associate director of the University of Wisconsin Institute on Aging. He has appeared often before legislative and congressional committees on aging issues and as a consultant to national and international organizations. A Fellow of the Gerontological Society, Sykes was awarded honorary memberships in five (Argentina, Brazil, Chile, Cuba, and Mexico) Latin American gerontological societies.

Sykes's photographs of older persons have appeared on the covers and inside a dozen journals and publications. Using these photographs, Sykes brings biographical and humanistic perspectives to his students and audiences.

He counts among his mentors Bernice L. Neugarten,* Carl Rogers, Arthur M. Flemming,* and (the late) Nelson Cruikshank.

T

PHILIP TAIETZ. Philip Taietz earned his Ph.D. from Cornell University in 1951, became professor emeritus of rural sociology in 1976, and remains at Cornell. His research in the sociology of aging has covered several important areas.

His first study, begun in 1950, explored the relationship between organizational characteristics and institutional quality. The study, ''Administrative Practices and Personal Adjustment in Homes for the Aged,'' came at a time when the art of measuring institutional quality was still in its infancy. Taietz found that previous studies had tended to cover up the variations among institutions and ignored the evaluations of the residents themselves. He therefore made the single institution his unit of analysis and sought both expert and resident input. See his ''Administrative Practices and Personal Adjustment in Homes for the Aged,'' *Cornell University Agriculture Experiment Station Bulletin,* 899 (July 1953).

Taietz's next major study was conducted with Paul Roman. The two men examined the role of the emeritus professor and found that those who were allowed role continuity exhibited a higher degree of continued engagement than those required to adopt new roles. See ''Organizational Structure and Disengagement: The Emeritus Professor,'' *The Gerontologist* 7 (September 1967, Part 1): 147–52.

Taietz has also made an effort to test the theory and practice of social gerontology. Taietz became aware that many supposedly ''private'' interviews were in fact conducted by researchers with a third person present. He found, for example, that interview responses changed when the subject's spouse or child was in the room. His findings are reported in "Conflicting Group Norms and the 'Third' Person in the Interview," *American Journal of Sociology,* 68 (July 1962): 97–104.

Taietz's 1976 study tested the accepted literature on the users of senior centers. Rather than view senior centers as programs designed to meet the needs of the elderly, he used a "voluntary organization model." He found that elderly people who are more active in voluntary organizations and who manifest strong community ties are most likely to use senior centers. See "Two Conceptual Models of the Senior Center," *Journal of Gerontology,* 31 (March 1976): 219–22.

Much of his work has been concerned with rural environments and aging. Here he has employed a macrostructural approach to uncover factors in a community that relate to the level of service provided. The two important predictors Taietz found were the variety of the community and its centrality. Institutions function well if they mimic the community structure, Taietz concluded. See, for example, "Community Complexity and Knowledge of Facilities," *Journal of Gerontology,* 30 (May 1975): 357–62.

In 1984 and 1987, Taietz conducted a study of one of the more intriguing, less recognized, and atypical patterns of aging and retirement, that of older Americans who are residing abroad. Taietz selected Paris as the site for the study and found that 70 percent of the older Americans had medium to high levels of sociocultural integration and 92 percent had a level of proficiency in French that enabled them to participate in the local culture. See "Sociocultural Integration of Older American Residents of Paris," *The Gerontologist,* 27 (August 1987): 464–70.

In 1990, Taietz and Nina Glasgow, in collaboration with the American Association of Retired Persons, conducted a national conference on successful aging. The purpose of the conference was to address the problem that Matilda White Riley* and John Riley* identified as the "imbalance between the strengths and capacities of the mounting number of long-lived people and the lack of opportunities in society to utilize and reward these strengths." See "Resourceful Aging: Today and Tomorrow," *Conference Proceedings, Vol. I Executive Summary* (AARP and Department of Rural Sociology, Cornell University).

In 1993 and in 1994, Taietz conducted a study to ascertain the individual and structural factors that are associated with continuing professional effectiveness of emeriti professors. The study, which was conducted at a large northeastern research university, measured the productivity of the emeriti before and after retirement in research teaching, publication, public service, and several other roles. Role continuity of the emeritus professor is facilitated through the provision of space and support services by the university, he found, but individual factors such as health and financial problems affect the ability of the emeritus professor to engage in activities that are necessary for role continuity. See "Factors Associated with Continued Productivity of Emeritus Professors at Cornell

University," *A Preliminary Report* (Ithaca, N.Y.: Department of Rural Sociology, Cornell University).

HANS THOMAE. Psychologist Hans Thomae was born in 1915, in Germany. He earned his Ph.D. from the University of Bonn in 1940. He was assistant at the Institute of Psychology of Leipzig University (1939–1945), lecturer in psychology at the University of Bonn (1950–1953) and professor of psychology at the University of Erlangen (1953–1959) and at Bonn University (1960–1983). As professor emeritus he continues doing research in different fields of psychology, especially theory of personality, of aging, and lifespan development. In addition to Robert J. Havighurst* and the Chicago gerontologists, Thomae traces his interest in the field to two German psychologists: Erich Rothacker's work on maturation and aging in *Die Schichten der Persönlichkeit* (Bonn: H. Bouvier, 1952, 5th edn.), and Charlotte M. Bühler's *Der Menschliche Lebenslauf als Psychologisches Problem* (Leipzig: S. Hirzel, 1933) directed his thinking.

His research has emphasized differential approaches to psychogerontology since 1967, and his most important works have been involved with a cognitive approach to aging. Thomae was part of the original team planning and performing the Bonn Longitudinal Study on Aging (BOLSA) in 1965. The team also included U. Lehr, R. Schmitz-Scherzer, and H. G. Tismer. Thomae edited the 1976 report, *Findings from the Bonn Longitudinal Study on Aging* (New York: Karger) and co-edited the 1987 report with U. Lehr (Stuttgart: Enke). In the first reports on this study, a differential approach was applied by analyzing the data in the context of physical, social, ecological, and personality influences on the aging process. In 1983, Thomae identified twelve "styles" respectively of various "fates" of aging (*Alternsstile and Altersschicksale, Fin Beitrag zur Differentiellen Gerontologie,* Bern: Huber.)

He has elaborated a cognitive theory of adjustment to aging, integrating the role of cognitive representations, motivational and emotional variables, and the restoration of balance between cognitive and motivational systems. He began this project in 1970 with "Theory of Aging and Cognitive Theory of Personality," *Human Development* 12 (1970): 1–16.

A follow-up study appeared in 1992, titled "Contributions of Longitudinal Research to a Cognitive Theory of Adjustment of Aging," *European Journal of Personality,* 6 (1992): 157–75. Based on a selection of the BOLSA findings, Thomae reported that the perceived rather than the objective situation directs behavior, and that perceptions of situations are related to an individual's dominant concerns. Proper adjustment to aging occurs when the cognitive and motivational systems of a person have been balanced.

When Thomae updated his BOLSA findings in 1990, his new focus on stress was evident. See, for example, his chapter, "Stress, Satisfaction, Competence," in *Clinical and Scientific Psychogeriatrics,* vol. 1, eds. M. Bergener and S. Finkel (New York: Springer, 1990), 117–34. He has developed the concept of a stress response hierarchy as a way to examine the consistency of reactions across time and differing situations. Underlying this concept is the notion of individuals and their world as an indivisible dynamic unit.

In collaboration with G. Rudinger, he analyzed the influences of gender, health, personality, socio-economic status, etc., on domain specific indexes of life satisfaction in old age (for example, satisfaction with spouse, children, home, income, neighborhood) and on global indexes. By use of different structural equation models, the need for a situation-specific conceptualization of life satisfaction in old age was demonstrated (Rudinger and Thomae, 1990). Since 1989, Thomae has been involved in a new longitudinal study in which the development of two cohorts that grew up under different political, social, and economic conditions is to be compared in middle and old age.

Thomae received honorary doctoral degrees from the universities of Leaven, Belgium (1970), Leipzig (1990), and Moscow (1993). In 1992 he was awarded (with Leonard Hayflick*) the Sandoz International Prize for gerontological research.

CLARK TIBBITTS. Clark Tibbitts was born in Chicago in 1903. After earning his B.S. from the Lewis Institute (now the Illinois Institute of Technology) in 1924, he did graduate work at the University of Chicago. There, he was a student of William Ogburn and collaborated with Ernest Burgess* on a study of parole violators. From 1928 to 1932, he served as an assistant on the President's Research Committee on Social Trends. After teaching (1932–1934) at the universities of Wisconsin and Michigan, Tibbitts became a research coordinator for urban projects in the Federal Emergency Relief Administration (1934–1935), and then directed a national survey for the U.S. Public Health Service (1935–1937).

In 1938, Tibbitts was invited to return to the University of Michigan to head a new Institute of Human Adjustment, which was to be supported through a $6 million bequest from the estate of Horace and Mary Rackham. Alexander Ruthven, a university president and zoologist by training, had been urged to focus on the biology of senescence. Ruthven, however, wanted "to begin our studies in those fields in which results could be obtained rather quickly and in which we could, therefore, gain experience." Accordingly, Tibbitts's first task was to survey the field. That he quickly seized on gerontology reflects his connections to ideas circulating at the University of Chicago at the time as well as his own Depression-era experiences. Tibbitts reported in a thirty-nine-page memorandum, "A Proposal for Research into Some of the Problems of Old Age" (1940),

It is mandatory that research, which has been so successful in prolonging life, be now directed to the objective showing how that latter years can be employed to the greatest satisfaction of all concerned. . . . The University appears to have an unequalled opportunity for initiating a program for experiment and research that could have great significance for the entire population of the State and of the country as well.

Tibbitts recommended that Michigan faculty and staff take a multidisciplinary approach to the problems of aging. He proposed capitalizing on the resources at hand—hence his emphasis on dealing with hearing loss in late life, because the Institute for Human Adjustment had an otology lab—and ways to retrain older workers. World War II intervened, and Tibbitts had to put his plans on hold while he directed the University War Board and Veterans Service Bureau.

After the war, Tibbitts decided to interview local older citizens to determine what they wanted. On the basis of his survey, he identified seven needs—financial security, health and physical care, adequate family and living arrangements, recognition and status, emotional relationships, recognized roles providing useful activity, and religion—that would remain central priorities throughout his career. With support from the University Extension Service, Tibbitts and his colleague, Wilma Donahue,* developed a course on "Aging and Living" in 1948 for older residents in Detroit. The following year, they taught the class at other sites and produced twenty-six radio broadcasts. The Institute for Human Adjustment staff also designed three conferences—"Living through the Older Years" (1948), "Planning for the Older Years" (1949), and "Growing in the Older Years" (1950)—to which nationally recognized experts, newcomers to the field, and older persons were invited to participate. These meetings became the foundation for annual conferences held in Ann Arbor over the next quarter-century, events that made gerontological activities on the University of Michigan campus a major hub in the national network.

In 1949, Tibbitts left Ann Arbor for Washington to coordinate aging-related activities in the Federal Security Agency. "The Federal Government should establish a clearing house for studies of and programs for the aging, with broad authority for research and promotion in this area," Tibbitts wrote shortly after his arrival. "National planning by public and private agencies and individuals should be comprehensive in scope and participation." Tibbitts coordinated the first National Conference on Aging (1950), which brought 816 delegates to the Capitol. The final set of recommendations, *Man and His Years* (Raleigh, N.C.: Health Publications Institute, 1951), served as a blueprint for the next decade. In 1951, Tibbitts became head of a Committee on Aging and Geriatrics created in the Federal Security Agency to gather information and to create programs for senior citizens.

As the new Department of Health, Education and Welfare took shape, Tibbitts's titles and visibility in the aging network grew. In 1956, for instance, as deputy director for the Special Staff on Aging, he assisted members of the Gerontological Society in obtaining support from the National Institute for Mental Health to train professionals in social gerontology. Tibbitts edited one of the three major volumes that emerged from this project, *The Handbook on Social Gerontology* (Chicago: University of Chicago Press, 1960). "This forecast of expanding research interest, along with the growing numbers of middle-aged and older people and the demands for social action, imply that there will be an increasing demand for training in that field," he noted. All the while, Tibbitts maintained his connections with Wilma Donahue and her associates at the University of Michigan. Through the university press, they co-edited several collections of papers from annual conferences, including *Social Contribution of the Aging* (Ann Arbor, Mich.: University of Michigan Press, 1952), *Aging in the Modern World* (Ann Arbor, Mich.: University of Michigan Press, 1957), and *New Frontiers of Aging* (Ann Arbor, Mich.: University of Michigan Press, 1958).

During the 1960s, Tibbitts's official titles often changed, but his strategic position in HEW assured him a prominent role as the federal government increased its promises and commitments to older Americans. From 1960 to 1966, he was deputy director of the U.S. Office on Aging. When the U.S. Administration on Aging was established as a result of the 1965 Older Americans Act, Tibbitts became director of training, a position he held until 1974. Keenly aware that other federal agencies, such as the National Institutes of Child Health and Human Development and of Mental Health, the Rehabilitation Services Administration, the Veterans Administration, and the U.S. Public Health Service supported advanced research and training in gerontology, Tibbitts chose to nurture program at sites that focused on particular policy issues, such as recreation and aging, and retirement housing management, and that studied planning and administration.

Although his federal responsibilities grew, Tibbitts nonetheless spent time in the trenches. From 1962 to 1969, he taught aging-related courses on public administration at George Washington University, inspiring talented graduate students such as Robert Atchley to pursue a career in gerontology. In 1972, with David Peterson and Wilma Donahue, he sketched in *The International Journal of Aging and Human Development,* 3 (1972): 253–60 the principles of a "Faculty Seminar in Social Gerontology: A Model for the Expansion of Gerontological Instruction," which happened to be found at the University of Michigan. The authors claimed success in training thirty-two faculty members to develop seventy-nine new instructional units, courses, workshops, and programs on gerontology in Michigan.

After leaving government service in 1974, Tibbitts became head of the National Clearinghouse on Aging in Washington. After his death, the Association for Gerontology in Higher Education established the Clark Tibbitts Award to recognize his extraordinary contributions to the field of aging.

SHELDON S. TOBIN. Sheldon S. Tobin was born in 1931 in Chicago. He earned a B.S. from the University of Illinois's College of Medicine in 1955 and then turned to the study of gerontology in 1959, completing his M.A. in human development at the University of Chicago in 1961. Working toward his Ph.D., Tobin included an internship in clinical psychology at the Psychosomatic and Psychiatric Institute at the Michael Reese Hospital in 1961 and 1962. He finished the Ph.D. in 1963, under the tutelage of Bernice L. Neugarten* and Robert J. Havighurst.*

Tobin quickly made important contributions to the field, beginning with the development of the life satisfaction rating system, originally conceived with Neugarten and Havighurst in 1961. The system is based on measuring the congruence between expected and achieved goals in aging. See "The Measurement of Life Satisfaction," *Journal of Gerontology* 16 (1961): 134–43; and S. Tobin and B. Neugarten, "Life Satisfaction and Social Interaction," *Journal of Gerontology* 16 (1961): 344–45.

Another important collaborator has been Morton A. Lieberman. With him, Tobin wrote *Last Home for the Aged* (San Francisco: Jossey-Bass, 1976), which examines the impact of institutionalization on the elderly. "Becoming what one has feared becoming explains waiting list effects during the process of becoming institutionalized when old," Tobin explains. They also collaborated on *The Experience of Old Age* (New York: Basic Books, 1982).

Tobin's recent research has been concerned with questions of support systems for the elderly—see his *Enabling the Elderly: Religious Institutions Within the Social Services* (Albany, N.Y.: State University of New York Press, 1981)—and with normative psychology and the oldest old. See his *Personhood in Advanced Old Age: Implications for Practice* (New York: Springer, 1991), which Tobin considers his most important work to date.

From 1963 until 1982, Tobin was on the faculty of the School of Social Service Administration and Committee on Human Development at the University of Chicago. Since 1982, he has been at the State University of New York at Albany. His titles suggest the range of his purview—professor of Social Welfare and Public Affairs and Policy in the Rockefeller College of Public Affairs and Policy, professor of psychology (since 1984), adjunct professor of Albany Medical College (since 1985), professor in the School of Public Health (since 1989), and from 1982 until 1990, director of Albany's Ringel Institute of Gerontology. His proudest professional service, though, was his four years as editor-in-chief of *The Gerontologist*. In that capacity, he tried to increase the quality and interdisciplinary range of articles accepted. He has served on a number of other editorial boards, including *Journal of Gerontological Social Work* (1979–present), *Research in Aging* (1979–1988), *Ageing and Society* (1980–1983), and the *Journal of the American Geriatrics Society* (1984–1988).

Tobin was awarded the 1987 Walter M. Beattie Jr. Award for Distinguished Service in Gerontology by the State Society on Aging of New York, the Donald Spence Research Award by the Northeastern Gerontological Society in 1991, and the Award for Excellence in Research from his university in 1992. He participates actively in the community and was chairman of the board of the Industries of the Blind of New York State, from 1990 to 1993.

T. WINGATE TODD. Thomas Wingate Todd was born in Sheffield, England, in 1855. He earned his bachelor degrees in chemistry and in medicine from the University of Manchester in 1907, where he began his academic career as a demonstrator and lecturer in anatomy and surgeon to the zoological collection.

In 1912, Todd emigrated to the United States, where he became Henry Wilson Payne Professor of Anatomy at Western Reserve University and director of the Hamann Museum of Comparative Anthropology and Anatomy. Over the course of his distinguished career, Todd was given memberships in British, Belgian, and French scientific societies.

Todd was best known for his work on clinical and veterinary anatomy, dental anatomy, anthropology, growth and repair, and child development. Representative of his scholarship is the *Atlas of Skeletal Malnutrition* and *An Introduction to Mammalian Dentition* (New York: Harper and Row, 1919). Todd is included in this volume because of his contribution, "Ageing of Vertebrates," to *Problems of Ageing,* ed. Edmund Vincent Cowdry* (Baltimore: Williams and Wilkins, 1939). On the basis of his study of fish, amphibia, reptiles, birds, and mammals, Todd distinguished between lifespan and duration of life. He confirmed Raymond Pearl's assertion that there was no universal law of mortality; each species differs in the age distribution of dying and mortality. In *The Atlas of Skeletal Maturation* (1937), Todd noted, "The maturation process, like growth, is a complex phenomenon and therefore, like growth depends for its full expression upon general constitution fitness rather than upon the influence of a single controlling factor."

Todd died in 1938.

FERNANDO TORRES-GIL. While a graduate student at Brandeis University, Fernando Torres-Gil attended the 1971 White House Conference on Aging, where he was struck by the lack of work being done on aging and minorities. He resolved to do his master's thesis, and subsequently his doctoral dissertation, on political issues facing Hispanic elders. This work was subsequently published as *The Politics of Aging Among Elder Hispanics* (Washington, D.C.: University Press of America, 1982).

However, he was no newcomer to the field. Torres-Gil earned a B.A. in political science from San Jose State University in 1970 and completed his M.S.W. at Brandeis in 1972. He continued for his Ph.D. with Robert H. Binstock* as his dissertation chairman, and finished in 1976. Throughout this period he was involved in labor organizing, Hispanic politics, and student politics. He continued putting theory into practice by helping to form the National Hispanic Council on Aging and the Asociacion Nacional Por Personas Mayores, which remain the principle advocacy groups for elderly Hispanics.

Torres-Gil's more recent work has been built from this base, and it has followed the path set out by Binstock, Bernice L. Neugarten,* Robert Hudson, and Andrew Achenbaum. He has sought out common issues facing members of all ethnic groups as they age, and issues for the United States as its diverse population ages. His approach to the subject can be found in a volume co-edited with Scott A. Bass* and Elizabeth Kutza, *Diversity in Aging: Challenges Facing Planners and Policymakers in the 1990s* (Glenview, Ill.: Scott, Foresman & Co., 1989).

He has put forth another approach to understanding issues of minority status and ethnicity that juxtaposes these issues with trends in the larger society. For example, Torres-Gil links the growth of the U.S. Hispanic population with the aging of the U.S. population and the generational issues affecting both trends. See "The Latinization of a Multigenerational Population: Hispanics in an Aging Society," *Daedalus*, 115 (Winter 1986): 325–48.

Expanding his research program, Torres-Gill wrote a seminal article with Jon Pynoos that examined the interest group struggles of older persons and younger disabled advocacy groups in the development of long-term care programs. See "Long Term Care Policy and Interest Group Struggles," *The Gerontologist*, 26 (1986): 488–95. He then turned to macro-political issues, and offered a prescription for ways that gerontology, as a field of study and a service profession, should respond to political change. For an overall look at Torres-Gil's diverse interest in the political process, public policy, and the future of aging, see his recent book, *The New Aging: Politics and Change in America* (Westport, Conn.: Greenwood Press, 1992).

In addition to his research, Torres-Gil served as staff director of the U.S. House of Representatives Select Committee on Aging from 1985 to 1987, as a White House Fellow in the Carter administration, and as president of the American Society on Aging (1990–1991). Since 1991 he has been a professor at the School of Social Welfare of the University of California at Los Angeles, and is serving as the (first) Assistant Secretary for Aging in the Clinton administration.

LILLIAN E. TROLL. Lillian E. Troll, born 1915, majored in psychology and pre-medicine studies as an undergraduate (B.S. 1937) at the University of Chicago and in human development as a graduate student there, leaving in 1941 half-way through a dissertation on a factor analysis of music ability tests to work in Washington during World War II. She returned to the university to complete a dissertation in 1965, and switched her topic to a study of personality similarities between college-age youth and their parents. Bernice L. Neugarten,* the chairwoman of this dissertation committee, interested her in gerontology. When her Ph.D. was awarded in 1967, Troll joined the faculty at the Merrill-Palmer Institute to round out its program in lifespan development. In 1970, she moved to the Psychology Department at Wayne State University, and in 1975 to Rutgers University, from where she retired as a Senior Professor in 1986.

Her primary interests since 1955, when she started working as a school psychologist in the Newton, Massachusetts, public schools, has been the study of modified extended families, focusing on generational relations and the roles of the older generations. On this subject, she has frequently interacted with Vern L. Bengtson,* Gunhild Hagestad, and Colleen Leahy Johnson.* Her doctoral research, in which she analyzed personal interviews with 100 white college-age youths and their parents, found similarities in personality and values unexplained by either family structure or gender. See "Similarities in Values and Other Personality Characteristics in College Students and Their Parents," *Merrill-*

Palmer Quarterly, 15 (1969): 323–36. She then studied three-generation same-sex adult lineages of grandparent, child, and grandchild, analyzed in terms of cognitive complexity, affect, achievement, and other variables, including, most recently, family connectedness. See, for example, "A Three-Generational Analysis of Change in Women's Motivation and Power" in *Social Power and Influence of Women,* eds. L. S. Stamm and C. D. Ryff* (Boulder, Colo.: Westview Press, 1984), 81–98; and "Family Connectedness of Old Women: Attachments in Later Life" in *Women Growing Older,* eds. B. F. Turner and L. E. Troll (Newport Beach, Calif.: Sage, 1994). Her general interests in the family and generations can be seen in "Generations in the Family" with Vern L. Bengston,* in the series *Contemporary Theories about the Family,* Vol. 1 (1979) and earlier in "The Family in the Second Half of Life: A Decade Review," *Journal of Marriage and the Family,* 2 (1971): 263–90; "Family of Later Life: A Decade Review" in *Social Problems of Aging,* eds. Sheila Miller and Robert C. Atchley* (Belmont, Calif.: Wadsworth, 1979); and *Gerontological Issues in the Family* (New York: Springer, 1986). Among her articles on grandparenting are "Grandparents: The Family Watchdogs" in 1983 in Timothy Brubaker's *Family Relationships in Later Life.*

Troll has long stressed the importance of gender differences in aging, editing the first book on that subject, *Looking Ahead: A Woman's Guide to the Problems and Joys of Growing Older* (Englewood Cliffs, N.J.: Prentice-Hall, 1977), with Joan and Kenneth Israel, and most recently, with Barbara Turner, *Women Growing Older* (New York: Springer, 1994).

Perhaps Troll's most important gerontological contribution has been to make research on families and human development accessible to students. She has written three adult development and aging textbooks, *Development in Early and Middle Adulthood* (Monterey, Calif.: Brooks/Cole, 1975, 1985), *Continuations: Development after 20* (Monterey, Calif.: Brooks/Cole, 1982), and *Families in Later Life* (Belmont, Calif.: Wadsworth, 1979). She also wrote a special edition on "Elders and their Families" for *Generations,* 1982. She participated with Nancy Schlossberg, Gunhild Hagestad, and Ilene Siegler to produce a television course on adult development in 1985.

An early interest in age norms and age bias appeared in several articles from 1971, and in a 1978 book, *Perspectives on Counseling Adults* (Monterey, Calif.: Brooks/Cole), with Nancy Schlossberg and Sandra Liebowitz. Her most recent work has been in collaboration with Colleen Johnson on the oldest old (see "Family-Embedded vs. Family-Deprived Oldest-Old: A Study of Contrasts," *International Journal of Aging and Human Development,* 38 (1994): 51–63; and with Vern L. Bengston on modified-extended families. See "The Oldest-Old in Families: An Intergenerational Perspective, Symbolic and Instrumental Links" in *Generations,* Summer 17 (1992): 39–44.

Troll is currently professor emerita at Rutgers University and is affiliated with the University of California in San Francisco.

V

CASSIUS JAMES VAN SLYKE. Cassius James Van Slyke was born in Benson, Minnesota, in 1890. He took his degrees at the University of Minnesota: B.S., 1923; M.B., 1927; M.D., 1928. Van Slyke then served as a medical officer with the U.S. Public Health Service (USPHS) in Washington (1928–1929), practiced medicine in Wisconsin (1929–1930), and then returned to the Public Health Service, where he essentially spent the rest of his career.

From 1936 to 1943, Van Slyke was associate director of the USPHS's veneral disease research laboratory. There he focused on sulfonade and penicillin therapy in gonococcal infections. He then moved to Washington, D.C., to supervise the grants program. After the war, he joined the National Institutes of Health. He became the director of the National Heart Institute in 1948. It was in this capacity that he developed an interest in research in aging: Nathan W. Shock's* Gerontology Research Center was one of the units under his supervision. In 1950, Van Slyke served as president of the Gerontological Society.

DAVID D. VAN TASSEL. David D. Van Tassel was born in Binghamton, New York, in 1928. After serving in the Army Signal Corps (1946–1947), he attended Dartmouth College, graduating in 1950. He then studied history under Merle Curti, then the dean of U.S. intellectual historians, at the University of Wisconsin. He earned his Ph.D. in 1955.

Van Tassel spent his early career at the University of Texas, becoming an associate professor in 1961 and a full professor four years later. There, he evinced his longstanding interest in historiography, with the publication of *Recording America's Past: An Interpretation of the Development of Historical*

Studies in America, 1607–1884 (Chicago: University of Chicago Press, 1960). Van Tassel also gained attention for two works he edited during this period: *Science and Society in the United States,* Michael G. Hall (Chicago, Ill.: Dorsey Press, 1966), and *American Thought in the Twentieth Century* (New York: Thomas Y. Crowell Company, 1967). In 1969, Van Tassel joined the faculty of Case Western Reserve University, serving as chair from 1976 to 1980 and from 1987 to 1992. Since 1993, he has been the Hiram C. Hayden Professor of History.

Van Tassel was probably the first senior U.S. historian to recognize the importance of developing humanistic perspectives on aging. In the early 1970s, he gained support from the National Endowment for the Humanities to invite distinguished scholars (such as Erik and Joan Erikson and Peter Laslett*) to Cleveland in 1975 to ''teach'' rising assistant professors (such as Daniel Scott Smith, David Stannard, and Maris Vinovskis in history) key concepts and useful strategies for thinking about growing older. Philosophers, literary critics, artists, and experts in non-western societies were invited to join the proceedings. Also in attendance were David Hackett Fischer, who would write the first history of aging in America, and several graduate students who would concentrate in this area. The group of scholars then reconvened in New York at a meeting of the Gerontological Society to discuss their papers. From this project came two major collections of essays. *Aging and the Elderly: Humanistic Perspectives in Gerontology* (Atlantic Highlands, N.J.: Humanities Press, 1978), which Van Tassel edited with Stuart Spicker and Kathleen Woodward, was cited as Book of the Year by the *American Journal of Nursing.* His *Aging, Death, and the Completion of Being* (Philadelphia: University of Pennsylvania Press, 1979) was cited as one of the outstanding books published by University Presses that year.

In 1984, Van Tassel once again invited a group of scholars to Case Western, though this time the guest list included mainly historians and some social scientists who were interested in comparing past and present trends in gerontology. From this symposium arose *Old Age in a Bureaucratic Society: The Elderly, the Experts, and the State in American History* (Westport, Conn.: Greenwood Press, 1986), which he edited with Peter N. Stearns. In addition to chairing panels and delivering papers on the history of old age at meetings of the American Historical Association and the Gerontological Society, Van Tassel has also chaired GSA's Arts and Humanities Committee and served on the editorial board of *The Gerontologist.* His importance as a gatekeeper is underscored in his serving as an editor (with Thomas R. Cole* and Robert Kastenbaum*) of the *Handbook of Aging and the Humanities* (New York: Springer Publishing, 1992) and as founding editor of the *Human Values and Aging Newsletter* (1975–present).

Van Tassel has also been a major force behind Case Western Reserve's program in the history of social policy. With Jimmy Meyer, he edited *Aging Policy Interest Groups* (Westport, Conn.: Greenwood Press, 1992). He also has served as senior editor of several works that recount the history of arts, sports, and lives of major figures in Cleveland. Perhaps best known in this series is his *Encyclopedia of Cleveland History* (Bloomington: Indiana University Press, 1987). Eager to share his enthusiasm for history with young people, Van Tassel was a major organizer of History Day programs.

For his many accomplishments, Van Tassel is listed in *Who's Who in America* and *Who's Who in the World.* He has served as a mentor to most of the historians of aging born after World War II, including W. Andrew Achenbaum, Brian Gratton,* and Carole Haber.*

LOIS M. VERBRUGGE. Lois M. Verbrugge was born in Massachusetts in 1945 but spent her childhood and teen years in Minnesota. After graduating *summa cum laude* from Stanford University with a major in French and a minor in mathematics (1967), she completed a master's degree in public health at the University of Michigan in 1969, where she studied population planning. Five years later, she completed her Ph.D. there.

Verbrugge's background in population studies and sociology led to early research in illness and mortality differences by gender. She contributed prominently to conceptual, theoretical, and empirical research that explained the paradox of higher morbidity but lower mortality among females. See, for example, her "Sex Differentials in Health," *Public Health Reports,* 97 (1982): 417–37. Verbrugge extended the logic of this work to research on aging when Richard C. Adelman* tapped her to join the University of Michigan's Institute of Gerontology.

Verbrugge's initial focus on aging stressed gender differences in health status. See (for its title no less than its contents), "From Sneezes to Adieux: Stages of Health for American Men and Women," *Social Science and Medicine,* 22 (1986): 1195–1212. Verbrugge conducted the first empirical analysis that demonstrated the increasing rates of chronic conditions and disability that correspond to mortality rate decreases in modern societies. See "Longer Life but Worsening Health? Trends in Health and Mortality of Middle-Aged and Older Persons," *Milbank Memorial Fund Quarterly/Health and Society,* 62 (1984): 475–519.

In the late 1980s, Verbrugge became interested in the ways that older people coped with physical disabilities. In particular, she has focused on arthritis because it is the leading chronic condition in middle and later life. Seeking to bridge the gap between medical research and social science, Verbrugge obtained formal training in rheumatology at the University of Michigan Medical School. The training was sponsored by the National Institute on Aging's Special Emphasis Research Career Award. More recently, she has been working with colleagues in the University of Michigan's School of Engineering on strategies for measuring musculoskeletal function in community-dwelling populations and also on musculoskeletal abilities and job demands of aging workers. Here, clearly, is an instance of someone in gerontology who is willing to pursue interdisciplinary research with the specialized training necessary.

Verbrugge's latest work is in the theory and measurement of disability. She has conceptualized disability as a gap between personal capability and environmental demand, and developed survey methods to assess changes in both. She has paid particular attention to co-morbidity and its impact on disability, comparative levels of disability for arthritic and non-arthritic persons, and disability transitions from functional to non-functional activities. In 1989 and 1990, Verbrugge participated in two pilot projects that developed innovative protocols and equipment to conduct in-home measurements of the musculoskeletal functions in order to detect osteoarthritis in older adults. In 1991 and 1992, she worked at the Gerontology Research Center, National Institute on Aging, analyzing time-use data in the Baltimore Longitudinal Study of Aging.

In addition to her work as a research scientist for the Institute of Gerontology, Verbrugge has been affiliated with the Johns Hopkins University as assistant professor and visiting professor, and at the University of Minnesota as a visiting professor. One of a handful of Distinguished Research Scientists at the University of Michigan, Verbrugge's work on gender was honored by the American Psychological Association in 1994.

W

ROY WALFORD. Roy Walford was born in 1924. According to a profile in *American Health* (September 1991): 18–21, he was in high school in San Diego when he first started thinking about the idea of living as long as possible. This early interest in prolongevity led him to medicine; he graduated from the University of Chicago (B.A., 1946; M.D., 1948). Upon graduation, his career took an unusual turn. With a friend he figured out a way to beat the roulette wheel; the pair won nearly $30,000 and spent the next eighteen months sailing around the Caribbean. Such eclecticism balanced with systematic thinking makes Walford one of the most original and controversial figures in research on aging today.

Early on, Walford was mainly associated with theories of immunology of aging. He believed that immune function and dysfunction, associated with built-in genetic controls, accounted for many aspects of aging discovered in the laboratory. See, for instance, his *Immunologic Theory of Aging* (Baltimore: Williams and Wilkins, 1969). Neither did Walford discount other possible ways of prolonging life that interacted with immunological processes. He and Robert Liu, a zoologist at UCLA where Walford has spent much of his career, studied "Increased Growth and Life-Span with Lowered Ambient Temperature in the Annual Fish, Cynolebias Adloffi," *Nature,* 212 (1966): 1277–78. Their experiments suggested that the suppression of auto-immune functions by lower ambient temperatures was responsible for augmenting lifespan.

Like other researchers on aging, Walford also stressed the importance of diet in promoting healthful longevity. With R. H. Weindruch, he published *The Retardation of Aging and Disease by Dietary Restriction* (New York: Harper and

Row, 1988). The message was popularized in *Maximum Life Span* (New York: Norton, 1983); his best-selling book, *The 120-Year Diet* (New York: Pocket Books, 1988); and more recently, *The Anti-Aging Plan* (San Francisco: Four Walls Eight Windows, 1994). There he stressed that gradually eating less, and then eating a selected diet that is high in nutrition and low in calories, so that one optimally weighed 10 percent to 25 percent less than the prescribed "normal" weight, would help to prolong life. Lest his suggestions for breakfast (¼ cup of rye flakes with 2.5 teaspoons of wheat bran and a teaspoon of yeast, accompanied by a glass of skim milk and a peach) sound as if Walford had traded the laboratory for talk shows, it is worth reading his essay (with Patricia Mote and Judith Grizzle), "Influence of Age and Caloric Restriction on Expression of Hepatic Genes for Xenobiotic and Oxygen Metabolizing Enzymes in the Mouse," *Journal of Gerontology*, 46 (1991): B995–B100, which found that catalase activity increased significantly with caloric restrictions in young and old hybrid strains of female mice.

Recently, Walford served as the medical officer of Biosphere 2, his laboratory for what he calls "biospheric medicine," which studies such things as the effects of oxygen depletion in humans. Inside Biosphere 2 he also carried out the first well-controlled calorie restriction with a nutrient-dense diet in humans (see Walford et al., *Proceedings of the National Academy of Science*, 89 (1992): 11533. An account of Walford's experiences appeared in "Science Under Glass," *Medicine on the Midway* (Winter 1993/94): 14–17.) Most of Walford's career has been spent at the University of California at Los Angeles; since 1966, he has been a professor of pathology.

RUSSELL A. WARD. Like many gerontologists, sociologist Russell A. Ward was drawn to studying age-related processes through other interests. He earned his B.A. with distinction from the University of Rochester in 1969. As a graduate student interested in medical sociology and deviance at the University of Wisconsin, where he completed his Ph.D. in 1974, Ward became interested in applying concepts in Erving Goffman's *Stigma: Notes on the Management of Spoiled Identity* (Englewood Cliffs, N.J.: Prentice-Hall, 1963) to aging and age-related stereotypes. In his emerging interests, he was greatly assisted by John Delamater, David Mechanic, and Geraldine Clausen. As Ward's subsequent interests in gerontology broadened, he was influenced by the work of Vern L. Bengtson,* M. Powell Lawton,* and Matilda White Riley.*

Ward's early analyses investigated patterns of "age identity." This work attended to the antecedents of an older age identity as "elderly" or "old," as well as the implications of age identity, or of "feeling old," for an individual's well-being. See his article, "The Impact of Subjective Age and Stigma on Older Persons," *Journal of Gerontology*, 32 (1977): 221–32. This early interest was more recently broadened to include "middle-aged" identities in a collaboration with John Loran and Glenna Spitze, "As Old As You Feel: Age Identity in Middle and Later Life," *Social Forces*, 71 (1992): 451–67.

Ward turned next to the dimensions of the informal support networks of older people. Much of this work has been done in collaboration with Mark LaGory and Susan R. Sherman*; see *The Environment for Aging: Social, Interpersonal, and Spatial Contexts* (Tuscaloosa, Ala.: University of Alabama Press, 1988). Ward's efforts include an emphasis on the differences between objective and subjective dimensions of networks, age structures in neighborhoods and communities, and the age-segregation process in the United States. This and his earlier work also contributed to a consideration of issues associated with age stratification. See, for example, Ward's article, "The Marginality and Salience of Being Old," *The Gerontologist*, 24 (1984): 221–32. These and other sociological issues related to aging were further elaborated in a textbook for undergraduate and graduate students, *The Aging Experience* (New York: Harper & Row, 2nd edn., 1984).

Ward's other gerontological work has reflected a variety of interests, including racial differences across age/cohort groups, sources of variation in attitudes toward euthanasia, and marital satisfaction among older couples. Several studies have explored health-related attitudes and behaviors, including provider choice and satisfaction. See, for example, "Health Care Provider Choice and Satisfaction," Ward's chapter in *The Legacy of Longevity*, edited by Sidney Stahl (Newbury Park, Calif.: Sage, 1990).

Most recently, Ward has been investigating patterns of co-residence between parents and adult children. Collaborative work with John Logan and Glenna Spitze has indicated the ways in which child needs lead to co-residence with both middle-aged and older parents. See their article, "The Influence of Parent and Child Needs on Co-Residence in Middle and Later Life," *Journal of Marriage and the Family*, 54 (1992): 205–21. Ward and Spitze have also investigated exchange patterns and outcomes among co-resident parents and children; see their article, "Consequences of Parent-Adult Child Co-Residence: A Review and Research Agenda," *Journal of Family Issues*, 13 (1992): 553–72.

Ward is currently a professor of sociology at the State University of New York at Albany.

ALDRED SCOTT WARTHIN. Aldred Scott Warthin was born in Greensburg, Indiana, in 1866. After earning a teacher's diploma from the Cincinnati Conservatory of Music in 1887, he received his B.A. and Phi Beta Kappa key from Indiana University a year later. Warthin did his graduate training at the University of Michigan, earning his M.D. in 1891 and his Ph.D. in 1893. He also did graduate medical work at the universities of Vienna, Freiburg, Munich, and Dresden.

Warthin spent his entire professional career in Ann Arbor. He established a practice in town, specializing in pathological research. Between 1892 and 1902, when not abroad, he held various junior positions at the University of Michigan. In 1903, he became a professor and director of the pathology laboratories in the university's medical school. In the course of his career, Warthin published over

1,000 articles in medical journals and textbooks. Among his areas of specialization were the pathology of the haemolymph gland, the pathology of diseases of the blood and blood-forming organs, cardiac syphillis, latent syphillis, and tuberculosis.

Active in many medical and historical societies, Warthin was president of the American Association of Pathologists and Bacteriologists (1908), the Association of Experimental Pathology (1924), and the American Association for Cancer Research (1927–1928).

Warthin merits inclusion in this book as the author of *Old Age, the Major Involution: The Physiology & Pathology of the Aging Process* (New York: P.B. Hoeber, 1930). The volume elaborated ideas Warthin first presented before the New York Academy of Medicine two years earlier. That these lectures were printed in the *Bulletin of the New York Academy of Medicine,* 4 (October 1928) and then reprinted in the *New York State Journal of Medicine,* 28 (1928) attests to their importance. The human "tragicomedy," he claimed, had three stages— evolution, maturity, and involution. The world-renowned pathologist went on to declare that aging was a physiological process: "Senescence is due primarily to the gradually weakening energy-charge set in action by the moment of fertilization." The decline could not be deferred much past the age of 75, he believed.

IRVING LEONARD WEBBER. Irving Leonard Webber was born in Luverne, Minnesota, in 1915. He served in the U.S. Navy from 1944 to 1947. After earning his M.A. from the University of Florida in 1950, Webber directed a retirement study for the Florida State Improvement Commission, a job that led to a full-time position on the commission. In 1953, he joined the Sociology and Anthropology Department of the University of Florida, and became a member of the University of Florida's Institute of Gerontology. Meanwhile, he completed his requirements for a Ph.D. from Louisiana State University in 1956.

Much of Webber's subsequent work focused on the retirees of St. Petersburg, and the relationship between social class, mental health, and age and aging. For instance, with E. Wilbur Bock, Webber wrote "Social Status and Relational System of Elderly Suicides," *Life-Threatening Behavior,* 2 (1972): 145–59, which analyzed 147 males over age sixty-five from a Florida county. The authors found that lower-class men were more likely to commit suicide.

With Albert J. Wilson, Webber wrote "Attrition in a Longitudinal Study of an Aged Population," in *Experimental Aging Research,* 2 (1976): 367–87, which traced the demographic characteristics of roughly 2,500 people in a Florida retirement community. Those who were around to be interviewed seemed to differ from those who dropped out in terms of age, sex, and prevalence of chronic conditions.

JACK WEINBERG. Jack Weinberg was born in Kiev, Russia, in 1910. He came to the United States in 1924, and became a naturalized citizen in 1937. After receiving his B.S. from the University of Illinois in 1934, he earned his M.D.

two years later. Weinberg did his internship at St. Elizabeth's Hospital in Chicago (1936–1937), and was a resident in psychiatry at the University of Illinois Medical School and Hospital (1938–1939). He did advanced studies at the Chicago Institute for Psychoanalysis (1941–1943) and then served as associate director for the residency teaching program at Michael Reese Hospital and Medical Center.

From 1950 to 1964, Weinberg was in private practice. In 1955, he became a lecturer at the University of Chicago's Industrial Relations Center and senior attending psychiatrist at Michael Reese's Psychosomatic and Psychiatric Institute. He then accepted a position as clinical director of the Illinois State Psychiatric Institute in 1964, becoming institute director in 1975. Concurrently, Weinberg served as a professor of psychiatry at the University of Illinois School of Medicine (1962) and at Rush Medical College (1972). In addition, he held a visiting professorship at the Andrus Gerontology Center at the University of Southern California and, in 1978, was invited to serve as distinguished senior scholar at the National Institute of Mental Health's Center for the Study of Mental Health of the Aging.

With Lawrence Lazarus, Weinberg summarized much of his clinical insights in two articles. In "Psychosocial Intervention with the Aged," *Psychiatric Clinics of North America*, 5 (April 1982): 215–27, the authors stressed the need for an interdisciplinary approach. At minimum, they argued, an integrated strategy required early intervention and frequent reassessments supervised by a designated patient coordinator. This bio-psychosocial approach also included family therapy, telephone psychotherapy, and home assessments. In "Training in Geropsychiatry: Problems and Process," *American Journal of Psychiatry*, 138 (October 1981): 1366–69, Lazarus and Weinberg suggested that the way to overcome medical school deans' resistance to incorporating substantive geropsychiatry training into curricula was to form alliances with department chairs and training directors, and to provide varied clinical experiences with both healthy and impaired elderly patients.

Weinberg was honored with the Edward B. Allen award from the American Geriatrics Society in 1970 and with the Kent Award four years later from the Gerontological Society of America. In 1980, he served as president of the American Medical Association's Group Advancement of Psychiatry. Weinberg was also active in several councils for the Jewish elderly.

WILLIAM G. WEISSERT. William G. Weissert graduated with an M.S. degree from Northwestern University in 1968 and a Ph.D. at California's Claremont Graduate School in 1972. He has since been studying the nature of long-term care problems here and abroad and the merits of approaches to solving them.

One of his continuing interests has been to describe geriatric care at the national level. An overview of this research can be found in Weissert et al., *Adult Day Care: Findings from a National Survey* (Baltimore: Johns Hopkins University Press, 1990).

He next turned to the cost-effectiveness of home care, which he describes as "a complement, not a substitute for nursing home care." Contrary to conventional wisdom, he argues, home care and community-based care serves a different population than do nursing homes. His views are summarized in "Seven Reasons Why it is So Difficult to Make Home Care Cost-Effective," *Health Services Research,* 20 (Summer 1985): 47–50. One of Weissert's missions has therefore been to find ways to improve the cost-effectiveness of home care. See, for example, "Strategies for Reducing Home Care Expenditures," *Generations* (Spring 1990): 42–44, and his chapter, "Targeting Home Care for Cost-Effectiveness" in *The Living-at-Home Program,* ed. Morton D. Bogdonoff (New York: Springer, 1991), 50–62. Weissert is best known for research in this area.

In addition, Weissert has proposed innovative funding mechanisms to make nursing home care affordable for patients and to improve the quality of care through financial incentives. He has further proposed public policy interventions to deal with the long-term care population, as well as demonstrated the inadequacy of private insurance schemes for long-term care.

His collaborators include colleagues Thomas Wan, Cynthia Cready, and Sidney Katz, and his students Jennifer Elston, Catherine Wilson, and Elise Bolda. Weissert is a professor of health management and policy with the University of Michigan School of Public Health and is a research scientist for Michigan's Institute of Gerontology.

ALAN TRAVISS WELFORD. A.T. Welford is one of the world's pioneers in the psychological study of human performance in relation to aging. He earned a bachelor's degree in 1935 and a senior doctorate (Sc.D.) in 1964 from the University of Cambridge. (The Sc.D. is awarded for major scientific research contributions over an extended period. Welford was only the third psychologist to earn this prestigious degree.)

Welford's interest in gerontology began when the late Sir Frederic Bartlett, who was the first professor of psychology at Cambridge and had been Welford's most significant teacher and mentor, invited him to lead a unit sponsored by the Nuffield Foundation at the Cambridge University Psychological Laboratory. This pioneering unit was the first in Britain to study the psychological aspects of aging performance.

The unit's research consisted of laboratory experiments on several aspects of cognitive and sensory-motor performance, and of field investigations in industry. The aim was to coordinate these two types of study so that each could benefit from the other. The work of the unit was described in Welford's immediately influential book, *Ageing and Human Skill* (Oxford, England: Oxford University Press, 1958). The work remains a classic in the field.

Since 1958, Welford has been concerned to bring together gerontological and general psychological research to further the understanding of human performance in relation to aging. Significant publications include "Motor Performance," in *Handbook of the Psychology of Aging,* eds. James E. Birren* and K. W. Schaie* (New York: Van Nostrand Reinhold, 1977), 450–96; and "Preventing Adverse Changes of Work with Age," *International Journal of Aging and Human Development,* 27 (1988): 283–91.

During the period that the Nuffield Unit was operating (1946–1956), colleagues in the Cambridge Laboratory developed the concept that performance depends on the relation between signal levels and randomness ("noise") within the sense organs and central nervous system. Welford saw in this concept a powerful model to account for several of the differences in performance with age, such as slowing of important changes in sensory-motor activity, lengthening of choice reactional times, and difficulty of recovering items from memory. He promoted the model in several published articles; see "Signal, Noise, Performance and Age," *Human Factors,* 23 (1981): 97–109.

In 1968 Welford moved from Cambridge to the University of Adelaide, South Australia. After retirement in 1979, he and his wife went to live in Honolulu, where he was given an honorary appointment by the University of Hawaii, before returning to England in 1987. His interest in gerontology continues.

TERRIE WETLE. Terrie Wetle earned a master of science degree from Portland State University in 1971 and her Ph.D. there five years later. Asked what drew her to the field, Wetle responds, "Robert Butler,* Robert Morris* and Robert Binstock* were the first 'names' whose work was of relevance." Her mentors include John O'Brien while at the Institute on Aging and Byron Gold at the Administration on Aging.

Wetle's principal contribution has been to bring a philosophically based understanding of ethics to the work-a-day practice of geriatric care through empirical research. She has improved understanding of the perceptions and experiences of older persons and professional caregivers as they relate to ethical choices. For example, she has examined the factors influencing the choices of caregivers as they relate to the distribution of scarce resources. See Julie Cwikel, Sue E. Levkoff, and Terrie Wetle, "Geriatric Medical Decisions: Factors Influencing Allocation of Scarce Resources and the Decision to Withhold Treatment," *The Gerontologist,* 28 (June 1988): 336–43.

Wetle has also described the ethical issues involved in protecting the bodily integrity, religious freedom, and self-determination of the elderly. "Frequently, these efforts have required questioning basic assumptions of advocates for aging issues and teasing out the multiple meanings of observed attitudes and decision processes," Wetle says. In a recent article she pointed out that the elderly in institutional settings are at particular risk of compromised autonomy. Caregivers are often faced with situations in which it is difficult to protect the individual's rights. The erosion of autonomy is often the result of paternalistic caregivers. See her "Ethical Issues in Long-Term Care of the Aged," *Journal of Geriatric Psychiatry,* 18 (1985): 63–75.

In her research, Wetle has found that age often stands as a proxy for other characteristics or risk factors, such as risk of a bad outcome, co-morbidities, social worth, and expected response to treatment. She has defined and articulated the concept of ethical risk in the particular way that it applies to older persons in health- and social-care decisions. See, for example, "Age as a Risk Factor for Inadequate Treatment," *The Journal of the American Medical Association,* 258 (July 1987): 41–42.

This research has informed her teaching of physicians. While at the Administration on Aging, Wetle developed a geriatric medicine fellowship program. At the Hastings Center in New York, she worked on a geriatric medicine program to improve the real-world experience of ethicists. Wetle is currently affiliated with the Hartford, Connecticut-based Braceland Center for Mental Health and Aging. John W. Rowe* and her husband, Richard W. Besdine,* have been important collaborators in this regard.

In 1995 Wetle became associate director of the National Institute on Aging.

NANCY ALVIS WHITELAW. Nancy Alvis Whitelaw completed her Ph.D. at the School of Public Health of the University of Michigan, in 1989. Like so many in the field, Whitelaw was attracted to gerontology by some of its most important figures, including Bernice L. Neugarten,* Ethel Shanas,* and M. Powell Lawton.* With her dissertation on "subjectively rated health among older men and women," Whitelaw entered the field as a full-time researcher. Her adviser was Jersey Liang. Actually her interest had been sparked earlier by her interventions with practitioners in the field.

Whitelaw noticed that despite the demonstrated usefulness of subjective health ratings as predictors of health services utilization, they were not clearly understood. Her doctoral research concluded that subjective health ratings are derived from older people's knowledge about their objective health status. Such ratings therefore provide valuable information about actual health status and are valuable in predicting service use and health care needs.

The Detroit-based Henry Ford Health System Center for Health System Studies hired Whitelaw first as a research associate, and two years later promoted her to her current position as associate director. There she continued her strong commitment to promoting interdisciplinary research and education, focusing on studies of models of care for older adults and urban, underserved populations.

In a 1991 article for the journal *Medical Care,* Whitelaw and Liang proposed and evaluated two models for integrating self-reported, subjective health status into dominant conceptualizations of physical health. Using the Older Americans Resources and Services Multidimensional Functional Assessment Questionnaire, they found a good correlation between the data and both models. See *Medical Care,* 29 (1991): 332–47.

BLOSSOM T. WIGDOR. Psychologist Blossom T. Wigdor studied at McGill University, earning her Ph.D. there in 1952. Like so many psychologists who did pioneering work in gerontology, Wigdor was first attracted by the research of James E. Birren.* She was also impressed by his development of a research and teaching center for the field.

Wigdor's own work has focused on the separation of retention issues from memory function. Simply put, she emphasized the need to ensure that material had in fact been learned before researchers could accurately test for memory. See her collaboration with R. E. Wimer, "Age Differences in Retention of Learning," *Journal of Gerontology,* 13 (1958): 291–95. More often, Wigdor has collaborated with V. A. Kral, beginning with a 1957 report on "Psychiatric and Psychological Observations in a Geriatric Clinic," *Canadian Psychiatric Association Journal,* 2 (1957): 185–89. For their work on memory function, see, for example, "Androgen Effect of Senescent Memory Function," *Geriatrics,* 14 (1959): 450–56.

Wigdor also contributed to the development of research and education in gerontology. She has developed curricula and directed the first all-university, multidisciplinary gerontology center in Canada. She has been affiliated with the Centre for Studies of Aging at the University of Toronto. Wigdor continues to shape aging research and policy in Canada. See, for example, "The Development of Gerontology in Canada," *Center Reports on Advances in Research,* 10 (1984): 1–8. She also has tried to translate scholarly findings into information for consumers. See her *Planning for Retirement: The Canadian Self-Help Guide,* 3rd edn. (Toronto: Grovenor House Press, 1988), and *Over-Forty Society's Issues for Canada's Aging Population,* written with David Foot (Toronto: Lorimer Press, 1989). Wigdor was the first editor-in-chief of the *Canadian Journal on Aging.*

Wigdor chaired the (Canadian) National Advisory Council on Aging (1990– 1993) and the Canadian Coalition on Medication Use of the Elderly (1991– 1993). She became a member of the Order of Canada (1989), and received honorary degrees from the University of Victoria (1990) and the University of Guelph (1994). In 1993, Wigdor received the 125th Anniversary of Canada Commemorative Medal.

SHERRY WILLIS. Sherry Willis earned a Ph.D. in educational psychology from the University of Texas at Austin in 1972. She was attracted to gerontology by her mentor Paul Baltes,* but sees her colleague and husband K. Warner Schaie* as a role model.

Willis's most important work to date has been in the study of cognitive training of older adults. Working with Schaie, Willis has examined the possibilities for enhancing the intellectual functioning of older adults through (brief) educational training programs. They reported findings in 1986 of a long-term longitudinal study of 229 older adults and efforts to reverse cognitive decline. Their results show that cognitive training techniques reliably reverse declines in spatial and reasoning abilities documented over a fourteen-year period in a substantial number of subjects. See Schaie and Willis, "Can Decline in Adult Intellectual

Functioning Be Reversed?'' *Developmental Psychology,* 22 (March 1986): 223–32.

The everyday life experiences of the elderly have been a more recent subject of interest for Willis. She has examined the intellectual abilities and processes in older adults' functioning on tasks of daily living. See her ''Cognitive and Everyday Competence,'' *Annual Review of Gerontology and Geriatrics* (Vol. 11), ed. K. W. Schaie (New York: Springer, 1991). See also, ''Everyday Cognition: Taxonomic and Methodological Considerations'' (with K. W. Schaie) in *Lifespan Developmental Psychology: Mechanisms of Everyday Cognition,* eds. J. M. Puckett and H. W. Reese (Hillsdale, N.J.: Erlbaum, 1991), 33–53. Willis's research was often cited in the late 1980s and early 1990s as educators, professors, and university administrators debated the opportunities and costs of uncapping mandatory retirement in higher education.

Willis is currently affiliated with Pennsylvania State University.

PHYLLIS M. WISE. Phyllis M. Wise was born in 1945. She earned her B. A. from Swarthmore College in 1967 and then studied at the University of Michigan, where she completed a master's degree (1969) and Ph.D. (1972) in zoology. From 1972 until 1974, Wise did postdoctoral work at Michigan.

Her next stop was the University of New Mexico's School of Medicine, where she worked as a research associate and later as an adjunct assistant professor in the Department of Physiology. In 1976, Wise joined the faculty at the University of Maryland, rising to full professor by 1987. She has been a visitor of the German University of Goettingen's Department of Obstetrics and Gynecology. In 1993, Wise accepted the position of professor and chairwoman of physiology at the University of Kentucky.

Neuroendocrine and neurochemical mechanisms have been Wise's primary research interests. She has studied how such mechanisms regulate the aging of neural function, with particular emphasis on their role in regulating the female reproduction system. Wise is interested in the daily rhythm of neurotransmitter function and its relationship to reproduction, and in prolactin as a regulator of reproduction. She has written more than six dozen peer-reviewed journal articles and two dozen chapters. Recent representative samples of her work include: J. M. Lloyd, G. E. Hoffman, and P. M. Wise, ''Decline in Immediate Early Gene Expression in Gonadotropin-Releasing Hormone Neurons During Proestrus in Regularly Cycling, Middle-Aged Rats,'' *Endocrinology,* 134 (1994): 1800–805; and N. G. Weiland, K. Scarbrough, and P. M. Wise, ''Aging Abolishes the Estradiol-Induced Suppression and Diurnal Rhythm of Propiomelanocortin Gene Expression in the Arcuate Nucleus,'' *Endocrinology,* 131 (1992): 2959–964.

The bulk of this research has been funded by the National Institutes of Health. Since 1980 Wise has been granted more than $2 million—including a MERIT Award—for work on neuroendocrine and neurochemical function research related to aging. She has in turn sponsored National Research Scientist Awards for I. R. Cohen-Becker, N. G. Weiland, G. H. Larson, and J. M. Lloyd, T. McShane and J. P. Harvey.

In addition to her teaching and research, Wise has taken on a number of professional responsibilities. At the University of Maryland she has chaired her share of search committees and worked briefly as the head of the graduate program in physiology. She has served on several National Institutes of Health advisory committees, and is a member of the board of the Nathan W. and Margaret T. Shock Aging Research Foundation. Wise was on the editorial board of *Neurobiology of Aging* from 1982 until 1988, at which time she joined the editorial board of the *Journal of Gerontology*. She will serve as chairwoman of the Biological Science Section of the GSA in 1995–1996.

ROSALIE S. WOLF. In 1964, Rosalie S. Wolf joined the first board of directors of the Age Center of the Worcester Area in her home town of Worcester, Massachusetts. The center was supported by a Ford Foundation grant and administered through Brandeis University's Heller Graduate School. So impressed was Wolf with the Brandeis students and their approach to social welfare problems that she decided to return to school after a twenty-one-year hiatus.

Wolf's earlier work had been in biochemistry. She earned a B.S. in chemistry from the University of Wisconsin and spent the next year at the Harvard Medical School studying biochemistry. During the years that followed, she was an active community volunteer, focusing on the development of policies and programs for the mentally ill and aging populations. She studied at Brandeis from 1971 until 1976, earning a Ph.D. in social welfare. Her dissertation examined the relationship between the availability of mental health services for the elderly and the use of long-term care facilities by the mentally impaired.

Wolf directed the Gerontology Planning Project for the University of Massachusetts Medical Center from 1977 until 1981 and then served as the associate director of its successor, the University Center on Aging. In 1989, she became the director of the Institute on Aging at the Medical Center of Central Massachusetts.

Wolf's most important work has been in the area of elder abuse. She has directed several projects supported by the Administration on Aging, including "An Evaluation of Three Model Projects on Elder Abuse," "Project IDEA: Information Dissemination about Elder Abuse," "Coalition Building for the Prevention of Elder Abuse," and "Synthesis and Dissemination of Title IV Research and Development Projects on Elder Abuse."

In collaboration with Karl A. Pillemer, she co-edited *Elder Abuse: Conflict in the Family* (Dover, Mass.: Auburn House, 1986) and co-wrote *Helping Elderly Victims: The Reality of Elder Abuse* (New York: Columbia University Press). She is currently president of the National Committee for the Prevention of Elder Abuse (NCPEA), which she founded, and has co-edited the *Journal of Elder Abuse and Neglect* since 1987. As president of NCPEA, Wolf serves on the management team for the National Center on Elder Abuse in Washington, D.C.

The National Council of Jewish Women honored Wolf with the Hannah G. Solomon Award for "outstanding service to the aging" in 1972. She became a Gerontological Society of America Fellow in 1985, and she earned first prize in the Retirement Research Foundation's National Media Awards educational film category in 1987.

ANNE MARBURY WYATT-BROWN. Anne Marbury Wyatt-Brown, born in 1939, graduated *cum laude* from Radcliffe College in 1961. She earned a master of arts in teaching degree (English) from Johns Hopkins the following year and completed her Ph.D. at Case Western Reserve in 1972. Her dissertation, written under the direction of Roger B. Solomon, was on "E. M. Forster and the Transformation of Comedy."

An expert in the British comedy of manners, Wyatt-Brown may seem an unlikely prospect for developing an interest in gerontology. But her research has focused on the relationship among aging, creativity, and literary style. Her interests were sparked by David Van Tassel, a historian at Case Western Reserve, who has tried to encourage experts from the humanities to do research on aging. For example, Wyatt-Brown's study of the late-life novels of Elizabeth Bowen has caused a re-examination of the connection between depression and loss in late middle age and the forging of a new literary style. Critics had dismissed Bowen's final works either as those of an old woman stuck in an earlier age or as the result of age-related decay. But, Wyatt-Brown argues, "by linking a psychodynamic understanding of depression with the theoretical perspectives of biography and literary gerontology, one can interpret Bowen's experimental novels in a much more favorable light." Her essay on Bowen can be found in a recent collection she edited with Janice Rossen, *Gender and Aging: Studies in Creativity* (Charlottesville, Va.: University Press of Virginia, 1993). She has also brought theories of aging to bear in *Barbara Pym: A Critical Biography* (Columbia, Mo.: University of Missouri Press, 1992).

Wyatt-Brown coined the term "literary gerontology" to describe her work and that of other critics interested in aging. She was certainly the first to review the newly labeled work in "Literary Gerontology Comes of Age," in the *Handbook of the Humanities and Aging,* edited by Thomas R. Cole,* David Van Tassel, and Robert Kastenbaum* (New York: Springer, 1992). See also "The Coming of Age of Literary Gerontology," *Journal of Aging Studies,* 4 (1990): 299–315.

Wyatt-Brown has served on the editorial board of the *Journal of Aging Studies* since 1989, *the International Journal of Aging and Human Development* since 1993, and the reviewers board of *The Gerontologist* since 1993. In 1993, she became founding editor of *Age Studies,* a book series at the Press of the University of Virginia. She is currently an assistant professor in the Program of Linguistics at the University of Florida.

Y _____

GWEN YEO. Gwen Yeo earned her Ph.D. from Stanford University in 1982, where she was "not fortunate enough to study under faculty in gerontology." She was influenced, however, by the work of James E. Birren,* Robert N. Butler,* and Robert C. Atchley.* Yeo has remained at Stanford's Geriatric Education Center (SGEC) ever since; she is currently the center's director. Her colleagues include Jose Cuellar, Nancy Morioka-Douglas, Julee Richardson, and Marita Grudzen.

Yeo is best known for her work in "ethnogeriatrics." The concept of ethnogerontology—the study of ethnic variations in aging—has been around for some time, but the application of this approach to geriatrics is fairly recent. It can be traced to the faculty of the SGEC, which in 1987 coined the term "ethnogeriatrics" to mean health care for elders of diverse populations.

Yeo's particular interest has been in the development of curriculum resources for training health care providers to serve ethnically diverse groups of elders. In many ways, Yeo is a promoter of the concept, which has gained wide use by organizers and writers. In 1991, she outlined and defined the field in "Ethnogeriatric Education: Need and Content," *Journal of Cross-Cultural Gerontology*, 6 (1991): 229–41.

With the concept fully established, Yeo is taking the next step—emphasizing the need to recognize heterogeneity within groups of elders in ethnic populations. The goal is to develop the "cultural competence" to provide effective health care. Yeo's approach can be summed up in her phrase, "Celebrate the diversity and appreciate the complexity." For more on Yeo's latest thinking, see "New Directions for Geriatric Education Centers for the 90s: Minority Involvement," *Workshop Report: Sixth Workshop for Key Staff of Geriatric Education Centers* (Tampa, Fla.: University of South Florida Geriatric Education Center, 1990).

THOMAS T. YOSHIKAWA. Thomas Toyokazu Yoshikawa was born in Los Angeles in 1941. He majored in zoology, receiving his B.A. in 1962 at the University of California at Los Angeles, and earned his M.D. from the University of Michigan Medical School four years later. He did his internship and residency (1966–1970) at the Harbor-UCLA Medical Center in Torrance. After two years of military service in the U.S. Public Health Service Hospital in San Francisco, where he was named teacher of the year, Yoshikawa returned to the Harbor-UCLA Medical Center and the Department of Veterans Affairs Wadsworth Medical Center to complete a fellowship in infectious diseases (1972–1974).

From 1974 to 1988, Yoshikawa was on the faculty of the School of Medicine at UCLA. In that capacity, he served as associate chief of the Division of Infectious Diseases at the Harbor-UCLA Medical Center and was an attending physician on general medical wards. In 1981, Yoshikawa became chief of the Division of Geriatric Medicine at the VA Medical Center in West Los Angeles and clinical director of its Geriatric Research, Education and Clinical Center (GRECC); he also served as an attending physician and was selected teacher of the year by the medical residents in 1981 and 1982. In 1983, Yoshikawa became medical director of the nursing home care unit in the West Los Angeles VA, and, in 1984, became director of the VA-UCLA Geriatric Medicine Fellowship Program. He was a member of the test committee that first board-certified geriatricians for the American Board of Internal Medicine.

Since 1988, Yoshikawa has headed the Office of Geriatrics and Extended Care in the VA's Central Office. In addition, he has been serving as a consultant physician in geriatrics, supervising Fellows in the George Washington University Medical Center. He has also been a consultant in infectious diseases and in geriatric medicine at the VA Medical Center in Washington. In this capacity, Yoshikawa has served on the liaison committee of the Association of American Medical Colleges and the VA, chaired several advisory committees on clinical and long-term care, and been a member of the research work group for VA's Health Care Reform and for planning the 1995 White House Conference on Aging.

Yoshikawa's research reflects his medical interests. He has explored topics in sepsis and endotoxin, antibiotic, aging and host defenses, aging and fever response, as well as urinary tract infection and tuberculosis. He has served on the editorial boards of the *Journal of Gerontology* (1984–1987) and the *Journal of the American Geriatrics Society* (1988–1991). He currently is section editor of the Geriatrics/Long-Term Care Section of *Infectious Diseases in Clinical Practice,* as well as a member of the board of *Drugs and Aging, Clinical Geriatrics,* and *Infectious Disease Practice.* He is also co-editor of the American Geriatrics Society's *Geriatric Review Syllabus* (3rd edn.).

Yoshikawa's success as a researcher, teacher, and administrator were recognized early in his career. In 1992, he won the Art Cherkin Award for his many contributions to the field of aging at UCLA. In 1994, Yoshikawa received the Milo Leavitt Award from the American Geriatrics Society for his work as an educator in geriatrics. That same year he also received the National Association of State Veterans Homes Distinguished Service Award.

Z

ZAHRA F. ZAKERI. Cell biologist Zahra F. Zakeri graduated *cum laude* from the City University of New York's York College with a B.S. in 1976. She earned an M.S. from Long Island University in 1979 and completed her Ph.D. at Jamaica, New York-based St. John's University in 1984. Her doctoral research with T. H. Garter was on the mechanism of enhancement of early gene expression in an adenovirus.

Zakeri did postdoctoral research at Columbia University's College of Physicians and Surgeons from 1984 to 1987 with D. J. Wolgemuth. There she continued work on gene expression in mammals. In 1987, Zakeri became an associate research scientist at Columbia and did her first research important to gerontology: She examined gene expression during embryogenesis and programmed cell death.

After a year as an assistant professor at the Robert Wood Johnson Medical School of Piscataway, New Jersey, Zakeri joined the faculty of Queens College and the Graduate Center, a City University of New York branch, as an assistant professor of biology. She has remained there since 1990 and is now an associate professor.

Much of Zakeri's work on programmed cell death has been done in collaboration with Richard A. Lockshin of St. John's University. Zakeri counts Lockshin as a primary mentor, role model, and collaborator. See their reviews of the literature, "Programmed Cell Death: New Thoughts and Relevance to Aging," *Journal of Gerontology,* 45 (1990): B135–140; and "Physiological Cell Death During Development and its Relationship to Aging," *Annual New York Academy of Science,* 719 (1993): 212–29. Zakeri is also co-chairing the First Gordon

Conference on Cell Death in 1995 and co-writing a section on programmed cell
death and aging in an upcoming encyclopedia of gerontology. Zackeri and Lockshin point out that recent data suggest that cell death is as tightly regulated as
mitosis. Therefore, they argue, cell death might be a manipulatable aspect of
aging.

NAME INDEX

SUBJECT INDEX ⎯⎯⎯⎯⎯⎯⎯

386 SUBJECT INDEX

About the Authors

W. ANDREW ACHENBAUM is Professor of History at the University of Michigan and deputy director of its Institute of Gerontology. He is the author of *Old Age in the New Land* (1978), *Images of Old Age in America, 1970 to the Present* (1978), *Shades of Gray* (1983), *Social Security: Visions and Revisions* (1986), and *Crossing Frontiers: Gerontology Emerges as a Science* (1995). Achenbaum, who earned his Ph.D. from the University of Michigan, is the editor, along with Carole Haber and Steven Weiland, of *Gerontological Keywords* (forthcoming).

DANIEL M. ALBERT is a doctoral candidate in History at the University of Michigan.

ISBN 0-313-29274-4

HARDCOVER BAR CODE